New Perspectives in Public Health

New Perspectives in Public Health

Edited by **Abby Calvin**

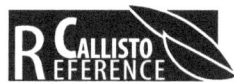

R CALLISTO
REFERENCE

New York

Published by Callisto Reference,
106 Park Avenue, Suite 200,
New York, NY 10016, USA
www.callistoreference.com

New Perspectives in Public Health
Edited by Abby Calvin

International Standard Book Number: 978-1-63239-773-7 (Hardback)

Printed in the United States of America.

Published by Callisto Reference,
106 Park Avenue, Suite 200,
New York, NY 10016, USA
www.callistoreference.com

New Perspectives in Public Health
Edited by Abby Calvin

International Standard Book Number: 978-1-63239-773-7 (Hardback)

Printed in the United States of America.

Contents

Preface

The purpose of the book is to provide a glimpse into the dynamics and to present opinions and studies of some of the scientists engaged in the development of new ideas in the field from very different standpoints. This book will prove useful to students and researchers owing to its high content quality.

The book aims to shed light on some of the unexplored aspects of public health and the recent researches in this field. It strives to provide a fair idea about this discipline and to help develop a better understanding of the latest advances within this area of study. Public health is mainly concerned with providing all round healthcare facilities. It aims at overall welfare rather than eradication of disease only. It is a multidisciplinary field that encompasses environmental health, community health, biostatistics, behavioral health, insurance medicine, etc. While understanding the long-term perspectives of the topics, this book makes an effort in highlighting their impact as a modern tool for the growth of the discipline. It will serve as a valuable source of reference for healthcare professionals, researchers and students associated with public health.

At the end, I would like to appreciate all the efforts made by the authors in completing their chapters professionally. I express my deepest gratitude to all of them for contributing to this book by sharing their valuable works. A special thanks to my family and friends for their constant support in this journey.

Editor

Body Mass Index in Clinic Attenders: Patient Self-Perception versus Actual Measurements

S. Pooransingh,[1] K. Ramgulam,[2] and I. Dialsingh[3]

[1] Department of Paraclinical Sciences, Faculty of Medical Sciences, The University of the West Indies, St. Augustine, Trinidad and Tobago
[2] South West Regional Health Authority, San Fernando, Trinidad and Tobago
[3] Department of Mathematics and Statistics, The University of the West Indies, St. Augustine, Trinidad and Tobago

Correspondence should be addressed to S. Pooransingh; shalini.pooransingh@sta.uwi.edu

Academic Editor: Guang-Hui Dong

Objectives. The objectives of the study were to measure actual BMI in patients attending chronic disease clinics in health centres and to relate this to the patients' own perceptions of their body image and the need to lose weight. *Study Design.* A cross sectional study. *Methods.* The actual BMIs in patients who attended chronic disease clinics in 14 health centres were measured. All participants were asked to state where they thought they were on a visual body image scale and were also asked if they thought they needed to lose weight. *Results.* All participants approached agreed to participate (RR 100%). 70% of patients were found to have a raised BMI. Approximately 73% of patients using the visual scale indicated that an overweight or obese BMI was ideal for them. *Conclusions.* Patients think they are thinner than they actually are, with obvious implications for health and health seeking behaviour. A whole of society approach is needed to change weight status perceptions and improve exercise and dietary behaviour.

1. Introduction

According to the World Health Organization, obesity has reached epidemic proportions globally, with more than 1 billion adults overweight and at least 300 million classified as clinically obese [1]. Obesity has been identified as the main contributor to the major causes of death [2, 3] and therefore presents an important global public health problem. Haslam and James in 2005 [4] reported that excess bodyweight is the sixth most important risk factor contributing to the overall burden of disease worldwide and that 1.1 billion adults and 10% of children were classified as overweight or obese.

In 2010, overweight and obesity accounted for 3.4 million deaths, 3.9% of years of life lost, and 3.8% of disability-adjusted life-years (DALYs) worldwide [5].

Obesity is associated with medical conditions such as diabetes, cardiovascular disease, pulmonary disease, metabolic syndrome, and obstructive sleep apnea. Obesity is being observed more frequently in orthopaedic patients. Orthopaedic patients with obesity-related comorbidities require specific preoperative and postoperative measures to improve their surgical outcomes. Furthermore, patients who are obese are at risk for increased perioperative complications [6].

Obesity impacts not only on the sufferers in terms of associated health effects but also on their families and society as a whole. The health effects associated with obesity result in healthcare costs to the state and costs in terms of the drop in productivity both at school and at work [7].

In two decades there has been a 400% increase in obesity in the Caribbean. The prevalence of obesity in Trinidad and Tobago, the setting of this study, is 16.8%, similar to that of neighbouring Caribbean countries, with a greater proportion of females (21.8%) obese compared to males (10.7%). Trinidad and Tobago ranked twentieth in a global study with a prevalence of overweight and obesity at 67.9% [8] with more than 25% of children aged between 5 and 18 years, obese [9].

The UK Health Secretary called for collective international action to tackle lifestyle related diseases. He stated "that we face new challenges from obesity.... These are inextricably linked to the way we live our lives. They are just as widespread, just as chronic and increasingly threaten early mortality and disability. We need a bold and determined 'whole government' approach looking at better outcomes and helping individuals to make better choices about their own health. With an emphasis on prevention, on physical activity, on personal and corporate responsibility and with unified government action, we can make a big difference" [10].

The body mass index (BMI) is a simple measurement of the ratio of weight (in kilograms) and height (metres squared) and is used in clinical medicine to categorise persons into overweight (BMI 25–29.9 kg/m^2) and obese (BMI > 30 kg/m^2). However, the influence on a person's BMI is multifactorial which includes genetic factors, behavioural and sociocultural factors, and economic and physical environments [11].

Given the list of contributory factors, it may seem obvious where to direct efforts to control BMI in the population but a lack of success stories in the literature suggests the solution may not be a simple one. Similar to other public health researchers, we decided to study BMI in patients. We decided to study self-perception of body image in patients and compare this to their actual measured BMI to determine if this would reveal areas for targeted interventions.

The aim of the study was therefore to record actual BMI in chronic disease clinic attenders and to ascertain individual patients' perceptions of their own body image in relation to their actual measured BMI.

2. Methods

Ethical approval was obtained from the University of the West Indies and from the South West Regional Health Authority where this work was carried out.

A cross-sectional study design was used. The study population comprised patients who attended the chronic disease clinics in the 14 health centres in a county in south Trinidad.

We used an estimate of the prevalence of obesity among Trinidadians at 60%. In order to be 95% confident of the results with a margin of error of 10%, we estimated our required sample size to be 150 participants.

Informed consent was obtained from all participants. Weight (kg) and height (m) were measured on all patients using a regularly calibrated SECA scale. The same scale was transported by one of the authors to all 14 clinics to measure the heights and weights of the patients. The same author performed all measurements. The BMI was calculated for all patients.

An interviewer administered questionnaire was used to obtain information on demographic characteristics and on patients' views about whether they thought they needed to lose weight and their perceptions of their body image using a pictorial representation of BMI, the Stunkard Scale. The questionnaire was pretested for face validity. The Stunkard Scale has 9 silhouette figures that increase in size from very thin (value = 1) to very obese (value = 9) [12].

Using the actual BMI of patients, patients were categorized into underweight, normal weight, overweight, and obese. Patients were asked if in their current state they thought they needed to lose weight. Patients were also asked

TABLE 1: Patients perceptions on whether they need to lose weight in relation to their actual BMI.

Patient BMI	Need to lose—yes	Need to lose weight—no	Total
Underweight	0	1 (100%)	1
Normal weight	15 (34.0%)	29 (65.9%)	44
Overweight	32 (53.3%)	28 (46.6%)	60
Obese	39 (86.6%)	5 (11.1%)*	44
Total	86	63	149

Fisher's exact test P value < 0.001.
N = 149 as complete data *not available on 1 patient.

to view the body images on the pictorial scale and identify which body image they thought correctly identified their present body image.

Patients were also asked to identify which body image on the scale they thought represented the normal/ideal body image for them.

Results from the questions posed to patients were tabulated against their actual BMIs. Statistical Analysis Software (SPSS, version 10) was used to perform descriptive analyses of data via frequency counts of responses and cross tabulations. Chi-squared tests were used to evaluate the significance of differences between response groups. In the cases where the chi-squared test was not reliable, we used the nonparametric Fisher's exact test. The P values for these tests were denoted by P and P < 0.05 was considered statistically significant.

3. Results

One hundred and fifty patients (N = 150) were invited to participate in the study and all agreed to participate leading to a response rate of 100%. The majority of patients (51.3%) were in the 41–60-year age group with females (74%) and Trinidadians of East Indian origin (73%) predominating.

All patients were asked if they thought they needed to lose weight. Table 1 shows the responses to this question tabulated against the actual BMI of the patient. Almost half of those who were measured to be overweight did not think they needed to lose weight, while 87% of those who were found to be obese said they needed to lose weight. Almost one-third of those who were found to have a normal BMI thought they needed to lose weight. Patients' perceptions on whether they need to lose weight and their actual BMI were significant (P < 0.001).

One hundred and five (70%) patients were measured as having a raised BMI (BMI > 25). Of the 60 patients who were overweight, 42 (70%) thought they were slightly overweight according to the visual scale. Of the 45 patients who were obese, 30 (67%) thought they were slightly overweight according to the visual scale. 71 out of 105 (67%) patients with a raised BMI thought they needed to lose weight.

Patients were asked to view the pictorial body images and identify which body image best matched their present shape. Table 2 shows that 85% of patients reported that they were at least overweight.

TABLE 2: Patients' perceptions of their body image using a visual scale.

Visual scale category	Patient number (%)
Underweight	7 (4.7)
Normal	16 (10.7)
Overweight	92 (61.3)
Obese	35 (23.3)
Total	150 (100)

TABLE 3: Patients perceptions on which body image was normal for them.

Visual scale category	Patient number (%)
Underweight	14 (9.3)
Normal	26 (17.3)
Overweight	63 (42.0)
Obese	47 (31.3)
Total	150 (100)

TABLE 4: Patients' perceptions on whether they need to lose weight according to where they see themselves on the visual scale.

Patients view on whether they need to lose weight	Underweight	Normal	Overweight	Obese
Yes	0	3	62	21
No	7	13	29	14
	7	16	91	35

Fisher's exact test P value < 0.001.

Patients were asked which body image was normal/ideal for them. Table 3 shows that 73% of patients identified body images that were at least overweight as ideal for them.

Patients were asked if they thought they needed to lose weight. These results were tabulated against the categories they put themselves into by viewing the visual scale (Table 4). Approximately one-third who categorised themselves as overweight and obese said they did not need to lose weight despite choosing the overweight and obese category for themselves on the visual body image scale. Patients' perceptions on whether they need to lose weight according to where they see themselves on the visual scale and their actual weight were associated ($P < 0.001$).

Approximately 30% of those who chose the overweight and obese categories as ideal for them said they did not need to lose weight; 64% said they needed to lose weight despite choosing that body image as ideal for themselves. Table 5 illustrates the findings. Patients perceptions on whether they need to lose weight according to where they think is normal for them on the visual scale are not associated (P value > 0.05).

Of 16 patients who thought a normal BMI body shape was where they were on the visual scale, 3 (19%) thought an overweight image was ideal for them. Of 91 who saw themselves as overweight on the visual scale, 37 (41%) thought overweight was normal/ideal for them while 39 (43%) thought obese was ideal for them.

TABLE 5: Patients' perceptions on whether they need to lose weight according to where they think is normal for them on the visual scale.

Patients view on whether they need to lose weight	Underweight	Normal	Overweight	Obese
Yes	5	11	39	31
No	9	15	24	15
	14	26	63	46

Chi-square test statistic = 7.524, df = 3, P value = 0.057.

In Table 6, where patients think they are on the visual scale is compared to what they think is normal for them on the visual scale. There is a significant association between these two variables (P value < 0.001).

4. Discussion

4.1. Main Findings. In patients who attend chronic disease clinics, 70% of patients sampled were found to have a raised BMI. Approximately 73.3% of patients, using the visual image scale [12], indicated that an overweight or obese BMI was ideal for them, while 85% said an overweight or obese body image was where they were presently at. Of 45 patients found to be obese on measurement, 30 (67%) thought they were slightly overweight. Furthermore 23 patients who saw themselves as obese thought overweight was normal for them; of concern is that 37 (41%) who were overweight thought this was normal for them and 39 (43%) who were overweight thought the obese image was normal for them. This is an important finding as self-perception and recognition of the problem has been reported to lead to weight loss attempts [13].

Approximately one-third of patients said they did not need to lose weight despite choosing the overweight and obese category for themselves on the visual body image scale.

In this study, there appears to be a misperception about what a healthy BMI should be and perhaps share the view that "men prefer women a little fat," for example [14]. Obesity has been associated with wealth and prosperity in men and health and reproductive abilities for women [15].

Addressing the challenge of overweight and obesity requires a multifaceted approach as there are several influencing factors. How patients perceive the weight of healthcare providers who give weight loss advice has also been shown to influence whether healthcare advice is accepted [16, 17].

Furthermore, health education messages are not effective when given to individuals who are not at the right stage for behaviour change [18].

4.2. What Is Already Known on This Topic? Obesity is a problem of developed and developing nations and is increasing. Traditionally overweight was associated with being healthy and wealthy. Ethnic variations in childhood obesity prevalence exist [19]. South Asian Americans underestimated their weight and had little knowledge of the link between their weight and the risk of chronic diseases [20]. Misperceptions

TABLE 6: Patients perception of where they are on the visual scale and what is normal for them on the visual scale.

Where patients think they are on visual scale	What patients think is normal for them on visual scale			
	Underweight	Normal	Overweight	Obese
Underweight	7	0	0	0
Normal	1	12	3	0
Overweight	4	11	37	39

Fisher's exact test P value < 0.001.

were also found in black and Hispanic female adolescents who underperceived their weight status [21]. A study revealed that female sex and older age group were associated with the thought that "men prefer women a little fat" [14].

4.3. What This Study Adds? This study adds that how patients identify themselves on a visual body image scale differs in relation to their actual measured BMI. In some instances what they think is normal for them is also outside of a healthy body image range. These findings strongly indicate that work is needed in the area of informing the public and patients about what is considered to be a healthy body shape and size and to inform them about the potential adverse effects of overweight and obesity. This is important given the association of central obesity with insulin resistance and the development of Type 2 diabetes mellitus and increased cardiovascular risk, common in persons of South Asian origin [22].

5. Conclusions

The majority of patients in this study were at least overweight. Some patients who were at least overweight did not think they needed to lose weight. In addition, there were differences in patient perceptions about body image compared to actual measured BMIs. As there is little doubt about the negative effects of overweight and obesity on health and that exercise and diet have a positive effect on obesity-related cardiovascular risk factors and cancers, the question of how to motivate persons to improve exercise and dietary habits arises. However this study strongly reveals that before motivating persons to increase exercise and improve their diet, patients need self-awareness that they are indeed overweight and obese with potentially serious implications for their health and well-being. This work suggests a role for health educators and promoters. Cultural factors can play a role in terms of body image perceptions and ethnicity [20, 23] and these factors need to be taken into account when targeting certain groups. The link with ethnicity has not been shown to be associated with deprivation but Asian and black school aged children in the UK have been shown to have more obesogenic lifestyles than their white counterparts [24].

Ng et al. state that national success stories addressing obesity have not been reported in the last 33 years and the prevalence of obesity continues to rise [5]. The whole of society approach is important [25] as governments need to make the living and working environments compatible with the health education messages being disseminated; citizens need to be able to access health information, healthy food items, and environments that are conducive to exercise.

Limitations of Methodology

The prevalence used to calculate the sample size was chosen as 60%. This is an estimate and will not be representative of the prevalence within the county (or country). The study was limited to one county in Trinidad and Tobago. Although the majority of patients were of East Indian ethnicity, this reflects the ethnic distribution of the county with a higher proportion of Indo-Trinidadians. Despite being limited to one county, most findings were significant. We do not make any claim that these results can be extended to the entire county and/or population of patients. However, the study presents results that may be used in designing a more comprehensive study. To date, no study has been done using comparisons of actual obesity measures using BMI and self-rating scales.

Ethical Approval

Ethical approval was obtained from the UWI Ethics Committee and the South West Regional Health Authority Ethics Committee.

Conflict of Interests

The authors declare that there is no conflict of interests regarding the publication of this paper.

References

[1] *Global Strategy on Diet Physical Activity and Health*, World Health Organization, Geneva, Switzerland, 2004.

[2] *Strategic Plan of Action for the Prevention and Control of Non-Communicable Diseases for Countries of the Caribbean Community 2011–2015*, Pan American Health Organization/World Health Organization/Caribbean Community Secretariat, 2011.

[3] E. D'Adamo and S. Caprio, "Type 2 diabetes in youth: epidemiology and pathophysiology," *Diabetes Care*, vol. 34, no. 2, pp. S161–S165, 2011.

[4] D. W. Haslam and W. P. T. James, "Obesity," *The Lancet*, vol. 366, no. 9492, pp. 1197–1209, 2005.

[5] M. Ng, T. Fleming, M. Robinson et al., "Global, regional, and national prevalence of overweight and obesity in children and adults during 1980–2013: a systematic analysis for the Global Burden of Disease Study 2013," *The Lancet*, vol. 384, no. 9945, pp. 766–781, 2013.

[6] W. M. Mihalko, P. F. Bergin, F. B. Kelly, and S. T. Canale, "Obesity, orthopaedics, and outcomes," *Journal of the American Academy of Orthopaedic Surgeons*, vol. 22, no. 11, pp. 683–690, 2014.

[7] M. Nestle and M. F. Jacobson, "Halting the obesity epidemic: a public policy approach," *Public Health Reports*, vol. 115, no. 1, pp. 12–24, 2000.

[8] F. J. Henry, "New strategies needed to fight obesity in the Caribbean," *Cajanus*, vol. 37, no. 1, pp. 1–54, 2004.

[9] M. Doughty, "New strategies for combating child obesity Trinidad and Tobago Guardian," 2012, http://www.guardian.co.tt/lifestyle/2012-03-21/new-strategies-combating-child-obesity.

[10] http://mediacentre.dh.gov.uk/2011/09/20/minister-calls-tough-international-action-obesity-smoking-cancer/.

[11] P. T. Campbell, "Obesity: a certain and avoidable cause of cancer," *The Lancet*, vol. 384, no. 9945, pp. 727–728, 2014.

[12] A. J. Stunkard, T. Sorensen, and F. Schulsinger, "Use of the Danish Adoption Register for the study of obesity and thinness," in *The Genetics of Neurological and Psychiatric Disorders*, S. Kety, L. Rowland, and R. Sidman, Eds., pp. 115–120, Raven Press, New York, NY, USA, 1983.

[13] J. Charles, H. Britt, and S. Knox, "Patient perception of their weight, attempts to lose weight and their diabetes status," *Australian Family Physician*, vol. 35, no. 11, pp. 925–928, 2006.

[14] O. P. Adams, J. T. Lynch-Prescod, and A. O. Carter, "Obesity in primary care in Barbados: prevalence and perceptions," *Ethnicity and Disease*, vol. 16, no. 2, pp. 384–390, 2006.

[15] Z. A. Memish, C. El Bcheraoui, M. Tuffaha et al., "Obesity and associated factors—Kingdom of Saudi Arabia, 2013," *Preventing Chronic Disease*, vol. 11, Article ID 140236, 2013.

[16] C. B. Ebbeling, D. B. Pawlak, and D. S. Ludwig, "Childhood obesity: public-health crisis, common sense cure," *The Lancet*, vol. 360, no. 9331, pp. 473–482, 2002.

[17] R. B. Hash, R. K. Munna, R. L. Vogel, and J. J. Bason, "Does physician weight affect perception of health advice?" *Preventive Medicine*, vol. 36, no. 1, pp. 41–44, 2003.

[18] J. O. Prochaska and C. C. DiClemente, "Stages and processes of self-change of smoking: toward an integrative model of change," *Journal of Consulting and Clinical Psychology*, vol. 51, no. 3, pp. 390–395, 1983.

[19] S. Karlsen, S. Morris, S. Kinra, L. Vallejo-Torres, and R. M. Viner, "Ethnic variations in overweight and obesity among children over time: findings from analyses of the Health Surveys for England 1998–2009," *Paediatric Obesity*, vol. 9, no. 3, pp. 186–196, 2014.

[20] J. W. Tang, M. Mason, R. F. Kushner, M. A. Tirodkar, N. Khurana, and N. R. Kandula, "South asian american perspectives on overweight, obesity, and the relationship between weight and health," *Preventing Chronic Disease*, vol. 9, no. 5, Article ID 110284, 2012.

[21] R. C. Krauss, L. M. Powell, and R. Wada, "Weight misperceptions and racial and ethnic disparities in adolescent female body mass index," *Journal of Obesity*, vol. 2012, Article ID 205393, 9 pages, 2012.

[22] P. M. McKeigue, B. Shah, and M. G. Marmot, "Relation of central obesity and insulin resistance with high diabetes prevalence and cardiovascular risk in South Asians," *The Lancet*, vol. 337, no. 8738, pp. 382–386, 1991.

[23] J. Heimuli, G. Sundborn, E. Rush, M. Oliver, and F. Savila, "Parental perceptions of their child's weight and future concern: the Pacific Islands Families Study," *Pacific Health Dialog*, vol. 17, no. 2, pp. 33–49, 2011.

[24] C. L. Falconer, M. H. Park, H. Croker et al., "Can the relationship between ethnicity and obesity-related behaviours among school-aged children be explained by deprivation? A cross-sectional study," *BMJ Open*, vol. 4, no. 1, Article ID e003949, 2014.

[25] P. Kopelman, "Symposium 1: overnutrition: consequences and solutions foresight report: The obesity challenge ahead," *Proceedings of the Nutrition Society*, vol. 69, no. 1, pp. 80–85, 2010.

2

Prevalence of Cardiovascular Disease and Associated Risk Factors among Adult Population in the Gulf Region: A Systematic Review

Najlaa Aljefree and Faruk Ahmed

Public Health, School of Medicine and Griffith Health Institute, Griffith University, Gold Coast Campus, QLD 4222, Australia

Correspondence should be addressed to Najlaa Aljefree; najlaa.aljefree@griffithuni.edu.au

Academic Editor: John Godleski

Background. CVD is a principal cause of mortality and disability globally. *Objective*. To analyse the epidemiological data on CHD, strokes, and the associated risk factors among adult population in the Gulf countries. *Methods*. A systematic review of published articles between 1990 and 2014 was conducted. *Results*. The analysis included 62 relevant studies. The prevalence of CHD was reported to be 5.5% in Saudi Arabia. The annual incidence of strokes ranged from 27.6 to 57 per 100 000 in the Gulf countries with ischaemic stroke being the most common subtype and hypertension and diabetes being the most common risk factors among stroke and ACS patients. The prevalence of overweight and obesity ranged from 31.2% to 43.3% and 22% to 34.1% in males and from 28% to 34.3% and 26.1% to 44% in females, respectively. In males, the prevalence of hypertension and diabetes ranged from 26.0% to 50.7% and 9.3% to 46.8%, respectively; in females these ranged from 20.9% to 57.2% and 6% to 53.2%, respectively. The prevalence of inactivity was from 24.3% to 93.9% and 56.7% to 98.1% in males and females, respectively. Relatively more males (13.4% to 37.4%) than females (0.5% to 20.7%) were current smokers. Available data indicate poor dietary habits with high consumption of snacks, fatty foods, sugar, and fast food. *Conclusion*. Effective preventative strategies and education programs are crucial in the Gulf region to reduce the risk of CVD mortality and morbidity in the coming years.

1. Introduction

Cardiovascular disease (CVD) is now recognized as the leading cause of death and disability worldwide [1]. The World Health Organization (WHO) estimated that in 2008, out of 17.3 million CVD deaths globally, heart attacks (myocardial infarction) and strokes were responsible for 7.3 and 6.2 million deaths, respectively [1]. According to the INTER-HEART and INTERSTROKE studies, hypertension, diabetes, dyslipidaemia, obesity, smoking, physical activity, poor diet, and alcohol consumption are the most common risk factors for myocardial infarction (heart attack) and strokes worldwide [2, 3].

The Gulf Cooperation Council (GCC) is cooperation between Saudi Arabia, Bahrain, Oman, Qatar, the United Arab Emirates, and Kuwait. In 1981, the GCC was created to encourage investment and to adopt free trade between member states. This agreement also contributed to several fields including: education, culture, tourism, social opportunities, and health among the GCC members. The discovery of oil and other natural resources such as gas in the GCC countries including Saudi Arabia led to rapid development and economic growth [4]. Along with the rapid socioeconomic growth in the Gulf countries, there has been a change in lifestyle such as an increased consumption of poor quality foods and the adoption of a sedentary lifestyle [5], and as a consequence the rates of CVD and associated risk factors among the Gulf population have also increased; the rates sometimes exceed that of developed countries [5]. Furthermore, the number of deaths resulting from ischemic heart disease and hypertensive heart disease in the Middle East and North Africa region (including the GCC countries) was 294/100,000 and 115/100,000 respectively. Also, the number of disability-adjusted life years (DALYs) resulting from

Cardiovascular disease

  (1) "Cardiovascular disease" OR "epidemiology of cardiovascular disease" OR
      "coronary heart disease" OR "epidemiology of coronary heart disease"

Strokes

  (2) "stroke" OR "epidemiology of stroke" OR "incidence of stroke"

Associated risk factors

  (3) "Cardiovascular risk factors" OR "coronary heart disease risk factors" OR
      "stroke risk factors" OR "diabetes mellitus" OR "epidemiology of diabetes
      mellitus" OR "NIDDM" OR "dyslipidaemia" OR "epidemiology of
      dyslipidaemia" OR "hypercholesterolemia" OR "high cholesterol" OR
      "smoking" OR "tobacco use" OR "epidemiology of smoking" OR
      "hypertension" OR "high blood pressure" OR "epidemiology of
      hypertension" OR "obesity" OR "overweight" OR "BMI" OR "epidemiology
      of obesity" OR "physical activity" OR "exercise" OR "epidemiology of
      physical activity" OR "Food consumption patterns" OR "eating habits" OR
      "dietary patterns" OR "food"

The Gulf region

  (4) "Gulf region" OR "Arab countries" OR "GCC" OR "Saudi Arabia" OR
      "Kuwait" OR "Oman" OR "Bahrain" OR "Qatar" OR "United Arab Emirates"
  (5) #1 AND #4
  (6) #2 AND #4
  (7) #3 AND #4
  (8) #1 AND #3 AND #4
  (9) #2 AND #3 AND #4

Box 1: Selected search terms.

ischemic and hypertensive heart disease is 3702/100,000 and 1389/100,000, respectively, in the same region [6]. The WHO estimated the total number of noncommunicable diseases resulting in death in the GCC states in 2008. CVD was estimated to account almost half of the deaths in Oman and Kuwait, 49% and 46%, respectively. The rate of CVD deaths was also high in Saudi Arabia, the UAE, Bahrain, and Qatar 42%, 38%, 32%, and 23%, respectively [7]. Although some systematic reviews on the prevalence of CVD and/or CVD risk factors in the Middle East region have been published [8, 9], these reviews were limited to either CVD risk factors only [8], or specific gender [9]. To our knowledge, this is the first systematic review that provides a comprehensive analysis on the prevalence of CHD, strokes, and associated risk factors in the Arabic Gulf countries. The aim of this paper was to review the epidemiology of CHD, strokes, and the related risk factors among the adult population in the GCC.

2. Methods

2.1. Data Sources. An extensive literature search was conducted on the prevalence of CHD and incidence of strokes and the burden of associated risk factors to identify articles or reports published between 1990 and 2014 using ProQuest Public Health, MEDLINE, PubMed, Google Scholar, and World Health Organization (WHO) website. A manual search of reference lists of original studies was searched. In addition, checking the review articles, contacting authors, the official website of the Gulf Heart Association were also searched http://www.gulfheart.org/ and the section labelled

"GHA studies" was specifically scanned. The search terms used were shown in Box 1.

2.2. Study Selection. A total of 7800 articles were identified in initial search. The titles and abstracts of all articles of potential interest were reviewed for inclusion and exclusion of studies. The criteria for selected studies aimed to include studies that indicated the prevalence of CHD and/or stroke and/or at least one of the associated risk factors: diabetes, hypertension, obesity, dyslipidaemia, dietary habits, smoking, and physical activity. All the included studies were required to only include individuals over 18. The CHD and stroke studies were not restricted by sample size due to the limited numbers of these studies in the GCC countries. However, all the included studies that examined the burden of the risk factors were restricted with a sample size that exceeded 500 except for diet studies. All selected studies were required to relate to at least one of the GCC populations. Only studies published in English and where full manuscripts were included. Studies were published in abstract form and those on congenital heart disease or other CVDs were excluded. A total of 190 full-text papers were identified and further reviewed. Finally, 62 articles including two articles by contacting authors directly were included in this review. Figure 1 summarizes the selection process of the reviewed studies.

2.3. Data Abstraction and Quality Assessment. Data extracted for each study included first author and publication year, sample size, demographic characteristics, the country of study, place of study, study objectives, year(s) of survey, response rate, study methods, the definition of CHD and/or

Potentially relevant titles and abstracts identified from database search ($n = 7800$)

Abstracts primarily excluded for no related data to the subjects of the study ($n = 7610$)

Studies retrieved for full-text evaluation ($n = 190$)

Full-text articles excluded ($n = 130$)

Reasons for exclusion:
- Studies among different populations
- Studies examined different age groups
- Not reporting the prevalence of CHD or stroke or related risk factors
- Data presented in other articles

Studies met the inclusion criteria ($n = 60$)

The final number of reviewed studies ($n = 62$)

Contacting authors $n = 2$

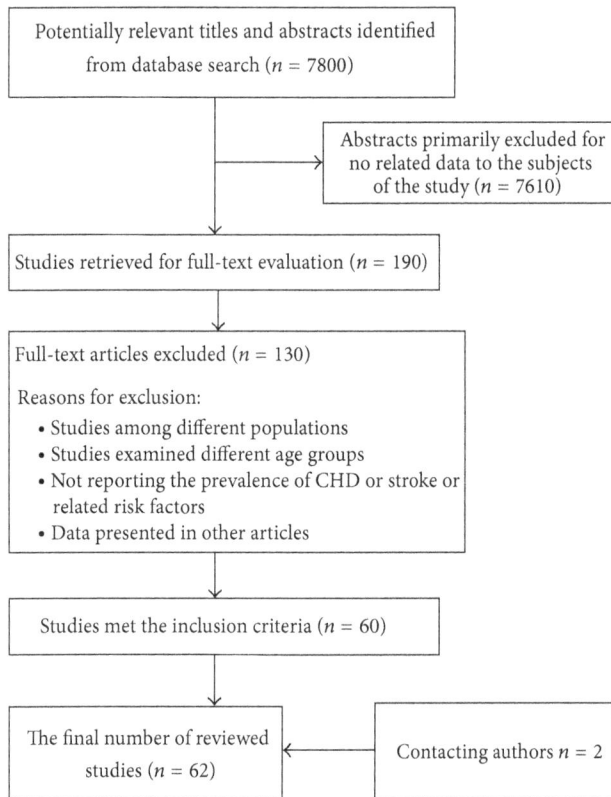

FIGURE 1: Study selection process.

stroke and/or associated risk factors, and the prevalence of CHD and/or stroke and/or associated risk factors. The quality of selected studies was assessed according to the Centre for Reviews and Dissemination guidelines [10]. Since there are few papers that addressed the study questions, no studies were excluded for their qualities. The quality assessment checklist of the included studies in the systematic review is shown in the far-right column of Tables 1 and 2.

2.4. Data Synthesis. A narrative synthesis was performed to identify the study questions. It included describing all the included papers, summarising the findings of the data extracted from each study, and exploring the relationships between the results of the different studies.

3. Results

Of the 62 articles that are reviewed in the present study, 13 were published in the 1990s, another 40 in the 2000s, and 9 in the last four years. Of the included studies, 4 reported data on CHD, 12 on stroke, and 46 on the prevalence of the associated risk factors. Further, of these 62 selected studies, 22 were carried out among Saudi, 8 in Bahraini, 10 in Kuwaiti, 5 in Omani, 6 in Qatari, and 8 in the UAE populations, and 3 were carried out in multiple GCC countries. Regarding the study design; 48 studies were cross-sectional, 7 were retrospective, and 7 were prospective observational studies. Seven studies looked at employees, 4 at university and college students,

8 at primary health care attendants, 14 at CHD and stroke patients, and 29 at the general population. The sample size in CHD and stroke studies ranged from 62 to 23,227 and in the burden of risk factors studies it ranged from 227 to 195,874. Response rates ranged from 59% to 99.8%. The summary of the included articles on CHD and strokes is shown in Table 1, whereas the summary of included articles on the burden of associated risk factors is shown in Table 2.

3.1. CHD and Strokes in the GCC Region. Overall, there is a lack of information on CHD and strokes in Arabic Gulf countries. The only nationally representative study conducted in Saudi Arabia reported the crude prevalence of CHD of 5.5% among the Saudi population [11]. This survey reported a higher prevalence of CHD in males (6.6%) compared to females (4.4%) and in urban Saudis (6.2%) than rural Saudis (4.0%). Further, the prevalence of CHD increased with age from 3.9% in 30–39-year olds to 9.3% in the 60–70-year olds [11].

The Gulf Registry of Acute Coronary Events (Gulf RACE), a project of Gulf Heart Association aimed to describe the characteristics, in-hospital outcomes, and associated risk factors of the acute coronary syndrome patients (ACS) and recruited patients from 64 hospitals in Bahrain, Oman, Qatar, Kuwait, the UAE, and Yemen [12, 13]. The Gulf RACE study reported ACS was more prevalent in male (74%) than female (24%) patients [12]. It also reported a high prevalence of diabetes (40%), hypertension (49%), dyslipidaemia (32%), smoking (38%), and obesity (27%) among ACS patients in the five Gulf countries [13]. The highest rates of the risk factors were in Bahrain and Kuwait, except for smoking, which has the highest rates in the UAE and Kuwait [13]. The prevalence of CVD risk factors was higher in females than males, including diabetes (55% versus 36%), hypertension (70% versus 43%), and dyslipidaemia (44% versus 28%), respectively [12]. Significantly more males (47%) than females (5%) were current smokers [13].

Similarly, the Saudi Project for Assessment of Coronary Events (SPACE) registry reported the characteristics and prevalence of risk factors among ACS patients in Saudi Arabia [14]. The SPACE registry reported that ACS was more frequent in males (77%) than females (23%) [14]. Ischemic heart disease was present in 32% of the study population. The study also reported diabetes to be the most common risk factor for CHD (56%) followed by hypertension (48%), being a current smoker (39%), and hyperlipidaemia (31%) [14].

The available data on strokes and the associated risk factors in the GCC were derived mostly from retrospective hospital-based studies but no population-based studies. The data on strokes and associated risk factors was reported in 12 studies: 4 in Saudi Arabia [15–18], 1 in Bahrain [19], 3 in Kuwait [20–22], 3 in Qatar [23–25], and 1 from multiple GCC countries [26].

Five studies reported the incidence of stroke in Saudi Arabia, Kuwait, Qatar and Bahrain [15, 17, 19, 20, 25]. The incidence of stroke ranged from 27.6 per 100 000 in Kuwait to 57 per 100 000 in Bahrain [15, 17, 19, 20, 25]. Further, the most common type of stroke in the region was ischemic

TABLE 1: The characteristics and the main outcomes of the included studies on CHD and strokes in the GCC region.

Reference country	Year(s) of survey	Total sample	Age, range, and mean	Sampling methods	Study design	Response rate (%)	Diagnostic criteria	The main outcomes (CHD/stroke/associated risk factors/mortality rates)	Quality assessment checklist (*)
					CHD studies				
[11] Saudi Arabia	1995–2000	17293 M: 47.3% F: 52.04%	30–70	Two-stage stratified cluster	National cross-sectional survey	NR	WHO MONICA (monitoring trends and determinant in cardiovascular disease)	Overall prevalence: 5.5% M: 6.6% F: 4.4%	1-Y, 2-Y, 3-Y, 4-Y, 5-Y, 6-N, 7-NA
[14] Saudi Arabia	2005–2006	435 M: 77% F: 23%	57.1	No sampling (all ACS patients included with no excluded patients)	Prospective study	NR	The Joint Committee of the European Society of Cardiology/American College of Cardiology (ACC)	Risk factors of ACS: DM 56%, HTN 48%, smoking 39%, and hyperlipidaemia 31%	1-Y, 2-Y, 3-Y, 4-Y, 5-N, 6-Y, 7-NA
[13] (Kuwait, Oman, Qatar, Bahrain, the UAE, and Yemen)	2007	6704 M & F = not clear	56	No sampling (all ACS patients included with no excluded patients)	Prospective multinational study	NR	The American College of Cardiology clinical data standards (ACC)/DM, hypertension, dyslipidaemia defined when patients known to have these risk factors and on treatment/regular smoking defined as 1 cigarette per day/nonsmoker after stopping 12 months ago	*Overall prevalence*: DM 40%, HTN 49%, dyslipidaemia 32%, and smoking 38% *In Oman*: DM 37%, HTN, 53%, smoking 18%, dyslipidaemia 35%, and obesity 22% *In the UAE*: DM 40%, HTN 50%, smoking 49%, dyslipidaemia 36%, and obesity 20% *In Qatar*: DM 46%, HTN 49%, smoking 37%, dyslipidaemia 29%, and obesity 23% *In Bahrain*: DM 51%, HTN 60%, smoking 32%, dyslipidaemia 45%, and obesity 28% *In Kuwait*: DM 50%, HTN 56%, smoking 40%, dyslipidaemia 37%, and obesity 37%	1-Y, 2-Y, 3-Y, 4-Y, 5-N, 6-Y, 7-NA
[12] (Kuwait, Oman, Qatar, Bahrain, the UAE, and Yemen)	2007	8166 M: 6183 F: 1983	M: 53 years F: 62 years	No sampling (all ACS patients included with no excluded patients)	Prospective multinational study	NR	The American College of Cardiology clinical data standards (ACC)/DM, hypertension, dyslipidaemia defined when patients known to have these risk factors and on treatment/regular smoking defined as 1 cigarette per day/nonsmoker after stopped 12 months ago	*Associated risk factors in men:* DM 36%, HTN 43%, dyslipidaemia 28%, and smoking 47% *In women:* DM 55% and HTN 70%, Dyslipidaemia 44% and smoking 5%	1-Y, 2-Y, 3-Y, 4-Y, 5-N, 6-Y, 7-NA

TABLE 1: Continued.

Reference country	Year(s) of survey	Total sample	Age, range, and mean	Sampling methods	Study design	Response rate (%)	Diagnostic criteria	The main outcomes (CHD/stroke/associated risk factors/mortality rates)	Quality assessment checklist (*)
					Strokes studies				
[15] Saudi Arabia	1982–1992	500 M: 342 F: 158	M: 65.2 years F: 62.2 years	Nonrandom sampling (500 medical records of stroke patients)	Retrospective study	NR	NA	*Incidence of stroke:* 43.8 per 100,000 *30-day mortality:* 12% *Stroke types:* ischemic strokes (76.2%) *Risk factors:* HTN 56%, DM 42%, and smoking 6%	1-Y, 2-Y, 3-Y, 4-Not well described, 5-N, 6-N, 7-NA
[20] Kuwait	1989, 1992 and 1993	Not clear	60.6 years	Nonrandom (all patients with first-ever stroke, patients with previous stroke were excluded)	Prospective study	NR	WHO definition for diagnosing stroke/HC defined as more than 5.78 mmol/L/smoking as any current use of cigarette/hypertension and DM were not clear	*Annual incidence:* 27.6 per 100,000 *The age-adjusted annual crude incidence:* 145.6 per 100,000 *30-day mortality:* 10% *Stroke types:* Carotid-territory large infarction (46.5%), *Risk factors:* HTN 53%/DM 42%/HC 61%/smoking 23%	1-Y, 2-Y, 3-Y, 4-Y, 5-N, 6-Y, 7-NA
[22] Kuwait	2008	151 M: 96 F: 55	60.5 years	Nonrandom (all ischemic stroke patients, there was an inclusion criterion)	Retrospective study	NR	Stroke defined according to WHO/stroke subtypes was defined according to the Trial of Org 10172 in Acute Stroke Treatment (TOAST) criteria	*Stroke types:* Ischemic stroke (90.1%) *Risk factors:* DM 56.3%/dyslipidaemia 57%/HTN 68.9%/smoking 40%	1-Y, 2-Y, 3-Y, 4-N, 5-N, 6-Y, 7-NA
[21] Kuwait	1995–1999	62 M: 30 F: 32	64.1 years	No random (all ischemic stroke patients included)	Retrospective study	NR	Stroke defined according to WHO criteria	*Risk factors:* HTN 72.5%/DM 69.4%, dyslipidaemia 30.6%/smoking 1.6% *30-day mortality:* 12.9%	1-Y, 2-Y, 3-Y, 4-Y, 5-N, 6-Y, 7-NA
[23] Qatar	2005–2008	116 M: 85% F: 15%	53 years	Nonrandom (all patients diagnosed with PCS stroke, there was an inclusion criterion)	Prospective study	NR	Stroke defined according to Kidwell and Warach/DM as fasting blood glucose >140 mg/dL or in medication/hypertension as >140/90 mmHg or on medication/dyslipidaemia as TC >5 mmol/L/smokers as currently smokers or during the last 12 months/obesity as BMI ≥30	*Risk factors:* HTN 61%, DM 44%, obesity 66%, smoking 20%, and dyslipidaemia 12% *30-day mortality rate:* 10%	1-Y, 2-Y, 3-Y, 4-Y, 5-Y, 6-Partly, 7-NA

TABLE 1: Continued.

Reference country	Year(s) of survey	Total sample	Age, range, and mean	Sampling methods	Study design	Response rate (%)	Diagnostic criteria	The main outcomes (CHD/stroke/associated risk factors/mortality rates)	Quality assessment checklist (*)
[17] Saudi Arabia	1989-1990 and 1991-1993	488 M: 314 F: 174	All	Nonrandom (all Saudi patients with first stroke were included, and there was excluded patients)	Prospective register	NR	The WHO multicentre Stroke Register/hypertension defined as BP >160/90 mmHg/DM defined as fasting blood sugar above 6.6 mmol/L.	*Incidence of stroke:* 29.8 per 100,000 *Age-adjustment incidence:* 125.8 per 100 000 *Stroke types:* ischemic stroke 69% *Risk factors:* HTN 38.1%/DM 37.1%/smoking 19.3%	1-Y, 2-Y, 3-Y, 4-Y, 5-Y, 6-N, 7-NA
[18] Saudi Arabia	1997–2000	71 M: 55 F: 16	63 years	Nonrandom (all stroke patients included, no excluded patients)	Retrospective study	NR	NR	*Stroke types:* cerebral infarction 80% *Risk factors:* DM 27%/HTN 61%/smoking 28%/dyslipidaemia 4%/Ischemic heart disease 8.5% *30-day mortality:* 31%	1-Y, 2-Y, 3-Y, 4-Y, 5-N, 6-N, 7-NA
[25] Qatar	1997	217 M: 72.4% F: 27.6%	57 years	Nonrandom (all stroke patients records were reviewed, and only first-ever stroke cases were included)	Retrospective study	NR	Stroke defined according to the WHO criteria	*Incidence of stroke:* 41 per 100,000 *Stroke types:* ischemic stroke (80%) *Risk factors:* HTN 63%/DM 42%/Ischemic heart disease 17% *30-day mortality rate:* 16%	1-Y, 2-Y, 3-Y, 4-Y, 5-N, 6-Y, 7-NA
[19] Bahrain	1995	144 M & F = not clear	≥20	Nonrandom (all stroke cases were reviewed)	Retrospective study	NR	Stroke defined according to the WHO criteria	*Incidence of stroke:* 57 per 100,000 *Stroke types:* cerebral infarction 60% *Risk factors:* HTN 52%/DM 20%/dyslipidaemia 29%/smoking 29%/Ischemic heart disease 50%	1-Y, 2-Y, 3- Y, 4-N, 5-N, 6-N, 7-NA

TABLE 1: Continued.

Reference country	Year(s) of survey	Total sample	Age, range, and mean	Sampling methods	Study design	Response rate (%)	Diagnostic criteria	The main outcomes (CHD/stroke/associated risk factors/mortality rates)	Quality assessment checklist (*)
[24] Qatar	2001	303 M: 72% F: 28%	61.2 years	Nonrandom (the data of all stroke patients were reviewed, and there were inclusion criteria)	Retrospective study	NR	Stroke: WHO criteria HTN: BP >140/90 mmHg or on medication/DM: past history or FPG (>7 mmol/L) or on medication/dyslipidaemia: TC > 5.2 mmol/L or TG > 2.0 mmol/L or HDL < 0.9 mmol/L LDL > 3.4 mmol/L/BMI ≥30 kg/m²/smokers: regular smoking within the last 5 years	*Risk factors:* HTN 69%/DM 51%/dyslipidaemia 57%/obesity 30%/smoking 26%/CAD 23%	1-Y, 2-Y, 3-Y, 4-Y, 5-N, 6-Y, 7-NA
[26] (Kuwait, Oman, Qatar, and the UAE)	2006-2007	780 M: 63.7% F: 36.3%	58.9 years	No sampling (all ischemic stroke patients were included, and there were inclusion criteria)	Prospective registry	NR	HTN: BP >160/90 mmHg or on medication/DM: past history or elevated A1c or on medication/dyslipidaemia: TC > 5.2 mmol/L or TG > 1.7 mmol/L or HDL > 1.0 mmol/L LDL < 3.4 mmol/L/BMI ≥30 kg/m²/smokers: regular smoking within the last 5 years	*Risk factors:* HTN 66.4%/DM 55.3%/current smokers 19.6%/dyslipidaemia 30.1% *90-day mortality:* 2.1%	1-Y, 2-Y, 3-Y, 4-Y, 5-Y, 6-Y, 7-NA
[16] Saudi Arabia	1993	23,227 M: 49.8% F: 50.2%	NR	No sampling (all Saudi living in the Thuqbah area were screened)	Community-based cross-sectional survey	NR	Stroke defined "sudden or rapid onset of focal or global brain dysfunction of vascular origin lasting for more than 24 h or leading to death especially if diagnosed by physicians"	*The overall prevalence of stroke survivors:* 186 per 100 000	1-Y, 2-Y, 3-Y, 4-N, 5-Y, 6-N, 7-NA

M, male; F, female; U, urban; R, rural; DM, diabetes; IFG, impaired fasting glucose; HC, hypercholesterolemia; TG, triglyceride; TC, total cholesterol; HDL, high-density lipoprotein; LDL, low-density lipoprotein; HTN, hypertension; SBP, systolic blood pressure; DBP, diastolic blood pressure; NR, not reported; ACS, acute coronary syndrome; BMI, body mass index; Y, yes; N, no; and NA, not applicable. (*) the quality assessment checklist assessed according to the Centre for Reviews and Dissemination guidelines (CRD) for nonrandomized studies: 1- Was the aim of the study stated clearly? 2- Was the methodology stated? And was it appropriate? 3- Were appropriate methods used for data collection and analysis? 4- Was the data analysis sufficiently rigorous? 5- Were preventive steps taken to minimize bias? 6- Were limitations of the study discussed? 7- In systematic review, was search strategy adequate and appropriate?

TABLE 2: Characteristics and prevalence data of the included studies on the burden of CVD risk factors in the GCC region.

Reference country	Year(s) of survey	Total sample	Age, mean, and min to max	Sampling methods	Study design	Response rate (%)	Diagnostic criteria and/or dietary assessment methods	The main findings and prevalence data	Quality assessment checklist (*)
[27] Saudi Arabia	1996-1997	1,649 M: 1,175 F: 474	≥40	Random stratified sampling	Cross-sectional study	76.6	HC: TC >6.2 mmol/L/overweight BMI for men ≥27.2 women ≥26.9/HTN: SBP ≥140 mmHg or DBP ≥95 or on medication	Overweight 49.8%/HTN 19.9%/current smoking 18.8%, HC: overall 10.1% M: 10.3% F: 9.7%	1-Y, 2-Y, 3-Y, 4-Y, 5-Y, 6-N, 7-NA
[28] Saudi Arabia	1990-1993	10,651 M: 50.8% F: 49.2%	≥20	Multistage stratified cluster sampling	National epidemiological cross-sectional survey	69	Overweight and obesity defined according to the WHO criteria	Overweight: overall 31.2% M 33.1%, F 29.4%, U 33.6%, R 28.3% Obesity: overall 22.1%, M 17.8%, F 26.6%, U 25.6%, and R 17.6%	1-Y, 2-Y, 3-Y, 4-Y, 5-Y, 6-N, 7-NA
[29] Saudi Arabia	1995-2000	16917 M: 8002 F: 8804	30-70	Two-stage stratified cluster sampling	National epidemiological cross-sectional survey	98.2	DM was defined according to the WHO	DM: overall 23.7%, M 26.2%, F 21.5%, U 25.5%, and R 19.5% The prevalence of IFG overall 14.1% M 14.4%, and F 13.9%	1-Y, 2-Y, 3-Y, 4-Y, 5-Y, 6-N, 7-NA
[30] Saudi Arabia	1996	647 M: 383 F: 264	18-26	Random sampling	Cross-sectional study	91	Current smokers: currently smoking at least 1 cigarette per day	Current smoking overall 29%, M 20%, F 9%	1-Y, 2-Y, 3-Y, 4-Y, 5-Y, 6-N, 7-NA
[31] Saudi Arabia	1990-1993	2049 M: 1033 F: 1016	30-64	Multistage stratified cluster sampling	National Cross-sectional survey	92	DM: the random serum glucose according to the WHO criteria or self-reported/HC: mild (5.2–6.2 mmol/L) severe (>6.2 mmol/L)/HDL: <0.9 mmol/L/HDL: WHO criteria	Overweight: M 38%, F 34% Obesity: M 23%, F 34% DM: M 16.4%, F 20% Smoking: M 21%, F 1% Moderate HC: M & F = 21.5% Severe HC: M & F = 9% LDL: M 6.6%, F 10.3% HDL: M 55%, F 47%	1-Y, 2-Y, 3-Y, 4-Y, 5-Y, 6-N, 7-NA
[32] Saudi Arabia	1995-2000	17,232 M: 8215 F: 9008	30-70	Two-stage stratified cluster sampling	National epidemiological cross-sectional survey	NR	Overweight and obesity defined according to the WHO	Overweight: Overall 36.9%, M 42.4%, F 31.8%, U 36.9%, R 36.9% Obesity: Overall 35.6%, M 26.4%, F 44% U 39.7%, R 27%	1-Y, 2-Y, 3-Y, 4-Y, 5-Y, 6-N, 7-NA
[33] Saudi Arabia	2001	1114 M: 442 F: 672	35-85	Cluster sampling	Cross-sectional study	NR	HTN: BP ≥140 mmHg systolic and 90 mmHg diastolic or self-reported with medication or both	HTN: Overall 30% M 33%, F 29%, U 29%, R 32%	1-Y, 2-Y, 3-Y, 4-Y, 5-Y, 6-N, 7-NA

TABLE 2: Continued.

Reference country	Year(s) of survey	Total sample	Age, mean, and min to max	Sampling methods	Study design	Response rate (%)	Diagnostic criteria and/or dietary assessment methods	The main findings and prevalence data	Quality assessment checklist (∗)
[34] Saudi Arabia	1996	1333 M: 100%	≥19	Random sampling	Cross-sectional study	75	Regular active: physically active for 30 or more minutes, 2 or more days a week	*Physically inactive* 53%, *irregularly active* 27.5%, and *physically active on a regular basis* 19%	1-Y, 2-Y, 3-Y, 4-Y, 5-N, 6-N, 7-NA
[35] Saudi Arabia	1995–2000	17,230 M: 47.7% F: 52.3%	30–70	Two-stage stratified cluster sampling	National epidemiological cross-sectional survey	NR	HTN: SBP ≥140 mmHg or DBP ≥90 mmHg	*HTN:* Overall 26.1% M 28.6%, F 23.9%, U 27.9%, R 22.4%	1-Y, 2-Y, 3-Y, 4-Y, 5-Y, 6-N, 7-NA
[36] Saudi Arabia	1995–2000	17,395 M: 8297 F: 9098	30–70	Two-stage stratified cluster sampling	National epidemiological cross-sectional survey	NR	Physically active: 30 minutes or more of at least moderate-intensity activity for three or more times per week/physical inactivity: participants who did not meet the physically active criteria	*Physical inactivity:* Overall 96.1% M 93.9%, F 98.1%	1-Y, 2-Y, 3-Y, 4-Y, 5-Y, 6-Y, 7-NA
[37] Saudi Arabia	1995–2000	16.819 M: 47.6% F: 52.4%	30–70	Two-stage stratified cluster sampling	National epidemiological cross-sectional survey	97	HC: TC ≥5.2 mmol/L/TG: ≥1.69 mmol/L	*HC:* overall 54% M 54.9%, F 53.2%, U 53.4%, R 55.3% *HG:* Overall 40.3% M 47.6%, F 33.7%	1-Y, 2-Y, 3-Y, 4-Y, 5-Y, 6-Y, 7-NA
[38] Saudi Arabia	1999–2000	1752 M & F = not clear	35.5	Random sampling	Cross-sectional study	70	Current smokers: those who regularly or occasionally smoke on a daily, weekly, or monthly basis/nonsmokers: those who never smoked.	*Current smokers* 52.3% U 55.9%, R 44.1%	1-Y, 2-Y, 3-Y, 4-Y, 5-Y, 6-Y, 7-NA
[39] Saudi Arabia	2004-2005	195,874 M: 99,946 F: 95,905	≥30	Nonrandom (all Saudis aged 30 and above who lived in the eastern region in SA were invited to participate in the screening programme)	Cross-sectional survey	99.1	Overweight and obesity defined according to the WHO	*Overweight:* overall 35.1% M 40.3%, F 29.7% *Obesity:* overall 43.8% M 36.1%, F 51.8%	1-Y, 2-Y, 3-Y, 4-Y, 5-Y, 6-Y, 7-NA

TABLE 2: Continued.

Reference country	Year(s) of survey	Total sample	Age, mean, and min to max	Sampling methods	Study design	Response rate (%)	Diagnostic criteria and/or dietary assessment methods	The main findings and prevalence data	Quality assessment checklist (*)
[40] Saudi Arabia	1993–1998	F: 1764	30–70 years	Multistage stratified cluster sampling	CSS	NR	NR/Structured questionnaire	(i) The consumption of black tea was 87.2%. (ii) Females who daily consumed >6 cups of tea (>480 mL) were significantly more likely to have lower rates of dyslipidaemia including, high (TC) (OR = 0.63, 95% CI: 0.41–0.97), high TG (OR = 0.56, 95% CI: 0.35–0.86), high (LDL) (OR = 0.70, 95% CI: 0.45–1.07), and high (VLDL) (OR = 0.61, 95% CI: 0.39–0.93).	1-Y, 2-Y, 3-Y, 4-Y, 5-Y, 6-Y, 7-NA
[41] Saudi Arabia	2008-2009	312 M: 132 & F: 180	21.1 years	Random selection	CSS	NR	BMI according to the National Institute of Health. HTN according to the Fourth Report on the Diagnosis, Evaluation, and Treatment of High Blood Pressure/Self-reported questionnaire (11 items)	(i) The % of total energy from carbohydrates and fats was (38% versus 39%) and (46.1% versus 46.8%) in both M and F. (ii) Unhealthy food habits were high consumption of snacks (42.5%), a low consumption of vegetables (30%), a high consumption of fatty foods (36% in F; 44% in M), a high consumption of salty foods (36% in F; 43% in M), and a high consumption of sugar (41% in F; 38% in M). (iii) A significant association between the high intakes of energy derived from fatty foods and BMI and HTN in both genders. (iv) A significant association was found between the high consumption of salty foods and HTN. (v) A negative association was found between the consumption of vegetables, grains, and beans and BMI and HTN in both genders.	1-Y, 2-Y, 3-Y, 4-Y, 5-Y, 6-N, 7-NA

TABLE 2: Continued.

Reference country	Year(s) of survey	Total sample	Age, mean, and min to max	Sampling methods	Study design	Response rate (%)	Diagnostic criteria and/or dietary assessment methods	The main findings and prevalence data	Quality assessment checklist (*)
[42] Saudi Arabia	2009	2789 M: 1806 F: 981	30–70 years	Random selection	CSS	NR	NR/Questionnaire and 24 h recall	(i) The most popular food was kabsa (80% in M and 65% in F), fresh fruits (63% in M and 45% in M and 47% in F), vegetables (62% in M and 47% in F) and dates (45%) in both genders and soft drinks (21% in M and 25% in F).	1-Y, 2-Y, 3-Y, 4-Y, 5-N, 6-Y, 7-NA
[43] The UAE	2008–2010	50138 M: 43% F: 57%	18–75	Nonrandom (all UAE nationals residing aged 18 to 75 who were living in Abu Dhabi city were enrolled in the CVD screening program)	Cross-sectional national survey	Measured data (98.7–99.9), self-reported data (86.1–99.8)	Obesity and overweight: according to WHO/DM: past history and on medication or HbA1c ≥6.5% or random glucose 11.1 mmol/L/HTN: self-reported and on medication or SBP ≥140 mmHg or DBP ≥90 mmHg/dyslipidaemia: self-reported on medication or LDL 4.1 mmol/L or HDL 1.0 mmol/L/current smokers: 1 cigarette per day during the last 12 months or 1 water pipe per month during the last 3 months	*Obesity:* overall 35.4% M 31.6%, and F 38.3% *Overweight:* overall 31.9% M 36.1%, and F 28.8% *Dyslipidaemia:* overall 44.2% M 57.7%, and F 33.9% *HTN:* overall 23.1% M 26%, and F 20.9% *Smoking:* overall 11.6% M 25.8%, and F 0.8% *DM:* overall 17.6% M 17.3%, and F 17.9%	1-Y, 2-Y, 3-Y, 4-Y, 5-Y, 6-Y, 7-NA
[44] The UAE	1997	3150 M: 1516 F: 1634	18–75	Stratified random sampling	Cross-sectional study	NR	HTN: SBP >140 mmHg and/or DBP >90 mmHg and/or self-reported with medication	*HTN:* overall 31.6% M 47%, F 53%	1-Y, 2-Y, 3-Y, 4-N, 5-Y, 6-N, 7-NA
[45] The UAE	1999–2000	5844 M: 2499 F: 3345	≥20	Stratified multistage cluster sampling	National epidemiological cross-sectional study	89	DM: fasting blood glucose ≥7.0 mmol/L or taking insulin or oral hypoglycemic agents	DM: overall 20% M 21.5%, F 19.2% IFG: overall 6.5% M 4.5%, F 8%	1-Y, 2-Y, 3-Y, 4-Y, 5-Y, 6-N, 7-NA
[46] The UAE	2000-2001	535 F: 100%	>19	Stratified random sampling	Cross-sectional survey	95	Overweight and obesity were defined according to WHO criteria	*Overweight* 27% *Obesity* 35%	1-Y, 2-Y, 3-Y, 4-Y, 5-Y, 6-Y, 7-NA
[47] The UAE	2002–2003	1104 M: 72% F: 28%	18–69	Multistage cluster random sample	Large cross-sectional survey	94.9	Physical inactivity: the person did not meet the following criteria: 3 or more days of various activities during the last week of at least 20 minutes per day or 5 or more days of moderate-intensity activity or walking during the last week of at least 30 minutes per day	*Physical inactivity* Overall 39.5% M 37.9%, F 56.7%	1-Y, 2-Y, 3-Y, 4-Y, 5-Y, 6-Y, 7-NA

TABLE 2: Continued.

Reference country	Year(s) of survey	Total sample	Age, mean, and min to max	Sampling methods	Study design	Response rate (%)	Diagnostic criteria and/or dietary assessment methods	The main findings and prevalence data	Quality assessment checklist (*)
[48] The UAE	2010	227 M: 74 F: 153	18–50 years	Convenience sampling	CCS	NR	MetS according to ATP III/24 h recall	(i) A high intake of total energy, carbohydrate, fat, and protein in M and F, (20971 versus 17180 kjoules/day), (627.3 versus 549.7 g/day), (207.5 versus 150.1 g/day), and (175.5 versus 151.5 g/day), respectively. (ii) The mean intake of total sugar and fibre was high (224.4 versus 202 g/day) and (44.4 versus 33.3 g/day), respectively.	1-Y, 2-Y, 3-Y, 4-Y, 5-Y, 6-Y, 7-NA
[49] The UAE	2001-2002	F: 400	18–25 years	Convenience sampling	CSS	NR	BMI according to WHO/self-administrated questionnaire	(i) The prevalence of overweight and obesity was 19.4% and 6.7%, respectively. (ii) Food habits include not having breakfast in 44.8%, fast food consumption once a day in 34.9%, and having only 1 or 2 meals/day in 52.3%. (iii) A low consumption of cereals, vegetables and fruits by 54.4%, 51.5%, and 49.5%, respectively. A high intake of fat in 46.7%. (iv) A significant association between obesity and low consumption of cereals and fruits.	1-Y, 2-Y, 3-Y, 4-Y, 5-N, 6-N, 7-NA
[50] The UAE	1993	2212 M: 1122 F: 1090	≥20	Random selection	CSS	NR	NA/pretested structured questionnaire	(i) A low consumption of fruits, vegetables, and milk in the study population. (ii) Elderly adults (≥50) were more likely to consume fruits, vegetables, fish, milk, and yoghurt than older adults. (iii) Young adult females were more likely to consume fruits, vegetables, and fish than young adult males.	1-Y, 2-Y, 3-Y, 4-Y, 5-N, 6-N, 7-NA

TABLE 2: Continued.

Reference country	Year(s) of survey	Total sample	Age, mean, and min to max	Sampling methods	Study design	Response rate (%)	Diagnostic criteria and/or dietary assessment methods	The main findings and prevalence data	Quality assessment checklist (*)
[51] Kuwait	1995-1996	3003 M: 1105 F: 1898	≥20	Convenience sampling (all Kuwaiti +20 in the survey area invited to participate)	Cross-sectional study	NR	DM according to the WHO diagnostic criteria for abnormal glucose tolerance	*DM:* overall 14.8% M 14.7%, F 14.8%	1-Y, 2-Y, 3-Y, 4-Y, 5-N, 6-N, 7-NA
[52] Kuwait	1996	3859 M: 1798 F: 2061	33.2	A three-stage stratified cluster sampling	Cross-sectional national study	96.5	Current smokers: if they were smoking at the time of the survey and had smoked more than 100 cigarette in their lifetime; former smokers: if they had smoked more than 100 cigarette in their life but no longer smoking, and never smokers: when they had never smoked or smoked less than 100 cigarettes in their life	*The prevalence of smoking:* Overall 17% M 34.4%, F 1.9%	1-Y, 2-Y, 3-Y, 4-Y, 5-Y, 6-Y, 7-NA
[53] Kuwait	1998–2009	32,811 M: 15,110 F: 17,701	20–69	**Convenience sampling** (Kuwaitis in health examination for Gov. and Hajj health check-ups and PHCCs)	National cross-sectional survey	NR	HC: moderate (5.2–6.22 TC mmol/L) severe (>6.23 TC mmol/L)	*HC* prevalence increased from 1998 to 1999 (M 35%; F 31%) until 2006-2007 (M 56%; F 53.6%) and then declined in 2008-2009 (M 33.7%; F 30.6%)	1-Y, 2-Y, 3-Y, 4-Y, 5-N, 6-Y, 7-NA
[54] Kuwait	2006	2280 M: 918 F: 1362	20–65	Systematic random sampling	National cross-sectional survey	77.6	Overweight and obesity were defined according to the WHO criteria	*Combined overweight* and *obesity:* 80.4% *Obesity:* M 39.2%, F 53%	1-Y, 2-Y, 3-Y, 4-Y, 5-Y, 6-N,7-NA
[55] Kuwait	1998–2009	38,611 M: 17,491 F: 21,120	20–69	convenience sampling (Kuwaitis in health examination for Gov. and Hajj health check-ups and PHCCs)	National cross-sectional survey	NR	Overweight and obesity defined according to the WHO criteria	*Obesity* increased from 1998 to 1999 (M 22.8%; F 28.4%) until 2008-2009 (M 34.1%; F 43%) *Overweight* increased from 1998 to 1999 (M 36.5%; F 33.4%) until 2008-2009 (M 43.3%; F 34.3%)	1-Y, 2-Y, 3-Y, 4-Y, 5-N, 6-Y, 7-NA

TABLE 2: Continued.

Reference country	Year(s) of survey	Total sample	Age, mean, and min to max	Sampling methods	Study design	Response rate (%)	Diagnostic criteria and/or dietary assessment methods	The main findings and prevalence data	Quality assessment checklist (*)
[56] Kuwait	2002–2009	6356 M: 2745 F: 3611	20–69	Convenience sampling (Kuwaitis in health examination for Gov. and Hajj health check-ups and PHCCs)	National cross-sectional survey	NR	Diabetes defined according to the WHO criteria	IFG decreased from 2002 to 2009 by (M: 7.4%, F: 6.8%) and DM decreased in the same period by (M 9.8%, F 8.9%) The prevalence in 2008-2009: IFG (M 6%, F 5.3%) DM (M 9.3%, F 6%) Physical activity (M 42.1%, F 19.2%)	1-Y, 2-Y, 3-Y, 4-Y, 5-N, 6-Y, 7-NA
[57] Kuwait	2006	761 M: 261 F: 500	M: 21 years F: 20.8 years	Random sampling	Cross-sectional study	84.5	Water-pipe smokers: a person who smoked sheesha and had smoked sheesha for at least one month, people who had not smoked sheesha were classified as sheesha nonsmokers	*Water-pipe smoking:* M 24.6%, F 5.5% *Cigarette smoking:* M 38.8%, F 7.9%	1-Y, 2-Y, 3-Y, 4-Y, 5-N, 6-N, 7-NA
[58] Qatar	2003	1208 M: 508 F: 700	25–65	A multistage stratified cluster sampling	Cross-sectional study	80.5	BP according to the WHO criteria	*HTN:* 32.1% M 32.6%, F 31.7%	1-Y, 2-Y, 3-Y, 4-Y, 5-Y, 6-N, 7-NA
[59] Qatar	2007–2008	1117 M: 571 F: 546	>20	A multistage stratified cluster sampling	Cross-sectional study	77.9	DM was defined according to the WHO expert group	*DM:* 16.7% M 15.2%, F 18.1%	1-Y, 2-Y, 3-Y, 4-Y, 5-Y, 6-Y, 7-NA
[60] Qatar	1992	603 F: 100%	18–67	Convenient sampling	Cross-sectional survey	NR	Obesity and overweight according to the WHO definition/self-reported of past history of DM and HTN	HTN: 12.3%, DM: 12.9% Smoking: 3.2%, overweight: 30%, obesity: 33.6%, regular exercise: 16%	1-Y, 2-partly; 3-not entirely appropriate, 4-Y, 5-N, 6-N, 7-NA
[61] Oman	2000	7011 M: 50% F: 50%	≥20	A multistage stratified probability-sampling	Cross-sectional national survey	83–91.5	Current smokers: people who were smoking at the time of the survey and had smoked more than 100 cigarette in their life/former smokers: if they had smoked more than 100 cigarette in their life but no longer smoking/never smokers: if they had never smoked or had smoked less than 100 cigarette in their life	*Current smoking:* 7% M 13.4%, F 0.5% *Former smokers:* 2.3% *Never smokers:* 90.7%	1-Y, 2-Y, 3-Y, 4-Y, 5-Y, 6-N, 7-NA

TABLE 2: Continued.

Reference country	Year(s) of survey	Total sample	Age, mean, and min to max	Sampling methods	Study design	Response rate (%)	Diagnostic criteria and/or dietary assessment methods	The main findings and prevalence data	Quality assessment checklist (*)
[62] Oman	2000	7179 M: 50% F: 50%	≥20	A multistage stratified probability-sampling design	Cross-sectional national survey	96	The WHO criteria for glucose intolerance, HC, and HTN	*DM*: overall 11.6% M 11.8%, F 11.3%, U 17.7%, R 10.5% *HTN*: overall 21.5% M 32.5%, F 22.7%, U 26.4%, R 20.2% *HC*: overall 50.6% M 50.8%, F 50.4%, U 50%, R 50.7%	1-Y, 2-Y, 3-Y, 4-Y, 5-Y, 6-N, 7-NA
[63] Oman	1991 and 2000	5086 M: 2128 F: 2958 6400 M: 3069 F: 3331	≥20	Convenient sampling A multistage stratified probability-sampling design	Cross-sectional surveys	92 91	Overweight and obesity were defined according to the WHO criteria	*Overweight*: in 1991 (M 28.8%, F 29.5%) in 2000 (M 32.1%, F 27.3%) *Obesity*: in 1991 (M 10.5%, F 25.1%) in 2000 (M 16.7%, 23.8%)	1-Y, 2-Y, 3-Y, 4-Y, 5-N, 6-N, 7-NA
[64] Oman	2001	1421 M: 49% F: 51%	≥20	A probabilistic random sampling	Community based cross-sectional study	75.5	DM: FPG ≥5.6 mmol/L or 2hG ≥11.1 mmol/L or on medication/HTN: SBP ≥130 mmHg and/or DBP ≥85 mmHg or on medication/TC: ≥5.2 mmol/L/TG: ≥1.69 mmol/L/HDL: <1.03 mmol/L or on medication for dyslipidaemia/current smokers: people who smoking at the time of the survey/physical activity at leisure time and/or at work	*HTN* (M 24.7%, F 13.8%) *DM* (M 12.9%, F 11.9%) *HC* (M 34.5%, F 34.5%) *TG* (M 24.4%, F 13%) *HDL* (M 75.9%, F 71.6%) *Inactivity* (M 24.3%, F 69.3%) *Smoking* (M 9.6%, F 0)	1-Y, 2-Y, 3-Y, 4-Y, 5-Y, 6-Y, 7-NA

TABLE 2: Continued.

Reference country	Year(s) of survey	Total sample	Age, mean, and min to max	Sampling methods	Study design	Response rate (%)	Diagnostic criteria and/or dietary assessment methods	The main findings and prevalence data	Quality assessment checklist (*)
[65] Oman	2008	40,179 M: 52% F: 48%	≥18	A multistage stratified cluster sampling design	Community-based national cross-sectional survey	93.5	The WHO criteria for diagnosis HTN, HC, BMI, and DM were used	*Overweight: overall 29.5%* M 31.2%, F 28% *Obesity: overall 24.1%* M 22%, F 26.1% *HTN: overall 40.3%* M 50.7%, F 31% *DM: overall 12.3%* M 12.4%, F 12.1% *HC: overall 33.6%* M 33.1%, F 33.9% *HDL: overall 35.2%* M 26.3%, F 42.7% *LDL: overall 32%* M 33%, F 31.2% *TG: overall 18%* M 21.6%, F 14.9%	1-Y, 2-Y, 3-Y, 4-Y, 5-Y, 6-Y, 7-NA
[66] Bahrain	1995-1996	2013 M: 1168 F: 845	40–69	Stratified sampling design	Cross-sectional national survey	70	Overweight and obesity: WHO criteria. Physical activity was assessed by walking and cycling information: walkkm = 5 × walkwk (walking/day in average week) + walkkm (walking in weekend). Cyclekm = 5 × cyclewk (cycling/day in average week) + cyclewe (cycling in weekend)	*Age-adjusted prevalence of overweight:* M 39.9%, F 32.7% *Age-adjusted prevalence of obesity:* M 25.3%, F 33.2% *Physical activity:* 21% of men and 6% of women aged 50–59 walked 1–3 km per day and 68% of men and 93% of women aged 50–59 walked less than 1 km per day	1-Y, 2-Y, 3-Y, 4-Y, 5-Y, 6-N, 7-NA
[67] Bahrain	2002	514 M: 298 F: 216	30–79	Probability cluster sampling design	Cross-sectional community-based survey	NR	DM was defined by self-reported past history of diabetes	*DM: 9%* M 41.3%, F 58.7%	1-Y, 2-Y, 3-not entirely appropriate, 4-Y, 5-N, 6-N, 7-NA
[68] Bahrain	2001	514 M: 298 F: 216	30–79	Probability cluster sampling design	Cross-sectional community-based survey	NR	Overweight and obesity were defined according to the WHO criteria	*Overweight:* Overall 31% M 35.2%, F 31% *Obesity:* Overall 48.7% M 21.2%, F 48.7%	1-Y, 2-Y, 3-Y, 4-Y, 5-Y, 6-N, 7-NA

TABLE 2: Continued.

Reference country	Year(s) of survey	Total sample	Age, mean, and min to max	Sampling methods	Study design	Response rate (%)	Diagnostic criteria and/or dietary assessment methods	The main findings and prevalence data	Quality assessment checklist (*)
[69] Bahrain	1995-1996	2090 M: 1192 F: 834	40-69	Stratified sampling design	Cross-sectional national survey	62	HTN: SBP ≥160 mmHg, DBP ≥95 mmHg or on antihypertensive	HTN: M: 21% in 40–49 years, 29% in 50–59 years F: 33% in 50–59 years, 43% in 60–69 years	1-Y, 2-Y, 3-Y, 4-Y, 5-Y, 6-N, 7-NA
[70] Bahrain	1995-1996	2029 M & F = not clear	40-69	Stratified sampling design	Cross-sectional national epidemiological	59–70	DM was defined according to WHO criteria	DM: M: 23% in 40–49 years, 29% in 50–59 years F: 36% in age groups 50–59 and 37% 60–69 years	1-Y, 2-Y, 3-Y, 4-Y, 5-Y, 6-N, 7-NA
[71] Bahrain	2000	516 M: 299 F: 217	30–79	Random cluster-sampling design	Cross-sectional study	NR	Current smokers: a person smoking at least 1 cigarette per day regularly/ex-smokers: person who gave up smoking at least 6 months previously/nonsmoker: person who had never smoked regularly	Overall cigarette smoking: (M 27.1%, F 3.2%) Overall sheesha smoking: (M 5%, F 17.5%) Overall total smoking: M 32.1%, F 20.7%	1-Y, 2-Y, 3-Y, 4-Y, 5-Y, 6-N, 7-NA
[72] Bahrain	1996	498 M: 174 F: 324	≥20	Random selection from health care centres attendances	Cross-sectional study	86.9	DM was defined according to WHO criteria OR if the person had a previous history of DM	The prevalence of known diabetes subjects: M: 18.4%/F: 16.7% The prevalence of unknown diabetes: M: 8%/F: 8.3% The overall prevalence of diabetes: 25.5% M: 26.4%/F: 25%	1-Y, 2-Y, 3-Y, 4-Y, 5-N, 6-Y, 7-NA

M, male; F, female; U, urban; R, rural; DM, diabetes; IFG, impaired fasting glucose; HC, hypercholesterolemia; TG, triglyceride; TC, total cholesterol; HDL, high-density lipoprotein; LDL, low-density lipoprotein; HTN, hypertension; SBP, systolic blood pressure; DBP, diastolic blood pressure; NR, not reported; ACS, acute coronary syndrome; BMI, body mass index; Y, yes; N, no; and NA, not applicable.
(*) the quality assessment checklist assessed according to the Centre for Reviews and Dissemination guidelines (CRD) for nonrandomized studies: 1- Was the aim of the study stated clearly? 2- Was the methodology stated? And was it appropriate? 3- Were appropriate methods used for data collection and analysis? 4- Was the data analysis sufficiently rigorous? 5- Were preventive steps taken to minimize bias? 6- Were limitations of the study discussed? 7- In systematic review, was search strategy adequate and appropriate?

ranging from 69 to 90.1% [15, 17, 22, 25]. There was no data available on the incidence of strokes in Oman and the UAE. Only one study in Saudi Arabia reported on the number of stroke survivors as 186/100,000 [16]. Further, in the majority of stroke studies, the incidence of strokes was higher in males than females across all age groups and it increased with age [15, 17–20, 25], although there was still relatively high stroke incidence in younger age groups (≤45 years) in the GCC region [15, 17, 19, 23]. Across all stroke studies, hypertension (38.1–72.5%) was the most common risk factor, followed by diabetes (20–69.4%) for stroke patients [15, 17–26]. Dyslipidemia was reported in 4–61% of stroke patients [18–24, 26]. Smoking was reported in 1.6–40% of stroke patients in the GCC [15, 17–24, 26].

3.2. The Burden of the CHD and Stroke Risk Factors in the GCC Region. The risk factors for CHD and stroke can be categorized into two groups: metabolic risk factors (obesity, hypertension, diabetes, and dyslipidaemia) and behavioural risk factors (diet, smoking, and physical activity). In this section, the burden of various risk factors among healthy population in the GCC states is described.

3.2.1. Overweight and Obesity. Prevalence of overweight and obesity has been reported in 13 studies: 4 in Saudi Arabia [28, 31, 32, 39], 2 in Bahrain [66, 68], 2 in Kuwait [54, 55], 2 in Oman [63, 65], 1 in Qatar [60], and 2 in the UAE [43, 46].

Based on the available national representative studies, the prevalence of overweight in males and females in the GCC region ranged from 28.8% to 42.4% and from 27.3% to 32.7%, respectively, while the prevalence of obesity in males ranged from 10.5% to 39.2% and in females ranged from 18.2% to 53%. The prevalence of overweight and obesity increased with age with the highest level in the middle age groups (30–39 and 40–49 years) [28, 31, 32, 39, 43, 46, 54, 55, 60, 63, 65, 66, 68]. The obesity rates in urban areas were higher than in rural areas [28, 31, 32, 63]. In general, the prevalence of overweight and obesity is remarkably high in the GCC states and Oman reported the lowest rates of obesity within the region.

3.2.2. Hypertension. The prevalence of hypertension was reported in 10 studies: 3 in Saudi Arabia [27, 33, 35], 1 in Bahrain [69], 2 in Oman [62, 65], 2 in Qatar [58, 60], and 2 in the UAE [43, 44].

The rate of hypertension in the GCC states ranged from 26% to 50.7% in males and from 20.9% to 31.7% in females [33, 35, 43, 44, 58, 62, 65, 69]. Across all studies, the prevalence of hypertension considerably increased with age with the highest rates in the 45–65 age groups. The prevalence of hypertension in Saudi Arabia was lower than Oman, Bahrain, and Qatar but close to the UAE. The lower rate of hypertension in Saudi Arabia may not be true reflection of the situation as the reported study was relatively old [35].

3.2.3. Diabetes Mellitus. The rates of diabetes mellitus in the GCC countries were addressed in 13 studies: 2 in Saudi Arabia [29, 31], 3 in Bahrain [67, 70, 72], 2 in Kuwait [51, 56], 2 in Oman [62, 65], 2 in Qatar [59, 60], and 2 in the UAE [43, 45].

The overall prevalence of diabetes ranged from 6% to 23.7% in the GCC. Three studies showed higher diabetes rates among females [31, 59, 67], while three studies indicated the opposite [29, 45, 56]. Four studies showed almost no difference in the prevalence of diabetes between genders [43, 51, 62, 65]. The prevalence of diabetes rose proportionally with age and reached the highest rates in both sexes among those aged 55-64 years and over [29, 31, 43, 45, 51, 56, 59, 62, 65, 67]. It was also considerably higher among the urban population [29, 62]. Overall, the available data on the prevalence of diabetes in this region indicated that Saudi Arabia, Bahrain, and the UAE have the highest rates of diabetes compared to the other Gulf countries especially Kuwait, where the rates of diabetes were relatively lower; however this might be due to the underestimation of the actual prevalence in one Kuwaiti study as it excluded diabetic subjects on medication [56].

3.2.4. Dyslipidaemia. The prevalence of dyslipidaemia was reported in 7 studies: 3 in Saudi Arabia [27, 31, 37], 1 in Kuwait [53], 2 in Oman [62, 65], and 1 in the UAE [43]. There was no consistent definition of dyslipidaemia within the region. The majority of the dyslipidaemia studies reported the prevalence rate based on total cholesterol and triglycerides levels.

Overall, dyslipidaemia levels were higher in males than females and increased with age gradually up to the age group of 50–59 when it became stable in some studies and slightly declined in others. The prevalence of hypercholesterolemia (HC) ranged from 17% to 54.9% in males and from 9% to 53.2% in females [27, 31, 37, 53, 62, 65]. There was no difference in HC between urban and rural residents [37, 62]. However, one study in Saudi Arabia showed higher rates of hypertriglyceridemia in the urban population (43.2%) than rural population (34.1%) [37]. Based on the available data on dyslipidaemia within the region, HC (≥5.2 mmol/L) was more prevalent in Saudi Arabia. The variation in definitions used in dyslipidaemia studies and the limited data in the GCC make it difficult to accurately compare between countries; however the levels of blood lipids appeared to be high in the Gulf region.

3.2.5. Diet. Six studies carried out in Saudi Arabia [40–42] and UAE [48–50] have determined the eating habits among adult population in these countries.

The dietary patterns presented in these studies are mainly characterized by a high consumption of snacks, fatty food, salty food, and sugar. A study in Saudi Arabia reported that more than half of the study population was consuming a high amount of snacks and fatty and salty foods in daily basis [41]. Similarly, a high consumption of sugar and fast food was reported in the UAE [48, 49]. Further, a low consumption of fruits, vegetable, and cereals was reported in several studies [41, 49, 50]. One study showed a high intake of fruits, vegetables, and dates [42]. The findings from these surveys also demonstrated a high intake of total energy, fats, and protein [41, 48]. A Saudi survey showed a high proportion of total energy derived from fat and carbohydrates (38% versus 39%) and (46.1% versus 46.8%) in both males and females, respectively [41]. Some of the popular unhealthy food habits reported were not having breakfast, consuming less than two meals per day, and a high consumption of fast food meals [41, 49]. A number of studies have examined the association between some food items and CVD risk factors [40, 41, 49]. One study showed an inverse association between consumption of black tea and serum lipids [40], while another study reported a significant association of high intake of energy derived from fatty foods with BMI and hypertension in both genders [41]. Further, low consumption of cereals and fruits was found to be associated with obesity [49].

3.2.6. Smoking.
The prevalence of smoking in the Gulf region was addressed in 9 studies: 3 in Saudi Arabia [27, 30, 38], 1 in Bahrain [71], 2 in Kuwait [52, 57], 1 in Oman [61], 1 in Qatar [60], and 1 in the UAE [43].

The rates of cigarette smoking in the GCC ranged from 13.4% to 37.4% in males and from 0.5% to 20.7% in females. Furthermore, the prevalence of smoking fluctuated from age group to age group. It was more common in males at younger ages (18–25 years); however some studies reported a high prevalence in the older age group (40–59 years). In females, the highest rates of smoking were in the older age group (40–49 years) [30, 43, 52, 57, 61, 71]. One study in Saudi Arabia reported higher rates of cigarette smoking in urban than rural subjects [38]. Overall, the prevalence of smoking was higher in Saudi Arabia, Kuwait, the UAE, and Bahrain in comparison to Oman.

3.2.7. Physical Activity.
The prevalence of physical activity in the GCC countries was presented in 7 studies: 2 in Saudi Arabia [34, 36], 1 in Bahrain [66], 1 in Kuwait [56], 1 in Oman [64], 1 in Qatar [60], and 1 in the UAE [47].

The prevalence of inactivity was found to be significantly higher among the younger population in the region, and across all age groups physical inactivity was higher in females than males. The rates of inactivity ranged from 24.3% to 93.9% in males and from 50% to 98.1% in females in the GCC [36, 47, 60, 64, 66]. In general, the rates of physical inactivity were considerably high in the GCC region especially Saudi Arabia.

4. Discussion

This review revealed that, in the GCC region, there is a lack of information on the prevalence of CHD with only exception in Saudi Arabia where one national survey reported 5.5% prevalence of CHD [11], which is lower than the prevalence rate reported in Egypt 8.3% [73], while it is higher than in India (3%), China (2%), and Europe (5%) [74, 75]. However, it is important to note that the Saudi report is relatively old and may not reflect the current situation. The rates of ACS and associated risk factors appeared to be very similar in Saudi Arabia (SPACE report) and other Gulf states (Gulf RACE report) except for diabetes, which is more prevalent in Saudi Arabia. However, the SPACE registry results came

from phase 1 (pilot study) and thus based on smaller sample size compared to that of Gulf RACE [13, 14].

In contrast to other ACS registries around the world, the prevalence rates of diabetes and current smoking are higher in the Gulf region, while a higher prevalence of hypertension and dyslipidaemia is observed in the Euro heart of the acute coronary syndrome survey and Canadian ACS registry [13, 14, 76, 77]. The rates of diabetes are ranged from 23.3% to 25.1% in the Euro heart survey, Canadian ACS registry, and the Global Registry of Acute Cardiac Events (GRACE) [76, 77], while the prevalence of diabetes is much higher among the ACS patients in the Gulf States especially in Saudi Arabia (56%) [13, 14]. One possible explanation for this high rate of diabetes could be due the high prevalence of obesity and physical inactivity in the GCC region, especially in Saudi Arabia. Furthermore, the mean age of presentation in the SPACE and Gulf RACE cohort is about ten years younger than that reported in the Euro heart survey and the GRACE cohort [13, 14, 78, 79]. This might be due to the high rates of uncontrolled risk factors in the Gulf region as well as the high percentage of younger populations in these countries.

The crude annual incidence of stroke in the Gulf countries was generally lower than the reported incidence in some Arabic countries, for example, Libya (63/100,000) [80] and Northern Palestine (51.4/100,000) [81]. The incidence is even much lower than that which is observed in some of the developed countries such as Scotland (280/100,000) [82] and the East Coast of Australia (206/100,000) [83]. The low rates of strokes in the GCC countries could be explained by the relatively younger age of patients in these countries. Further, the majority of stroke studies in the region had no record on the number of patients who died before reaching hospital, thus underestimating the actual incidence rate.

Several studies in the Gulf States have reported a high incidence of stroke at a younger age. Of the stroke patients, 9.8% to 25% were less than 45 years old [17, 23, 25]. The higher proportion of undiagnosed hypertension and diabetes might be a reason for younger stroke patients. One study in Saudi Arabia showed that only half of the hypertensive stroke patients were actually on medication [17]. Further, lack of awareness about stroke in the Gulf countries might have led to an increase in the incidence of strokes as well as the rates of associated risk factors [84].

When looking at the burden of risk factors among healthy subjects in the GCC region, the prevalence of obesity in adult females is one of the highest amongst females worldwide. This review found that almost half of the females in Kuwait and Bahrain and around 35% of females in Saudi Arabia, the UAE, and Qatar were obese. The overall prevalence of overweight and obesity in the GCC is higher than that which was reported in other Middle Eastern countries such as Lebanon and Turkey [85, 86]. The prevalence was even higher than in many developed countries such as the USA and in developing countries such as India [87, 88]. The food customs in the Gulf region, such as weddings and religious events, might be an important contributory factor for such a high rate of obesity as they serve food that is rich in fat, usually "Kabsa," which includes meat (from sheep or small camel) with rice. Even socialising with friends and family is usually around eating meals and snacks.

Likewise, more than half of the GCC population are physically inactive, with only a small proportion of people being active on a regular basis. Furthermore, the rate of inactivity appeared to be remarkably higher in Saudi Arabia than in other Gulf countries. The reviewed studies also indicated that males are more likely to be physically active than females, a finding similar to that was reported in Turkey and Pakistan [47]. The unique social, cultural, and environmental factors of the GCC states, such as hot climate, lack of outdoor facilities, the limited number of health clubs, high cost of attending such clubs especially for females, high level of employment of domestic helpers, and the high dependency on automobiles are blamed on the increased levels of physical inactivity in both genders but more noticeably in females. Also, females have more social barriers that make it difficult for them to exercise outside the home without a family member [5, 89].

In the Gulf region, males start smoking cigarettes at an early age (before 18 years), while females generally start after 30s. Cigarette smoking by younger and unmarried females is viewed as culturally unacceptable and can potentially destroy their reputation. However, the case is different when smoking sheesha (water-pipe) as Arabic societies in general accept sheesha smoking by females irrespective of their age and/or social status.

Hypertension and diabetes are the two major risk factors associated with CHD and stroke patients in all studies in the Gulf region; this might be related to the high rates of undiagnosed hypertensive and diabetic patients within the region. In Saudi Arabia, about 70% of the hypertensive people were unaware of their disease [35]. A similar situation was reported in Oman, the UAE, and Bahrain [44, 65, 69]. Likewise, a large number of diabetic subjects in Saudi Arabia (28%) and the UAE (41%) were unaware of their disease [29, 45]. The high rates of uncontrolled diseases such as hypertension and diabetes could be a reason for the relatively young age of CHD and stroke patients in the Gulf region.

The prevalence of dyslipidaemia in general is high in the GCC countries. The available national surveys indicated that half the Saudi population have high level of total cholesterol and almost half of the males and one-third of Saudi females have high level of hypertriglyceridemia [37]. The rates of HC in Saudi Arabia are similar to that reported in USA (53.2%) [90]. Dyslipidaemia is a major risk factor for CHD and plays a central role in the development of atherosclerosis. The high rates of dyslipidaemia in the GCC countries may be due to the high prevalence of physical inactivity, obesity, and diabetes among the Gulf populations. Also, as mentioned before, food customs and the consumption of high fatty foods might be contributing factors.

This review has a number of limitations. First, there was a lack of recent nationally representative reports in the GCC countries, and thus it is difficult to compare the data between GCC countries. Second, there was significant heterogeneity between studies with respect to definitions of the risk factors, design, and population characteristics. Third, only a few studies reported stroke incidence and the majority of them were hospital-based studies with an absence of data on Oman and the UAE. Fourth, there were only a few studies focusing on hypertension, dyslipidaemia, and physical activity. Moreover, the number of included studies relating to the prevalence of risk factors in Qatar and Bahrain were also relatively low. However, the strength of this review was that the literature search was conducted on multiple databases including personal contact of the authors to capture all relevant documents.

5. Conclusion

The present review revealed lower incidence of strokes in the GCC countries than in developed countries and that those affected were younger than in some developing and developed countries. Although there was lack of nationally representative data on the prevalence of CHD in the region, high prevalence of key risk factors was observed. Further, the patterns of risk factors were very similar between the Gulf countries; this may be due to the similarity in culture, religion, cuisine, lifestyle, and environmental factors between these countries. With the rapid urbanization in the Gulf region and the relatively young population, the prevalence of CHD and strokes is expected to increase in the next few decades, which in turn will raise the rate of CVD mortality and morbidity in the region. Well-designed population-based nationally representative surveys focusing on CVD and its associated risk factors are crucial in the Gulf States. Furthermore, there is a need to increase the awareness of the high prevalence of CVD and associated risk factors among the public along with education programs on nutrition and healthier lifestyles including increase in physical activity levels in both men and women. In addition, there is also a need for preventative strategies, especially for type 2 diabetes, to be used in the region and the cooperation in management strategies, especially in obesity and diabetes is also crucial across the region. Moreover, addressing some of the cultural and social barriers that were mentioned previously is also important for reducing the risk of CVD and related risk factors among the GCC population.

Conflict of Interests

The authors declare that they have no competing interests.

Authors' Contribution

Najlaa Aljefree designed the concept of study and prepared the paper draft. Faruk Ahmed has provided guidance on the study design and critically reviewed the paper. All authors read and approved the final paper.

Acknowledgments

Mrs. Najlaa Aljefree is supported by a scholarship from King Abdul Aziz University for Nutrition and Dietetics. The King Abdul Aziz University had no role in the design, analysis, or writing of this paper.

References

[1] S. Mendis, P. Puska, and B. Norrving, *Global Atlas on Cardiovascular Disease Prevention and Control*, World Health Organization, 2011.

[2] M. J. O'Donnell, X. Denis, L. Liu et al., "Risk factors for ischaemic and intracerebral haemorrhagic stroke in 22 countries (the INTERSTROKE Study): a case-control study," *The Lancet*, vol. 376, no. 9735, pp. 112–123, 2010.

[3] S. Yusuf, S. Hawken, S. Ôunpuu et al., "Effect of potentially modifiable risk factors associated with myocardial infarction in 52 countries (the INTERHEART study): case-control study," *The Lancet*, vol. 364, no. 9438, pp. 937–952, 2004.

[4] The Cooperation Council for the Arab States of the Gulf, http://www.gcc-sg.org/.

[5] R. M. Mabry, M. M. Reeves, E. G. Eakin, and N. Owen, "Evidence of physical activity participation among men and women in the countries of the gulf cooperation council: a review," *Obesity Reviews*, vol. 11, no. 6, pp. 457–464, 2010.

[6] C. M. Lawes, S. V. Hoorn, and A. Rodgers, "Global burden of blood-pressure-related disease, 2001," *The Lancet*, vol. 371, no. 9623, pp. 1513–1518, 2008.

[7] WHO, *Noncommunicable Diseases Country Profiles 2011*, World Health Organization, Geneva, Switzerland, 2011.

[8] B. Motlagh, M. O'Donnell, and S. Yusuf, "Prevalence of cardiovascular risk factors in the middle east: a systematic review," *European Journal of Cardiovascular Prevention and Rehabilitation*, vol. 16, no. 3, pp. 268–280, 2009.

[9] N. M. Shara, "Cardiovascular disease in Middle Eastern women,' ' *Nutrition, Metabolism and Cardiovascular Diseases*, vol. 20, no. 6, pp. 412–418, 2010.

[10] *Systematic Reviews: CRD's Guidance for Undertaking Reviews in Health Care*, University of York, Centre for Reviews and Dissemination, York, UK, 2009.

[11] M. M. Al-Nozha, M. R. Arafah, Y. Y. Al-Mazrou et al., "Coronary artery disease in Saudia Arabia," *Saudi Medical Journal*, vol. 25, no. 9, pp. 1165–1171, 2004.

[12] A. El-Menyar, M. Zubaid, W. Rashed et al., "Comparison of men and women with acute coronary syndrome in six Middle Eastern countries," *The American Journal of Cardiology*, vol. 104, no. 8, pp. 1018–1022, 2009.

[13] A. El-Menyar, M. Zubaid, A. Shehab et al., "Prevalence and impact of cardiovascular risk factors among patients presenting with acute coronary syndrome in the Middle East," *Clinical Cardiology*, vol. 34, no. 1, pp. 51–58, 2011.

[14] K. F. AlHabib, A. Hersi, H. AlFaleh et al., "The Saudi Project for Assessment of Coronary Events (SPACE) registry: design and results of a phase I pilot study," *Canadian Journal of Cardiology*, vol. 25, no. 7, pp. e255–e258, 2009.

[15] S. Al Rajeh, A. Awada, G. Niazi, and E. Larbi, "Stroke in a Saudi Arabian National Guard community: analysis of 500 consecutive cases from a population-based hospital," *Stroke*, vol. 24, no. 11, pp. 1635–1639, 1993.

[16] S. Al Rajeh, O. Bademosi, H. Ismail et al., "A community survey of neurological disorders in Saudi Arabia: the Thugbah study," *Neuroepidemiology*, vol. 12, no. 3, pp. 164–178, 1993.

[17] S. Al-Rajeh, E. B. Larbi, O. Bademosi et al., "Stroke register: experience from the eastern province of Saudi Arabia," *Cerebrovascular Diseases*, vol. 8, no. 2, pp. 86–89, 1998.

[18] F. A. Qari, "Profile of stroke in a teaching university hospital in the western region," *Saudi Medical Journal*, vol. 21, no. 11, pp. 1030–1033, 2000.

[19] A. Al-Jishi and P. Mohan, "Profile of stroke in Bahrain," *Neurosciences*, vol. 5, no. 1, pp. 30–34, 2000.

[20] N. U. A. M. A. Abdul-Ghaffar, M. R. El-Sonbaty, M. S. El-Din Abdul-Baky, A. A. Marafie, and A. M. Al-Said, "Stroke in Kuwait: a three-year prospective study," *Neuroepidemiology*, vol. 16, no. 1, pp. 40–47, 1997.

[21] S. Al-Shammri, Z. Shahid, A. Ghali et al., "Risk factors, subtypes and outcome of ischaemic stroke in Kuwait—a hospital-based study," *Medical Principles and Practice*, vol. 12, no. 4, pp. 218–223, 2003.

[22] A. Ashkanani, K. A. Hassan, and S. Lamdhade, "Risk factors of stroke patients admitted to a general hospital in Kuwait," *International Journal of Neuroscience*, vol. 123, no. 2, pp. 89–92, 2013.

[23] N. Akhtar, S. I. Kamran, D. Deleu et al., "Ischaemic posterior circulation stroke in State of Qatar," *European Journal of Neurology*, vol. 16, no. 9, pp. 1004–1009, 2009.

[24] D. Deleu, A. A. Hamad, S. Kamram, A. El Siddig, H. Al Hail, and S. M. K. Hamdy, "Ethnic variations in risk factor profile, pattern and recurrence of non-cardioembolic ischemic stroke," *Archives of Medical Research*, vol. 37, no. 5, pp. 655–662, 2006.

[25] A. Hamad, T. E. O. Sokrab, S. Momeni, B. Mesraoua, and A. Lingren, "Stroke in Qatar: a one-year, hospital-based study," *Journal of Stroke and Cerebrovascular Diseases*, vol. 10, no. 5, pp. 236–241, 2001.

[26] D. Deleu, J. Inshasi, N. Akhtar et al., "Risk factors, management and outcome of subtypes of ischemic stroke: a stroke registry from the Arabian Gulf," *Journal of the Neurological Sciences*, vol. 300, no. 1-2, pp. 142–147, 2011.

[27] B. A. Abalkhail, S. Shawky, T. M. Ghabrah, and W. A. Milaat, "Hypercholesterolemia and 5-year risk of development of coronary heart disease among university and school workers in Jeddah, Saudi Arabia," *Preventive Medicine*, vol. 31, no. 4, pp. 390–395, 2000.

[28] A. A. Al-Nuaim, E. A. Bamgboye, K. A. Al-Rubeaan, and Y. Al-Mazrou, "Overweight and obesity in Saudi Arabian adult population, role of sociodemographic variables," *Journal of Community Health*, vol. 22, no. 3, pp. 211–223, 1997.

[29] M. M. Al-Nozha, M. A. Al-Maatouq, Y. Y. Al-Mazrou et al., "Diabetes mellitus in Saudi Arabia," *Saudi Medical Journal*, vol. 25, no. 11, pp. 1603–1610, 2004.

[30] T. J. Hashim, "Smoking habits of students in College of Applied Medical Science, Saudi Arabia," *Saudi Medical Journal*, vol. 21, no. 1, pp. 76–80, 2000.

[31] A. Rahman Al-Nuaim, "High prevalence of metabolic risk factors for cardiovascular diseases among Saudi population, aged 30–64 years," *International Journal of Cardiology*, vol. 62, no. 3, pp. 227–235, 1997.

[32] M. M. Al-Nozha, Y. Y. Al-Mazrou, M. A. Al-Maatouq et al., "Obesity in Saudi Arabia," *Saudi Medical Journal*, vol. 26, no. 5, pp. 824–829, 2005.

[33] K. A. Kalantan, A. G. Mohamed, A. A. Al-Taweel, and H. M. Abdul Ghani, "Hypertension among attendants of primary health care centers in Al-Qassim region, Saudi Arabia," *Saudi Medical Journal*, vol. 22, no. 11, pp. 960–963, 2001.

[34] S. A. Al-Refaee and H. M. Al-Hazzaa, "Physical activity profile of adult males in Riyadh City," *Saudi Medical Journal*, vol. 22, no. 9, pp. 784–789, 2001.

[35] M. M. Al-Nozha, M. Abdullah, M. R. Arafah et al., "Hypertension in Saudi Arabia," *Saudi Medical Journal*, vol. 28, no. 1, pp. 77–84, 2007.

[36] M. M. Al-Nozha, H. M. Al-Hazzaa, M. R. Arafah et al., "Prevalence of physical activity and inactivity among Saudis aged 30-70 years: a population-based cross-sectional study," *Saudi Medical Journal*, vol. 28, no. 4, pp. 559–568, 2007.

[37] M. M. Al-Nozha, M. R. Arafah, M. A. Al-Maatouq et al., "Hyperlipidemia in Saudi Arabia," *Saudi Medical Journal*, vol. 29, no. 2, pp. 282–287, 2008.

[38] N. S. Al-Haddad, T. A. Al-Habeeb, M. H. Abdelgadir, Y. S. Al-Ghamdy, and N. A. Qureshi, "Smoking patterns among primary health care attendees, Al-Qassim region, Saudi Arabia," *Eastern Mediterranean Health Journal*, vol. 9, no. 5-6, pp. 911–922, 2003.

[39] N. A. Al-Baghli, A. J. Al-Ghamdi, K. A. Al-Turki, A. G. El-Zubaier, M. Al-Ameer, and F. A. Al-Baghli, "Overweight and obesity in the eastern province of Saudi Arabia," *Saudi Medical Journal*, vol. 29, no. 9, pp. 1319–1325, 2008.

[40] I. A. Hakim, M. A. Alsaif, A. Aloud et al., "Black tea consumption and serum lipid profiles in Saudi women: a cross-sectional study in Saudi Arabia," *Nutrition Research*, vol. 23, no. 11, pp. 1515–1526, 2003.

[41] F. Y. Abdel-Megeid, H. M. Abdelkarem, and A. M. El-Fetouh, "Unhealthy nutritional habits in university students are a risk factor for cardiovascular diseases," *Saudi Medical Journal*, vol. 32, no. 6, pp. 621–627, 2011.

[42] F. Midhet, A. R. Al Mohaimeed, and F. Sharaf, "Dietary practices, physical activity and health education in qassim region of Saudi Arabia," *International Journal Of Health Sciences*, vol. 4, no. 1, pp. 3–10, 2010.

[43] C. Hajat, O. Harrison, and Z. Al Siksek, "Weqaya: A population-wide cardiovascular screening program in Abu Dhabi, United Arab Emirates," *The American Journal of Public Health*, vol. 102, no. 5, pp. 909–914, 2012.

[44] Y. El-Shahat, S. Z. Bakir, N. Farjou et al., "Hypertension in UAE citizens-preliminary results of a prospective study," *Saudi Journal of Kidney Diseases and Transplantation*, vol. 10, no. 3, pp. 376–381, 1999.

[45] M. Malik, A. Bakir, B. Abi Saab, G. Roglic, and H. King, "Glucose intolerance and associated factors in the multi-ethnic population of the United Arab Emirates: results of a national survey," *Diabetes Research and Clinical Practice*, vol. 69, no. 2, pp. 188–195, 2005.

[46] A. O. Carter, H. F. Saadi, R. L. Reed, and E. V. Dunn, "Assessment of obesity, lifestyle, and reproductive health needs of female citizens of Al Ain, United Arab Emirates," *Journal of Health, Population and Nutrition*, vol. 22, no. 1, pp. 75–83, 2004.

[47] R. Guthold, T. Ono, K. L. Strong, S. Chatterji, and A. Morabia, "Worldwide variability in physical inactivity: a 51-Country Survey," *The American Journal of Preventive Medicine*, vol. 34, no. 6, pp. 486–494, 2008.

[48] T. Al-Sarraj, H. Saadi, J. S. Volek, and M. L. Fernandez, "Metabolic syndrome prevalence, dietary intake, and cardiovascular risk profile among overweight and obese adults 18–50 years old from the united arab emirates," *Metabolic Syndrome and Related Disorders*, vol. 8, no. 1, pp. 39–46, 2010.

[49] A. Kerkadi, "Evaluation of nutritional status of united arab emirates university female students," *Emirates Journal of Food and Agriculture*, vol. 15, no. 2, pp. 42–50, 2003.

[50] A. O. Musaiger and N. M. Abuirmeileh, "Food consumption patterns of adults in the United Arab Emirates," *The Journal of The Royal Society for the Promotion of Health*, vol. 118, no. 3, pp. 146–150, 1998.

[51] N. Abdella, M. Al Arouj, A. Al Nakhi, A. Al Assoussi, and M. Moussa, "Non-insulin-dependent diabetes in Kuwait: prevalence rates and associated risk factors," *Diabetes Research and Clinical Practice*, vol. 42, no. 3, pp. 187–196, 1998.

[52] A. Memon, P. M. Moody, T. N. Sugathan et al., "Epidemiology of smoking among Kuwaiti adults: prevalence, characteristics, and attitudes," *Bulletin of the World Health Organization*, vol. 78, no. 11, pp. 1306–1315, 2000.

[53] F. Ahmed, C. Waslien, M. Al-Sumaie, and P. Prakash, "Trends and risk factors of hypercholesterolemia among Kuwaiti adults: National Nutrition Surveillance Data from 1998 to 2009," *Nutrition*, vol. 28, no. 9, pp. 917–923, 2012.

[54] I. Al Rashdan and Y. Al Nesef, "Prevalence of overweight, obesity, and metabolic syndrome among adult Kuwaitis: results from community-based national survey," *Angiology*, vol. 61, no. 1, pp. 42–48, 2010.

[55] F. Ahmed, C. Waslien, M. A. Al-Sumaie, and P. Prakash, "Secular trends and risk factors of overweight and obesity among Kuwaiti adults: National Nutrition Surveillance System data from 1998 to 2009," *Public Health Nutrition*, vol. 15, no. 11, pp. 2124–2130, 2012.

[56] F. Ahmed, C. Waslien, M. A. Al-Sumaie, P. Prakash, and A. Allafi, "Trends and risk factors of hyperglycemia and diabetes among Kuwaiti adults: National Nutrition Surveillance Data from 2002 to 2009," *BMC Public Health*, vol. 13, no. 1, article 103, 2013.

[57] H. R. Mohammed, I. M. Newman, and R. Tayeh, "Sheesha smoking among a sample of future teachers in Kuwait," *Kuwait Medical Journal*, vol. 38, no. 2, article 107, 2006.

[58] A. Bener, J. Al-Suwaidi, K. Al-Jaber, S. Al-Marri, and I. E. A. Elbagi, "Epidemiology of hypertension and its associated risk factors in the Qatari population," *Journal of Human Hypertension*, vol. 18, no. 7, pp. 529–530, 2004.

[59] A. Bener, M. Zirie, I. M. Janahi, A. O. A. A. Al-Hamaq, M. Musallam, and N. J. Wareham, "Prevalence of diagnosed and undiagnosed diabetes mellitus and its risk factors in a population-based study of Qatar," *Diabetes Research and Clinical Practice*, vol. 84, no. 1, pp. 99–106, 2009.

[60] A. O. Musaiger, F. A. Al-Khalaf, and N. E. Shahbeek, "Risk factors for cardiovascular disease among women attending health centers in Qatar," *Emirates Journal of Food and Agriculture*, vol. 6, no. 1, pp. 188–200, 1994.

[61] A. A. Al Riyami and M. Afifi, "Smoking in Oman: prevalence and characteristics of smokers," *Eastern Mediterranean Health Journal*, vol. 10, no. 4-5, pp. 600–609, 2004.

[62] S. Al-Moosa, S. Allin, N. Jemiai, J. Al-Lawati, and E. Mossialos, "Diabetes and urbanization in the Omani population: an analysis of national survey data," *Population Health Metrics*, vol. 4, article 5, 2006.

[63] J. A. Al-Lawati and P. J. Jousilahti, "Prevalence and 10-year secular trend of obesity in Oman," *Saudi Medical Journal*, vol. 25, no. 3, pp. 346–351, 2004.

[64] J. A. Al-Lawati and P. Jousilahti, "Body mass index, waist circumference and waist-to-hip ratio cut-off points for categorisation of obesity among Omani Arabs," *Public Health Nutrition*, vol. 11, no. 1, pp. 102–108, 2008.

[65] A. Al Riyami, M. A. Abd Elaty, M. Morsi, H. Al Kharusi, W. Al Shukaily, and S. Jaju, "Oman World Health Survey: part 1—methodology, sociodemographic profile and epidemiology of non-communicable diseases in Oman," *Oman Medical Journal*, vol. 27, no. 5, pp. 425–443, 2012.

[66] F. Al-Mahroos and K. Al-Roomi, "Obesity among adult Bahraini population: impact of physical activity and educational level," *Annals of Saudi Medicine*, vol. 21, no. 3-4, pp. 183–187, 2001.

[67] A. O. Musaiger and M. A. Al-Mannai, "Social and lifestyle factors associated with diabetes in the adult Bahraini population," *Journal of Biosocial Science*, vol. 34, no. 2, pp. 277–281, 2002.

[68] A. O. Musaiger and M. A. Al-Mannai, "Weight, height, body mass index and prevalence of obesity among the adult population in Bahrain," *Annals of Human Biology*, vol. 28, no. 3, pp. 346–350, 2001.

[69] F. Al-Mahroos, K. Al-Roomi, and P. M. McKeigue, "Relation of high blood pressure to glucose intolerance, plasma lipids and educational status in an Arabian Gulf population," *International Journal of Epidemiology*, vol. 29, no. 1, pp. 71–76, 2000.

[70] F. Al-Mahroos and P. M. Mckeigue, "High prevalence of diabetes in bahrainis: associations with ethnicity and raised plasma cholesterol," *Diabetes Care*, vol. 21, no. 6, pp. 936–942, 1998.

[71] R. R. Hamadeh and A. O. Musaiger, "Lifestyle patterns in smokers and non-smokers in the state of Bahrain," *Nicotine & Tobacco Research*, vol. 2, no. 1, pp. 65–69, 2000.

[72] F. I. Al Zurba and A. Al Garf, "Prevalence of diabetes mellitus among Bahrainis attending primary health care centres," *Eastern Mediterranean Health Journal*, vol. 2, no. 2, pp. 274–282, 1996.

[73] W. Almahmeed, M. S. Arnaout, R. Chettaoui et al., "Coronary artery disease in Africa and the Middle East," *Therapeutics and Clinical Risk Management*, vol. 8, pp. 65–72, 2012.

[74] S. S. Anand, S. Yusuf, V. Vuksan et al., "Differences in risk factors, atherosclerosis, and cardiovascular disease between ethnic groups in Canada: the Study of Health Assessment and Risk in Ethnic groups (SHARE)," *The Lancet*, vol. 356, no. 9226, pp. 279–284, 2000.

[75] R. Gupta, P. Joshi, V. Mohan, K. S. Reddy, and S. Yusuf, "Epidemiology and causation of coronary heart disease and stroke in India," *Heart*, vol. 94, no. 1, pp. 16–26, 2008.

[76] A. T. Yan, P. Jong, R. T. Yan et al., "Clinical trial-derived risk model may not generalize to real-world patients with acute coronary syndrome," *American Heart Journal*, vol. 148, no. 6, pp. 1020–1027, 2004.

[77] A. Rosengren, L. Wallentin, M. Simoons et al., "Cardiovascular risk factors and clinical presentation in acute coronary syndromes," *Heart*, vol. 91, no. 9, pp. 1141–1147, 2005.

[78] D. Hasdai, S. Behar, L. Wallentin et al., "A prospective survey of the characteristics, treatments and outcomes of patients with acute coronary syndromes in Europe and the Mediterranean basin: the Euro Heart Survey of Acute Coronary Syndromes (Euro Heart Survey ACS)," *European Heart Journal*, vol. 23, no. 15, pp. 1190–1201, 2002.

[79] K. A. A. Fox, S. G. Goodman, F. A. Anderson Jr. et al., "From guidelines to clinical practice: the impact of hospital and geographical characteristics on temporal trends in the management of acute coronary syndromes: the Global Registry of Acute Coronary Events (GRACE)," *European Heart Journal*, vol. 24, no. 15, pp. 1414–1424, 2003.

[80] P. P. Ashok, K. Radhakrishnan, R. Sridharan, and M. A. El-Mangoush, "Incidence and pattern of cerebrovascular diseases in Benghazi, Libya," *Journal of Neurology Neurosurgery and Psychiatry*, vol. 49, no. 5, pp. 519–523, 1986.

[81] W. M. Sweileh, A. F. Sawalha, S. M. Al-Aqad, S. H. Zyoud, and S. W. Al-Jabi, "The epidemiology of stroke in northern palestine: a 1-year, hospital-based study," *Journal of Stroke and Cerebrovascular Diseases*, vol. 17, no. 6, pp. 406–411, 2008.

[82] P. D. Syme, A. W. Byrne, R. Chen, R. Devenny, and J. F. Forbes, "Community-based stroke incidence in a Scottish population: the Scottish borders stroke study," *Stroke*, vol. 36, no. 9, pp. 1837–1843, 2005.

[83] A. G. Thrift, H. M. Dewey, R. A. L. Macdonell, J. J. McNeil, and G. A. Donnan, "Stroke incidence on the east coast of Australia: the North East Melbourne Stroke Incidence Study (NEMESIS)," *Stroke*, vol. 31, no. 9, pp. 2087–2092, 2000.

[84] S. Kamran, A. B. Bener, D. Deleu et al., "The level of awareness of stroke risk factors and symptoms in the Gulf Cooperation Council countries: Gulf Cooperation Council stroke awareness study," *Neuroepidemiology*, vol. 29, no. 3-4, pp. 235–242, 2008.

[85] A. M. Sibai, N. Hwalla, N. Adra, and B. Rahal, "Prevalence and covariates of obesity in Lebanon: findings from the first epidemiological study," *Obesity Research*, vol. 11, no. 11, pp. 1353–1361, 2003.

[86] C. Erem, C. Arslan, A. Hacihasanoglu et al., "Prevalence of obesity and associated risk factors in a Turkish population (Trabzon City, Turkey)," *Obesity Research*, vol. 12, no. 7, pp. 1117–1127, 2004.

[87] C. L. Ogden, M. D. Carroll, L. R. Curtin, M. A. McDowell, C. J. Tabak, and K. M. Flegal, "Prevalence of overweight and obesity in the United States, 1999–2004," *The Journal of the American Medical Association*, vol. 295, no. 13, pp. 1549–1555, 2006.

[88] A. Misra, R. M. Pandey, J. R. Devi, R. Sharma, N. K. Vikram, and N. Khanna, "High prevalence of diabetes, obesity and dyslipidaemia in urban slum population in northern India," *International Journal of Obesity*, vol. 25, no. 11, pp. 1722–1729, 2001.

[89] A. M. Sibai, L. Nasreddine, A. H. Mokdad, N. Adra, M. Tabet, and N. Hwalla, "Nutrition transition and cardiovascular disease risk factors in middle East and North Africa countries: reviewing the evidence," *Annals of Nutrition & Metabolism*, vol. 57, no. 3-4, pp. 193–203, 2011.

[90] E. S. Ford, C. Li, W. S. Pearson, G. Zhao, and A. H. Mokdad, "Trends in hypercholesterolemia, treatment and control among United States adults," *International Journal of Cardiology*, vol. 140, no. 2, pp. 226–235, 2010.

3

Severity of Burn Injury and the Relationship to Socioeconomic Status in Nova Scotia, Canada

Jeffrey Le,[1] Sarah Alyouha,[1] Lihui Liu,[2] Michael Bezuhly,[1] and Jason Williams[1]

[1]*Division of Plastic and Reconstructive Surgery, Dalhousie Department of Surgery, Dalhousie University, Halifax, NS, Canada*
[2]*Department of Mathematics and Statistics, Dalhousie University, Halifax, NS, Canada*

Correspondence should be addressed to Jeffrey Le; htjle@dal.ca

Academic Editor: Guang-Hui Dong

Objective. Few Canadian studies have examined the relationship between socioeconomic status (SES) and incidence of burn injury. We seek to evaluate this relationship using median income as a measure of SES in Nova Scotia, Canada. *Methods.* Nova Scotia residents admitted to the Queen Elizabeth II burn unit in Halifax, Nova Scotia, from 1995 to 2012, were included in the study. SES was estimated by linking the subject's postal code to median family household income via Canadian population census data at the level of dissemination areas. Four equal income groups ranging from lowest to highest income quartile were compared (average total burn percentage). Likelihood ratio was calculated to evaluate the effect of median family income burn injury in each income quartile. *Results.* 302 patients were included in the analysis. Average percent total burn surface area was 19%, 15%, 15%, and 14% ($p = 0.18$) per income quartile (Q1: lowest, Q4: highest), respectively. Likelihood ratios for income quartile Q1–Q4 were 1.3 (0.8–1.6), 1.2 (0.6–1.4), and 0.7 (0.6–1.2), respectively. *Conclusion.* Contrary to findings in other geographic regions of the world, severity or incidence of burn injury in Nova Scotia, Canada, does not change in relation to SES when using family median income as a surrogate.

1. Introduction

Burns are a significant public health issue due to their associated morbidity and mortality. Globally, an estimated 265,000 deaths occur yearly from burn injury [1]. However, this burden is not equally shared, with 95% of burns occurring in low- and middle-income countries [2]. Low-income and middle-income countries are defined as nations whose gross national income per capital is less than 1045$ and 12,476, respectively [3].

Socioeconomic status (SES) is a risk factor for both the burn incidence and burn severity [4, 5] and can be measured using a variety of epidemiological markers including GDP median household income, property values, and housing quality [6].

The relation median household income to the incidence of severe burns in the province of Nova Scotia is unknown.

Nova Scotia is Canada's second smallest but second most densely populated province, with an area of 55,284 km^2 and a population of 921,727. Out of the ten provinces and three

territories, Nova Scotia ranked second to last in GDP per capita in 2013 [7]. Nova Scotia is similar to other Canadian provinces in terms of other established risk factors for burns such as education level (high school diploma or equivalent) and percentage of low-income individuals by province [8, 9].

The objective of this study is to perform an analysis of the relationship between percentage total burn surface area (TBSA) and socioeconomic status of patients using median family income as a method of assessment. The Halifax Infirmary Burn Unit is the largest tertiary care unit in the Maritime Provinces. It is dedicated to the treatment and rehabilitation of patients with severe thermal injuries from Nova Scotia. Data for this study was obtained from the Burn Unit Database.

2. Methods

Patient information was collected retrospectively from 1995 to 2012 on all patients who were admitted to the Halifax Infirmary Burn Unit, Nova Scotia, Canada. Patients were excluded

TABLE 1: Average % of total burns from lowest to highest adjusted median family income.

Variable	Q1 income: <$49377 (n = 75)	Q2 income: ≥$49377 to <$55885 (n = 77)	Q3 income: ≥$55885 to <$60323 (n = 75)	Q4 income: >$103564 (n = 75)	p value
Average % TBSA	19	15	15	14	0.18

Q: quartile, TBSA: total burn surface area.

from final analysis if they did not possess a postal code from Nova Scotia or if postal codes were not obtainable from patients charts.

2.1. CPI Adjusted Annual Income. Socioeconomic status was estimated by linking the subject's postal code to median family household income via Canadian population census at the level of dissemination areas (a dissemination area (DA) is a small, relatively stable geographic unit composed of one or more adjacent dissemination blocks; it is the smallest standard geographic area for which all census data are disseminated [10]) from 1995 to 2012. In order to remove the economic inflation factor, we adjusted the annual income by incorporating consumer price index (CPI) reported by Statistics Canada. Year 2005 was used as the base year and all observations from the year other than 2005 were adjusted accordingly.

Median family income was divided into 4 equal income groups ranging from lowest to highest income quartiles. Percentage of total burn surface area (TBSA) per each income quartile was compared. Kruskal-Wallis chi-squared test was used to evaluate significance of the results.

2.2. Beta Regression. A beta regression model was generated to analyze the effect of median income on likelihood of causing burn injury. The statistical analysis was implemented by software R (Version 3.1.1).

3. Results

Three hundred and two patients were included in the study, with one-quarter of the patient population in each income quartile ranging from lowest income (<$49377) to highest income (>$103564). Adjusted for inflation, total average percentage TBSA was 19%, 15%, 15%, and 14% ($p = 0.18$) for each income quartile (Q1–Q4), respectively (Table 1).

A beta regression model was created to evaluate the effect of median family income on likelihood of causing burn injury. Likelihood ratios for income quartiles Q1–Q4 were 1.3 (0.8–1.6), 1.2 (0.6–1.4), and 0.7 (0.6–1.2) with Q4 being the reference value (Figure 1).

4. Discussion

Socioeconomic status is often measured using a combination of education, health, income, and occupation variables to define the social standing or class of an individual or group [11]. In rural settings specifically, median income alone is an unreliable measure of SES. A study examining a population from western Canada reports the relationship between low

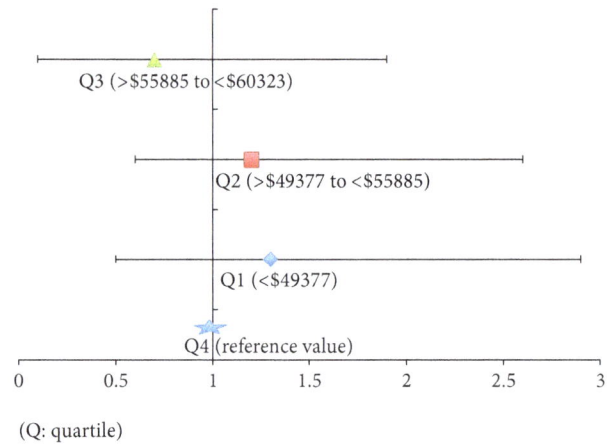

(Q: quartile)

FIGURE 1: Adjusted odds ratio for prediction of burn injury based on median family income quartile.

SES and incidence/severity of burns was less pronounced and in many cases absent with individuals living in rural areas [12]. A similar study analyzing a population from the Republic of Korea concluded income was not a meaningful descriptor of the relationship between low SES and burn severity for the self-employed and those with job instabilities [13]. In Nova Scotia, 43% of its population lives in a rural setting. Rural setting is defined as towns and villages with less than 1000 individuals that lie outside population centers [14, 15].

Nova Scotians experience difficulty in obtaining stable employment (unemployment rate 8.4%; national average 6.6%; seasonal employment 5.8%; national average 2.4%) [16, 17]. This difficulty is further compounded by a weak economic performance relative to the rest of Canada [18].

The incidence of burns is most influenced by poverty, lack of education, and unemployment according to a meta-analysis of 34 studies. In addition, substandard housing and family dynamics (large families or single parent families) emerged as risk factors [19]. Perhaps one of the aforementioned variables or available alternative proxies of wealth and social strata would be more representative to the unique economical and geographical landscape.

It should be noted that though we found that percentage of TBSA does not change in relation to median income in the context of a rural community setting, it does not imply that data on household income is not a potentially valuable measure. In Canada, low-income cut-off (LICO) equation calculates if a family needs to spend a greater proportion of its income on necessities than the average family of the same size. Low-income status is based on the calculated LICO [20].

Perhaps an approach in which the LICO equation is utilized in rural communities as a surrogate for low socioeconomic status would result in a greater accuracy in reporting.

Beta regression modeling showed decreasing income does not increase burn risk (Figure 1). These results suggest that, in Nova Scotia, median income (as surrogate for SES) is not associated with burn risk.

The authors recognize that this study has limitations. With a population of 940,000, the amount of burn-injured patients admitted from 1995 to 2012 in Nova Scotia may not constitute a large enough sample size to properly power the study. The Halifax Infirmary Burn Unit is the only tertiary care unit in the Maritime Provinces and thus constitutes the only collection of burn patient data available in Nova Scotia. In contrast, a larger study conducted in the Republic of Korea involving 870,411 burn cases demonstrated that patients arising from low-income households or areas with high poverty were at increased risk of burns [13].

5. Conclusion

Severity of burn injury in Nova Scotia, Canada, does not change in relation to increasing socioeconomic status when using family median income as a surrogate. Our statistical model demonstrated no decrease in likelihood of burn injury relative to increasing median family income.

Conflict of Interests

The authors declare that there is no conflict of interests regarding the publication of this paper.

References

[1] World Health Organization, BURNS, 2014, http://www.who.int/entity/mediacentre/factsheets/fs365/en/index.html.

[2] WHO Burns Fact Sheet #365, 2012, http://www.who.int/mediacentre/factsheets/fs365/en/index.html.

[3] Updated Income Classifications, 2014, http://data.worldbank.org/news/2015-country-classifications.

[4] M. D. Peck, "Epidemiology of burns throughout the world. Part I: distribution and risk factors," *Burns*, vol. 37, no. 7, pp. 1087–1100, 2011.

[5] R. F. Mullins, B. Alarm, M. A. H. Mian et al., "Burns in mobile home fires—descriptive study at a regional burn center," *Journal of Burn Care & Research*, vol. 30, no. 4, pp. 694–699, 2009.

[6] S. Mallonee, G. R. Istre, M. Rosenberg et al., "Surveillance and prevention of residential-fire injuries," *The New England Journal of Medicine*, vol. 335, no. 1, pp. 27–31, 1996.

[7] Gross domestic product, expenditure-based, by province and territory, 2014, http://www.statcan.gc.ca/tables-tableaux/sum-som/l01/cst01/econ15-eng.htm.

[8] Education in Canada: Attainment, Field of Study and Location of Study, 2011, http://www12.statcan.gc.ca/nhs-enm/2011/as-sa/99-012-x/99-012-x2011001-eng.cfm#a6.

[9] Employment and Social Development, 2011, http://www4.hrsdc.gc.ca/.3ndic.1t.4r@-eng.jsp?iid=23#M_4.

[10] Dissemination area (DA), 2012, http://www12.statcan.gc.ca/census-recensement/2011/ref/dict/geo021-eng.cfm.

[11] S. R. Psaki, J. C. Seidman, M. Miller et al., "Measuring socioeconomic status in multicountry studies: results from the eight-country MAL-ED study," *Population Health Metrics*, vol. 12, no. 1, article 8, 2014.

[12] N. J. Bell, N. Schuurman, and S. Morad Hameed, "A small-area population analysis of socioeconomic status and incidence of severe burn/fire-related injury in British Columbia, Canada," *Burns*, vol. 35, no. 8, pp. 1133–1141, 2009.

[13] J. O. Park, S. D. Shin, J. Kim, K. J. Song, and M. D. Peck, "Association between socioeconomic status and burn injury severity," *Burns*, vol. 35, no. 4, pp. 482–490, 2009.

[14] Population, urban and rural, by province and territory (Nova Scotia), 2011, http://www.statcan.gc.ca/tables-tableaux/sum-som/l01/cst01/demo62d-eng.htm.

[15] Rural Area (RA), 2012, https://www12.statcan.gc.ca/census-recensement/2011/ref/dict/geo042-eng.cfm.

[16] Labour force characteristics, seasonally adjusted, by province (monthly) (Newfoundland and Labrador, Prince Edward Island, Nova Scotia, New Brunswick), 2015, http://www.statcan.gc.ca/tables-tableaux/sum-som/l01/cst01/lfss01a-eng.htm.

[17] Seasonal workers, by province, 2015, http://www.statcan.gc.ca/pub/71-222-x/2008001/sectioni/i-seasonal-saisonniers-eng.htm.

[18] Painting the Landscape of Rural Nova Scotia, Economy, 2003, Low income cut-offs, 2013, http://www.ruralnovascotia.ca/RCIP/PDF/RR_final_full.pdf, http://www.statcan.gc.ca/pub/75f0002m/2012002/lico-sfr-eng.htm.

[19] L. S. Edelman, "Social and economic factors associated with the risk of burn injury," *Burns*, vol. 33, no. 8, pp. 958–965, 2007.

[20] Low income cut-offs, 2013, http://www.statcan.gc.ca/pub/75f0002m/2012002/lico-sfr-eng.htm.

4

Seroprevalence of Leptospiral Antibodies among Healthy Municipal Service Workers in Selangor

Suhailah Samsudin,[1] Siti Norbaya Masri,[2] Tengku Zetty Maztura Tengku Jamaluddin,[2] Siti Nor Sakinah Saudi,[1] Umi Kalsom Md Ariffin,[3] Fairuz Amran,[4] and Malina Osman[2]

[1]*Department of Community Health, Faculty of Medicine and Health Sciences, Universiti Putra Malaysia (UPM), 43400 Serdang, Selangor, Malaysia*
[2]*Department of Medical Microbiology and Parasitology, Faculty of Medicine and Health Sciences, Universiti Putra Malaysia (UPM), 43400 Serdang, Selangor, Malaysia*
[3]*Department of Urban Services and Health, Ampang Jaya Municipal Council (MPAJ), Jalan Pandan Utama, Taman Pandah Indah, 55100 Ampang, Selangor, Malaysia*
[4]*Institute of Medical Research, Jalan Pahang, 50588 Kuala Lumpur, Malaysia*

Correspondence should be addressed to Malina Osman; malinaosman@upm.edu.my

Academic Editor: Guang-Hui Dong

Introduction. Municipal service workers have been found to have an occupational risk of leptospirosis. Study among municipality workers shows high seropositivity of leptospiral antibodies detected among town cleaners and garbage collectors. *Objective*. Aims of this study were to determine seroprevalence of leptospiral antibodies and distribution of serovars detected in samples among municipal service workers. *Methodology*. Cross-sectional study involved 89 municipal service workers in Selangor. Blood samples were taken and serological test was done using MAT following standard procedures. *Results*. Seropositivity of leptospiral antibodies among municipal service workers was 34.8%. Serovars identified were strains of *Sarawak, Copenhageni, Hardjobovis, Lai, Bataviae, Patoc, Celledoni, Hardjoprajitno, Tarrasovi*, and *Pomona*. There were 31 workers with positive leptospiral antibodies. All of them were frequently exposed towards leptospirosis. Significant associations have been reported between seropositivity of leptospiral antibodies with job category ($P = 0.021$) and worker's nationality ($P = 0.014$) among municipal service workers. *Conclusion*. High seropositivity of leptospiral antibodies detected among municipal service workers which was associated with job category and nationality of workers. The significant findings from this study suggest that health education programs and safe work practice should be considered to prevent leptospirosis among municipal service workers in future.

1. Introduction

Leptospirosis is an infectious disease that affects humans and animals. It is considered as the most widespread reemerging zoonotic disease in the world [1–3]. The high prevalence of leptospirosis in humans is of great public health concern, particularly in tropical and subtropical regions. Recent data have shown that human leptospirosis is an endemic infection in Malaysia [2, 4]. An increasing trend of cases occurs in this country between 2005 and 2009, starting with 263 cases in 2004 and up to 1418 in 2009 [5, 6]. Cases continually rise in 2010 with 1876 cases followed by 2268 cases in 2011 and 3665 cases in 2012 [7, 8].

Human infections may be acquired through occupational, recreational, or environmental exposures [2]. Occupational outdoor job involved direct contact with soil, mud, or water during work putting individuals at risk. Environmental exposure through environmental sanitation and hygiene is a proven factor being responsible for the disease [9]. Positive result of leptospiral antibodies was reported among sanitation workers in Brazil. Majority of them had job exposure towards environmental sanitation concerned with water supply, drains and drainage, galleries, sewers, garbage collection, and road sweeping [10].

Rampant urbanization of cities can lead to improper garbage management system in urban areas, creating favourable conditions for animal carriers [11]. The most important animals associated with human leptospirosis are peridomestic rodents which are rats and mice [12, 13]. This may pose a health risk for leptospirosis as animal reservoir might contaminate environmental waters and soils via their excreta and urine [11].

Ampang Jaya Municipal Council was facing unrelieved problems regarding high number of rat population especially in residential areas. Furthermore, urban rats are prolific breeders with average weight up to one kilogram and may produce up to fifteen rats a year [14]. The council had created a method to control this issue such as rat elimination campaigns in their authority areas. Furthermore, eradication of rats indirectly may prevent spreading of *Leptospira* which is commonly transmitted by rats. This situation becomes crucial for any work activities which involve environmental sanitation and rat catching campaign. Thus, the council as the employer and local authority has to ensure safe working environment and proper procedures are followed by workers and individuals with high probability of exposure towards leptospirosis. In order to address this issue, the study of seroprevalence of leptospiral antibodies among municipal service workers was performed.

The purpose of this study was to determine seroprevalence of leptospiral antibodies and distribution of *Leptospira* serovars presented in sample of municipal service workers. Furthermore, the association between seropositivity of leptospiral antibodies with job category and nationality of municipal service workers was also determined in this study.

2. Materials and Methods

2.1. Study Design and Population. A cross-sectional study was conducted in December 2012 until May 2013 at Ampang Jaya Municipal Council (MPAJ) which is located in an urban area of Selangor. The study population was healthy municipal service workers with no recent signs and symptoms related to leptospirosis within 2-3 weeks during the period of data collection and working as garbage collector, town cleaner, public worker, and public health assistant in MPAJ. Workers who did not meet these inclusive criteria were excluded from this study. The study used a nonprobability sampling. The total of workers participating in this study was 89 healthy workers, who fulfilled all the inclusive criteria.

2.2. Sample Collection and Serological Test. Respondents were identified from a list provided from the MPAJ Health Office. Informed written consent was obtained from all respondents based on approved study protocol by the Medical Research Ethics Committee, Universiti Putra Malaysia. Blood samples from workers were obtained by using venepuncture technique. Five milliliters of venous blood was drawn by medically trained personnel and collected into sterile blood containers. The blood in plain tube was centrifuged for 10

minutes by using the Powerspin MX centrifuge machine at 3000 rpm (round per minute) to obtain the serum. The serum was kept at $-20°C$ in a freezer until it is further processed [2, 15].

The microscopic agglutination test (MAT) was performed to determine the presence of *Leptospira* antibodies among municipal service workers. The MAT was performed with a panel of 20 live reference serovars, representing 20 serogroups that were used as antigen, as recommended by WHO [16]. Each serum sample was subjected to serial dilution by using phosphate buffered saline (PBS). Then, the microtitre plates were incubated at room temperature in the dark for two (2) hours. Agglutination was determined by slide agglutination method which gives an agglutination of at least 50% of the leptospires which is considered positive in this study.

Leptospira reference serovars were obtained for local (Malaysian Serovar) and WHO from Institute Medical Research, Malaysia. The serovars used in the MAT were divided into local and WHO. Serovars for local were *Melaka, Terengganu, Sarawak, Copenhageni, Hardjobovis,* and *Lai.* Serovar for WHO consists of *Australis, Autumnalis, Bataviae, Canicola, Celledoni, Grippotyphosa, Hardjoprajitno, Icterohaemorrhagiae, Javanica, Pyrogenes, Tarrasovi, Djasiman, Patoc,* and *Pomona.*

In this study, we used titre of $1 \geq 50$ as cut-off value because respondents were healthy workers without any symptoms related to leptospirosis. Furthermore, there is no standard cut-off titre in this local geographical area as a baseline in the community [2]. Some studies used cut-off titre of $1 \geq 100$ but there is controversy on the single diagnostic titre as it is dependent on endemicity [17]. In this study, we used titre of $1 \geq 50$ to avoid probability in underestimation of seroprevalent [2]. Study by Shivakumar and Krishnakumar also used cut-off titre of $1 \geq 50$ on serosurveys in the asymptomatic high risk group [17].

2.3. Statistical Analysis. Data were entered and analyzed by using Statistical Packages for Social Sciences (SPSS) Version 21.0. Analysis was done by using this software at different levels. The level of significance in this study was set up at $P < 0.05$. Descriptive analysis was limited to identify sociodemographic characteristics of respondents.

3. Result

3.1. Sociodemographic Characteristics. Eighty-nine workers were recruited into the study based on the list of workers provided by the municipal office. The distribution of respondents by gender showed there were 84 (94.4%) male workers and only 5 (5.6%) female workers. Most of respondents participated in this study were foreigners, 79 (88.8%) and Malaysians, 10 (11.2%). The distribution of respondents by job category was divided into two parts which were frequently exposed to leptospirosis and infrequently exposed to leptospirosis. Frequently exposed group consists of fifty-three (59.6%) garbage collectors and twenty-six (29.2%) town cleaners, while infrequently exposed group consists of

TABLE 1: Sociodemographic characteristic of municipal service workers.

Variable	Study group $n = 89$	
	n	(%)
Gender		
Male	84	94.4
Female	5	5.6
Nationality		
Malaysian	10	11.2
Foreign	79	88.8
Job category		
Frequently exposed		
Garbage collector	53	59.6
Town cleaner	27	30.3
Infrequently exposed		
Public worker	6	6.7
Public health assistant	3	3.3

$n = 89$, total number of respondent in the study.

TABLE 2: Prevalence of leptospiral antibodies among municipal service workers.

Variable	Study group $n = 89$
	n (%)
Leptospiral antibodies	
Positive	31 (34.8)
Negative	58 (65.2)

$n = 89$.

TABLE 3: Prevalence of leptospiral antibodies according to job category.

Variable	Leptospiral antibodies	
	Positive (%)	Negative (%)
Job category		
Garbage collector	22 (41.5)	31 (58.5)
Town cleaner	9 (33.3)	18 (66.7)
Public worker	0 (0.0)	6 (100.0)
Public health worker	0 (0.0)	3 (100.0)
Total	**31 (34.8)**	**58 (65.2)**

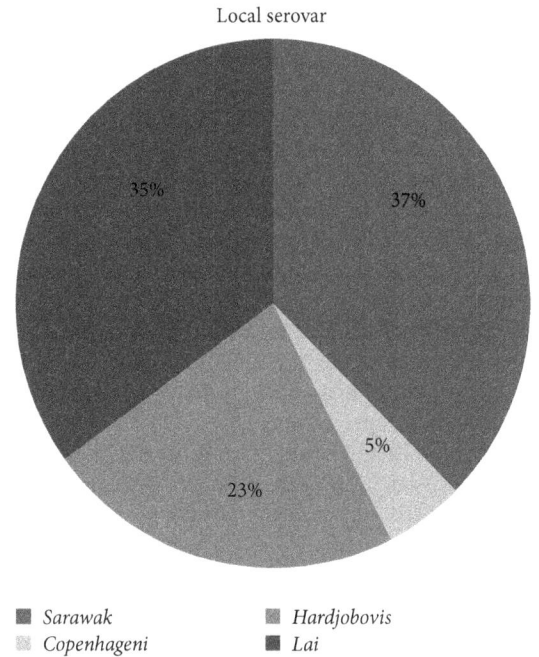

FIGURE 1: Serovar (local) among seropositive municipal service workers.

seven (7.9%) public workers and three (3.3%) public health assistants (Table 1).

3.2. Prevalence of Leptospiral Antibodies. For distribution of seroprevalence of leptospiral antibodies, thirty-one (34.8%) respondents involved in this study were seropositive and fifty-eight (65.2%) respondents were seronegative of leptospiral antibodies (Table 2). The highest seropositivity of leptospiral antibodies was detected among garbage collectors, twenty-two (41.5%) workers followed by nine (33.3%) town cleaners. All public workers and public health assistants were seronegative of leptospiral antibodies in this study (Table 3).

For local *Leptospira* serovar, positive samples were identified as serovars *Sarawak*, *Copenhageni*, *Hardjobovis*, and *Lai*. The highest local serovar was *Sarawak* (37.0%) and the lowest serovars present for local serovar were *Copenhageni* (5.0%) (Figure 1), while in WHO *Leptospira* serovar positive samples were serovars *Bataviae*, *Celledoni*, *Hardjoprajitno*, *Tarrasovi*, *Patoc*, and *Pomona*. Mainly serovars present were *Bataviae* (57.0%), followed by *Patoc* (27.0%), and only 4.0% was identified in each serovar, *Celledoni*, *Hardjoprajitno*, *Tarrasovi*, and *Pomona* (Figure 2).

Only eleven of respondents had monoserovar antibody. The highest frequency of serovars was pentaserovars,

detected from a Burmese (Myanmar) working as garbage collector in MPAJ (Figure 3). The study found 26 of serovars at titre of $1 \geq 50$ and 17 serovars at titer of $1 \geq 100$ while 12 serovars were found at titer of $1 \geq 200$ and 11 of serovars at $1 \geq 400$ (Table 4). In addition, 16 from 31 workers who are positive of leptospiral antibodies had both local and WHO serovars, four workers had positive leptospiral antibodies with more than one local serovar, and one worker had positive four WHO serovars.

3.3. Association between Seropositivity of Leptospiral Antibodies with Job Category and Nationality among Municipal Service Workers. In this study, thirty-one workers (38.8%) in the frequently exposed group had positive leptospiral antibodies, while forty-nine (61.3%) had negative result. All nine respondents who were infrequently exposed towards leptospirosis were negative leptospiral antibodies. There was significant association between seropositivity of leptospiral antibodies and job category of municipal service workers ($P = 0.021$). Furthermore, there was also a significant

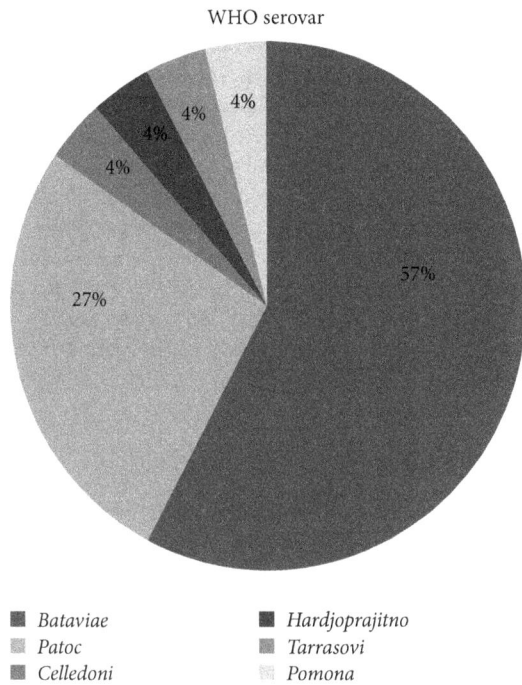

FIGURE 2: Serovar (WHO) among seropositive municipal service workers.

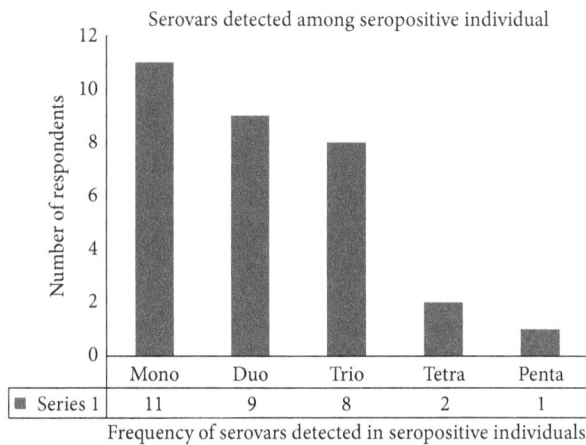

FIGURE 3: Frequency of serovars in seropositive samples.

TABLE 4: Leptospiral antibody titres of local and WHO serovars.

Local serovar	Titres			
	1 : 50	1 : 100	1 : 200	1 : 400
Melaka (*IMR LEP 1*)	0	0	0	0
Terengganu (*IMR LEP 115*)	0	0	0	0
Sarawak (*IMR LEP 175*)	5	3	4	3
Copenhageni (*IMR LEP 803/11*)	0	1	0	1
Hardjobovis (*IMR LEP 27*)	0	2	3	4
Lai (*IMR LEP 22*)	11	3	0	0
WHO serovar				
Australis	0	0	0	0
Autumnalis	0	0	0	0
Bataviae	6	4	3	2
Canicola	0	0	0	0
Celledoni	1	0	0	0
Grippotyphosa	0	0	0	0
Hardjoprajitno	1	0	0	0
Icterohaemorrhage	0	0	0	0
Javanica	0	0	0	0
Pyrogenes	0	0	0	0
Tarrasovi	0	1	0	0
Djasiman	0	0	0	0
Patoc	1	3	2	1
Pomona	1	0	0	0
Total	**26**	**17**	**12**	**11**

TABLE 5: Association between seropositivity of leptospiral antibodies with job category and nationality among municipal service workers.

Variable	Leptospiral antibodies		P
	Positive (%)	Negative (%)	
Job category			
Frequently exposed to leptospirosis infection	31 (38.8)	49 (61.2)	
Infrequently exposed to leptospirosis infection	0 (0.0)	9 (100.0)	0.021[a]
Nationality			
Malaysian	0 (0.0)	10 (0.0)	
Foreign	31 (39.2)	48 (60.8)	0.014[a]
Total	**31**	**58**	

n = 89.
[a]Chi-square test.

association between seropositivity of leptospiral antibodies and nationality of municipal service workers (P = 0.014) (Table 5).

4. Discussion

4.1. Leptospiral Antibodies Status among Municipal Service Workers. Findings in this study showed a high prevalence (34.8%) of leptospiral antibodies among municipal service workers. All respondents who are involved in this study did not have any signs and symptoms suggestive of *Leptospira* infection. Asymptomatic infection of leptospirosis is common and has been reported in many studies. In 2012, Nazri et al. [2] reported that there was 24.8% seroprevalence of leptospirosis among town service workers in Kelantan. Another local study in north-eastern Malaysia reported 31.0% of confirmed leptospirosis case at titre of $1 \geq 400$ by MAT

[18]. Even though both previous studies [2, 18] were from the same locality, seroprevalence of leptospiral antibodies showed distinct values as cut-off value for titre used was different. As our study showed higher seroprevalence (34.8%) compared with previous study (24.8%) in similar study population in Kelantan probably due to different locality of study, Ratnam et al. [19] showed sanitation workers in urban areas had the highest risk of leptospiral infection with seroprevalence recording 32.9%.

Ampang Jaya is an urban area with high population density. Rapid development of infrastructure such as construction of new houses and commercial buildings makes the area more complex and crowded. High positivity in seroprevalence of leptospiral antibodies in this study probably related to urbanization and improper waste disposal. Swapna et al. [13] reported similar association between urbanization and seroprevalence of leptospirosis. In Calicut, India, the rapid urbanization and man-made ecoenvironmental disturbances may have contributed to water logging condition which increase in leptospirosis cases in this region [13].

Moreover, there is an abundance of food premises such as stalls, restaurants, and markets to cater for its dense population resulting in more conducive environments and solid waste deposited in Ampang Jaya, thus contributing to the increasing of rat population in Ampang Jaya these past years. Workers who are involved in sanitation activity such as garbage collectors and town cleaners have a higher tendency to be exposed to leptospiral infection.

4.2. Distribution of Local and WHO Serovar among Municipal Service Workers. In this study, the most common serovar detected among local serovar was *Sarawak* (37.0%) while WHO serovar was *Bataviae* (57.0%). Similarly, Nazri et al. [2] reported that serovar *Bataviae* was the predominant pathogenic serovars in his study in Kelantan. In addition to this, Swapna et al. [13] also verified serovar *Bataviae* as one of the predominant serovars among workers in North Kerala, India. Similar findings were also documented by Van et al. [20] in the Mekong Delta, Vietnam, which documented fifty-seven cases of *Bataviae* among seropositive subjects. Other than that, there was presence of serovar *Patoc* in seven respondents. The study by Nazri et al. [2] also found that serovar *Patoc* was the most common serovar identified among town service workers with twenty-nine serovar detected.

4.3. Distribution of Serovar Frequencies among Seropositive Municipal Service Workers. This study shows a frequency of serovars detected among seropositive respondents. Majority of respondents had monoserovar leptospiral antibody. Throughout the study, we have identified pentaserovars (*Sarawak, Hardjobovis, Lai, Bataviae*, and *Patoc*) from a Burmese (Myanmar) garbage collector who had been working in Malaysia for the past 10 years.

Besides, there were four respondents from Myanmar who had double serovars detected with titre of $1 \geq 400$ during this study. The study among environmental sanitation workers in the southern region of Brazil reported that 10.4% was positive

to one or more serovars [10]. Higher frequency of serovars detected in this population is probably due to their routine jobs and poor hygiene practices. This finding indicates that workers involved in waste management such as garbage collectors have higher risk of getting leptospirosis. From our observations during sample collection, personal protective equipment usage was inadequate among the garbage collectors. None of the garbage collectors wore gloves while working and only few of them wore long sleeve shirts and boots while working. These might contribute to the high exposure towards *Leptospira* hence contributing to the high seroprevalence and frequency of serovars among this population.

5. Conclusion

This study had determined a high seroprevalence (34.8%) of leptospiral antibodies among municipal service workers. Seropositivity among municipal service workers was associated with job and nationality. These findings show that municipal service workers have occupational risk of contracting leptospirosis infection. This may be due to the daily exposure in managing solid waste which may be contaminated with *Leptospira*. In order to handle this issue, proper health program and training in using personal protective equipment should be initiated among municipal service workers to reduce risk of infection.

There were two predominant serovars detected among seropositive municipal service workers which are *Sarawak* and *Bataviae*. Many other studies on leptospirosis included study on animal reservoirs. However, this study did not include leptospirosis among animal reservoirs. Thus, we could not conclude if WHO serovar or local serovar was contracted during the course of work. Hence, we were unable to compare the serovar frequency between humans and reservoirs.

In this study, one of the seropositive respondents had five different serovars detected in his sample, probably due to frequent exposure and poor hygiene practices. The findings indicate that workers involved in waste management such as garbage collectors have higher risk of getting leptospirosis. The result shows an alarming sign of public health problem to initiate leptospirosis control program. Health education to the public regarding leptospirosis should be done, so that the public can be more aware of the risk of infection. Collaborative approach by local authorities, government, and private agencies should be done to reduce favourable environment for the rats. Proper approach should be planned towards this type of occupation in avoidance of leptospirosis in future.

Study Limitation

The study was performed in a single population, among municipal service workers in Ampang Jaya; future findings may not be generalized to other populations. The study was a cross-sectional study; therefore, it could only determine the antibody level at the present time of blood sampling. It could not determine the temporal relationship between leptospiral infection and the leptospiral antibodies. There was a sampling bias in this study. Sampling bias can be minimized through randomly chosen respondent from a listing of workers.

Ethical Approval

Ethical approval had been obtained from Medical Research Ethics Committee, Universiti Putra Malaysia (JKEUPM), and permission from Ampang Jaya Municipal Council (MPAJ) prior to the commencement of this study.

Conflict of Interests

The authors declare that there is no conflict of interests regarding the publication of this paper.

Acknowledgments

The authors would like to express their deepest gratitude and thanks to Ampang Jaya Municipal Council (MPAJ) and their workers for their support and contribution in this study. They personally thank Dr. Saliza Mohd Elias for guidance through the study and staff from the Department of Medical Microbiology and Parasitology, Faculty of Medicine and Health Sciences, UPM, for their great assistance.

References

[1] M. Sapian, M. T. Khairi, S. H. How et al., "Outbreak of melioidosis and leptospirosis co-infection following a rescue operation," *Medical Journal of Malaysia*, vol. 67, no. 3, pp. 293–297, 2012.

[2] S. M. Nazri, S. M. Rahim, N. Y. Azwany et al., "Seroprevalence of leptospirosis among town service workers in Northeastern state of Malaysia," *International Journal of Collaborative Research on Internal Medicine and Public Health*, vol. 4, no. 4, pp. 395–403, 2012.

[3] A. P. Sugunan, P. Vijayachari, S. Sharma et al., "Risk factors associated with leptospirosis during an outbreak in Middle Andaman, India," *The Indian Journal of Medical Research*, vol. 130, no. 1, pp. 67–73, 2009.

[4] I. M. El Jalii and A. R. Bahaman, *A Review of Human Leptospirosis in Malaysia*, 2006.

[5] MOH, *Guidelines for the Diagnosis, Management, Prevention and Control of Leptospirosis in Malaysia*, Disease Control Division Department of Public Health, Ministry of Health Malaysia, Putrajaya, Malaysia, 1st edition, 2011.

[6] J. K. Lim, V. A. Murugaiyah, A. Ramli et al., *A Case Study: Leptospirosis in Malaysia*, 2011.

[7] S. Khairani-Bejo, *Leptospirosis and Environment. Prosiding Kolokium Leptospirosis Pendekatan 'One Health' Dalam Pengawalan Leptospirosis*, PICC, Putrajaya, Malaysia, 2012.

[8] E. Fernandez, "Keep clean: Health Ministry advises against patronizing dirty outlets," 2013, http://www2.nst.com.my/nation/general/2-775-leptospirosis-cases-23-deaths-this-year-1.340149.

[9] R. Kamath, S. Swain, S. Pattanshetty, and N. S. Nair, "Studying risk factors associated with human leptospirosis," *Journal of Global Infectious Diseases*, vol. 6, no. 1, pp. 3–9, 2014.

[10] L. P. de Almeida, L. F. Martins, C. S. Brod, and P. M. Germano, "Seroepidemiologic survey of leptospirosis among environmental sanitation workers in an urban locality in the Southern region of Brazil," *Revista de Saude Publica*, vol. 28, no. 1, pp. 76–81, 1994.

[11] D. Benacer, P. Y. Who, S. N. M. Zain, F. Amran, and K. L. Thong, "Pathogenic and saprophytic *Leptospira* species in water and soils from selected urban sites in peninsular Malaysia," *Microbes and Environments*, vol. 28, no. 1, pp. 135–140, 2013.

[12] A. R. M. Mohan and D. D. Chadee, "Knowledge, attitudes and practices of Trinidadian households regarding leptospirosis and related matters," *International Health*, vol. 3, no. 2, pp. 131–137, 2011.

[13] R. N. Swapna, U. Tuteja, L. Nair, and J. Sudarsana, "Seroprevalence of leptospirosis in high risk groups in Calicut, North Kerala, India," *Indian Journal of Medical Microbiology*, vol. 24, no. 4, pp. 349–352, 2006.

[14] R. A. Ismail, *Bukan habuan "ternak" tikus*, 2011, http://www.hmetro.com.my/myMetro/articles/Bukanhabuan__8216_ternak__8217_tikus/Article/index_html.

[15] WHO, *Human Leptospirosis: Guidance for Diagnosis, Surveillance and Control*, 2003, http://whqlibdoc.who.int/hq/2003/WHO_CDS_CSR_EPH_2002.23.pdf.

[16] WHO, *Leptospirosis: Laboratory Manual*, World Health Organization, 2007.

[17] S. Shivakumar and B. Krishnakumar, "Diagnosis of Leptospirosis—role of MAT," *Journal of Association of Physicians of India*, vol. 54, pp. 338–339, 2006.

[18] A. A. Noor Rafizah, B. D. Aziah, Y. N. Azwany et al., "Leptospirosis in Northeastern Malaysia: misdiagnosed or coinfection?" *International Journal of Collaborative Research on Internal Medicine & Public Health*, vol. 4, no. 7, p. 1419, 2012.

[19] S. Ratnam, C. O. R. Everard, J. C. Alex, B. Suresh, and P. Thangaraju, "Prevalence of leptospiral agglutinins among conservancy workers in Madras City, India," *Journal of Tropical Medicine and Hygiene*, vol. 96, no. 1, pp. 41–45, 1993.

[20] C. T. B. Van, N. T. T. Thuy, N. H. San, T. T. Hien, G. Baranton, and P. Perolat, "Human leptospirosis in the Mekong delta, Viet Nam," *Transactions of the Royal Society of Tropical Medicine and Hygiene*, vol. 92, no. 6, pp. 625–628, 1998.

5

Children's Oral Health: The Opportunity for Improvement Using the WHO Health Promoting School Model

Andrew J. Macnab[1,2]

[1]Department of Pediatrics, University of British Columbia, Room C323, 4500 Oak Street, Vancouver, BC, Canada V6H 3N1
[2]Stellenbosch Institute for Advanced Study, Wallenberg Research Centre, 10 Marais Street, 7600 Stellenbosch, South Africa

Correspondence should be addressed to Andrew J. Macnab; amacnab@cw.bc.ca

Academic Editor: Haiying Chen

The health and quality of life of a large proportion of the world's children are compromised by dental caries and periodontal disease. Those in developing countries and from disadvantaged populations suffer disproportionately from these forms of poor oral health; however, much of the primary disease and secondary pathology is preventable by simple and inexpensive measures that children can readily learn. WHO health promoting schools (HPS) are an established model for addressing public health issues through education of children in a manner that achieves acquisition of knowledge and health practices that promote behaviours that positively impact determinants of health. HPS programs that address poor oral health have achieved improvement in oral health practices and reduction in caries rates among disadvantaged populations of children. WHO has called for more programs to address the "epidemic" of poor oral health worldwide, and the WHO HPS model appears to be a relevant and applicable way forward. Health care professionals and educators who want to improve the health and quality of life of children related to caries and periodontal disease now have an opportunity to collaborate to initiate, deliver, and evaluate community-based HPS interventions using proven concepts, content, and process.

1. Introduction

Dental caries and periodontal disease have a worldwide impact on the health of children [1, 2]. The negative effects on their wellbeing, quality of life, and overall health during childhood are well documented [3], and in addition the literature reports the association of chronically compromised oral health and a growing number of significant systemic conditions that manifest later in life. These include adverse pregnancy outcomes, cardiovascular disease, stroke, and diabetes [4–7], hence the relevance to public health intervention, although the causal relationships linking periodontal disease to these conditions have not yet been established [8, 9]. Importantly children in developing countries and disadvantaged populations in the developed world are known to suffer disproportionately from the burden of caries and periodontal disease [10]. And while the majority of such children lack adequate formal dental care because of multiple factors, including cost and limited access, much of the poor oral health from which they suffer is largely preventable when they have access to simple knowledge and are taught inexpensive health care practices. Although risk factors like poverty, dietary habits, and poor nutrition also contribute, even specific local sociobehavioural and environmental factors that play a role in caries and periodontal disease can be addressed in programs that provide health promotion focussed on improvement of oral health.

Many such programs now exist, but strengthening and increasing their availability has been called for, particularly in developing countries, and amongst disadvantaged special populations [11]. Such calls include ones from the World Health Organization (WHO), and WHO advocates the use of Health Promoting Schools (HPS) as an effective avenue for promoting and protecting health in children [12, 13]. In addition, WHO defines a health promoting school as one that "constantly strengthens its capacity to as a healthy setting for living, learning and working," recognizing the broader impact where effective HPS programs alter the ethos of the whole school [14]. HPS provide classroom education and school-based activities that increase knowledge and develop behaviors that benefit the health of children. Such schools are also an investment in the wellbeing of the larger community, and HPS programs can be targeted to address health issues of particular relevance to a given community. Because children's oral health is one public health issue where improvement has been achieved through HPS programs this paper summarizes the negative impact of poor oral health on children, explains the concept of school-based health promotion using the WHO HPS model, and describes the content incorporated and methods used for evaluation of HPS programs to improve oral health.

2. Poor Oral Health in Children

Caries is regarded as the commonest preventable infectious disease affecting children [15], and periodontal diseases are estimated to affect up to 90% of the world's population [8]. Caries develops when tooth surfaces are damaged by acids produced when bacteria present in the mouth ferment carbohydrates and food debris. The risk factors for caries and periodontal disease are well described [16–18], but in children dietary intake of sugars and carbonated soft drinks combined with poor oral hygiene are important factors that promote an environment conducive to bacterial activity and biofilm (plaque) formation [15]. Gingivitis develops as dental plaque accumulates in proximity to the gingiva. Plaque harbours bacteria such as *Streptococcus mutans* and causes inflammation of the gingival (gum) margins, which is the first stage of periodontal disease [19]. Periodontitis results in loss of connective tissue and tooth loss. Undernutrition increases a child's susceptibility to dental caries; however, diets common in developing countries that contain predominantly starchy foods, fruits, and vegetables are also linked to low levels of dental caries [20].

Children with poor oral health experience pain and tooth loss which compromise normal eating and negatively impact their nutrition, self-esteem, speech, socialization, quality of life, and school attendance. Worldwide it is estimated that >51 million school hours are lost annually from dental-related illness [2, 17, 21–23]. The consequences of established disease also place a considerable economic burden on children's families and society [24], yet caries can be arrested, and the early stages potentially reversed, by employing measures that are inexpensive and simple to teach [18], principally by the maintenance of oral hygiene through regular removal of food deposits and related measures to reduce dental plaque formation and the negative impact of gingivitis [25, 26].

Importantly, children's oral health can be improved through school-based intervention programs that are simple and inexpensive to implement and are readily evaluated [11, 18, 27, 28]. A significant reduction in caries rates and improvement in quantitative measures such as the decayed, missing, and filled teeth scores have been documented in several child populations including Canadian aboriginal children and rural primary school pupils in Africa [11, 15, 27–30]. Even though oral hygiene measures are long established practices in most cultures [26], it is possible to improve children's oral hygiene through simple additions to their knowledge

and learning improved health practices. Importantly, these two elements of health education, knowledge provision, and teaching/reinforcing healthy practices are the components central to the WHO health promoting school model. Also, in the context of the worldwide need for improvement of children's oral health, none of the interventions necessary to achieve positive change are difficult, expensive, or controversial. Even the use of tooth brushes can be replaced by readily available and acceptable local alternatives such as tooth sticks, in situations where even the modest cost of tooth brushing is not financially viable or is not accepted as an intervention, as is the case in some Muslim countries [31].

3. Health Promoting Schools (HPS)

The concepts underlying the WHO HPS model for health promotion in schools have been well described previously, as have their history and evolution, initiatives implemented in a range of different countries, and the methods used to document impact and processes that contribute to success or failure [12, 32–38]. And a 2014 structured review evaluated the evidence for improvement of student health and wellbeing and academic achievement [39]. In HPS health education curriculum content is included in classroom teaching and school-based "healthy practice" activities are provided that together increase knowledge and develop and reinforce behaviors that benefit the health of children.

While many schools begin by addressing a single health topic [40] (poor oral health is an example) WHO also advocates for a broader "whole-school" approach where the health and educational outcomes of children and adolescents are enhanced by a broad range of approaches and learning experiences that effectively alter the ethos of the school towards health. HPS activities benefit the individual children in the program but there is also a "trickle-down" effect which benefits siblings and parents, and even the broader community has been shown to benefit through dissemination of new knowledge, changes in attitudes, and adoption of healthier behaviours. Hence, such schools are an investment in the health and future wellbeing of the community as a whole.

The current consensus on implementation strategies and the potential of HPS to achieve behavioural change has been summarized in recent publications [13, 41, 42]. Essential first steps and engagement and implementation components central to effective programs have been identified [12, 13, 37, 43–45]. These include the following:

(i) dialogue to identify the health issue(s) to be addressed—it is important that any issue chosen has "relevance" for the community and its importance "resonates" with those who will deliver the HPS program,

(ii) achievement of "buy in" to the need for health education and of the concepts central to HPS,

(iii) planning of the educational content and health practices to be offered,

(iv) definition of the roles of teachers and collaborating health professionals/educators/agencies,

(v) agreement on support to be provided for HPS program delivery and the evaluation mechanisms to be used to examine impact and effect,

(vi) Professional development for teachers—this has been shown to aid the process of HPS delivery by improving participation by school staff and sustaining their commitment.

A body of evidence exists on the effect of HPS programs implemented to address a variety of health issues, in various populations and different countries; this has been summarized by Tang et al. [12] and systematically reviewed by Langford et al. [39]. However, as with other approaches to health promotion there is still a call for more comprehensive evaluation and in particularly for long term studies on the duration of behavioural change [12, 13]. Also it is clear that not only do the children, whole school, and broader community benefit from effective HPS programs, those collaborating to initiate and deliver them also derive benefits from the experience, and many report increased awareness of "real world" challenges and solutions related to public health issues such as the prevalence of poor oral health amongst children [28, 46]. Effective HPS programs can be established in individual schools or local communities and in many countries national agencies exist for HPS-based health promotion [42].

4. Content and Evaluation of HPS Oral Health Programs

Factual teaching around oral health is added to classroom curriculum and visual aids are prepared and displayed that highlight key facts and beneficial behaviours. While the children learn the association between caries formation and acid production from sugars in the mouth by bacteria and the importance of oral hygiene to break this cycle, their attention can be drawn to relevant dietary practices [15, 20, 46]. These include the sources of sugar in the diet, especially the addition of sugar to food and drinks, and the high sugar content of carbonated beverages. Candy and chocolate consumption, snacking practices, and less healthy food preferences driven by advertising can also be addressed, and emphasis is placed on the choice of local alternatives that are healthier and available in individual communities. In many developing countries such alternatives include fruit, nuts, and sugar cane. Although cane contains sugar, it is naturally fibrous. Consequently chewing and sucking it cleans teeth and gums effectively, and the cleansing effect outweighs the potential risk of the sugar content as a potential cause of caries [47].

Healthy practices taught in the context of improving oral health include methods to effectively cleanse the mouth and in particular how and when to remove food debris and accumulations of sugars, acids, and forming biofilm [11, 15, 27]. The principal practice in this regard is tooth brushing [25, 46] but in many developing countries will also incorporate the use of tooth sticks as an acceptable alternative. Tooth sticks can be as effective in removing plaque as tooth brushes

[48], and WHO advocates their use in oral health programs. An additional benefit of incorporating their use in HPS programs is that no cost is involved if suitable sticks are harvested locally by participating children, or very low cost if supplies are purchased in village markets. In many countries suitable sticks can be sourced from a variety of local trees and shrubs that have a suitably fibrous structure, and some of these are known containing agents that inhibit the activity of oral bacteria including *Streptococcus mutans*, the bacteria principally responsible for caries formation [26, 49, 50]. However, regardless of the method used to clean the teeth instruction on what constitutes a good technique must be explained and demonstrated carefully, and conduct of the "healthy practice" must be checked and reinforced in daily oral hygiene sessions that in most schools are instituted after the daily lunch break. In our programs we have found it particularly important to ensure that children are taught to clean their posterior teeth and interdental surfaces effectively [15].

Teaching should also address any local practices that are potentially harmful to the teeth or gums, such as the use of ash as cleaning agents, and where possible suggest healthy alternative measures [46]. Positive practices that can be done at home and shared with siblings and parents should also be addressed. In some communities incentive programs enhance interest and compliance related to desired changes in behaviour. In class quizzes keep knowledge current and maintain focus on oral health as an issue, and health messages disseminated amongst participants using social media are a recent addition to the medium of health promotion [28, 51].

An evaluation process should monitor program effectiveness and enable both the curriculum "knowledge" and "healthy practices" content taught to be refined and improved where necessary.

Processes for evaluation depend on the resources available and desired outcome criteria [36, 37, 42]. Examples include surveys, interviews, and self-report questionnaires; such tools can provide numeric data on participation and with the use of open ended questions can provide relevant information on what works and what needs to be improved [15, 39]. Responses can be content coded or used as qualitative data. For example, when asked what changes children noted in their oral health the commonest response was that their mouths no longer "smelled bad." Though subjective, this observation is valuable as it equates with the reduced incidence of halitosis secondary to gingivitis documented by Quirynen et al. [52]. Other social consequences of poor oral health and evidence of behavioral impact of HPS programs are also captured in this way.

Quantitative indices, and particularly those documenting the effects of caries, are the "gold standard" measures of oral health. An example is the decayed missing filled teeth (DMFT) index [52], an established measure performed according to criteria described by WHO [53], by a health care provider trained to do a standard oral examination. The surfaces of each tooth are examined and the presence or absence of caries is recorded. A tooth is considered as filled where it has permanent restoration and missing due to caries if pain or a cavity was noted prior to extraction [54]. Cohorts of children in HPS oral health promotion programs can be evaluated before programs begin and then annually thereafter [28, 39]. These data are robust validated quantitative measure that allows valid comparisons to be made within and between national cohorts and even with international data sets [15]. However, DMFT and comparable quantitative scores do require trained personal to conduct them and provision of examination gloves and disposable dental instruments; therefore a significant cost is involved that may be beyond the scope of some intervention programs. While all HPS oral health initiatives should have some element of evaluation to ensure the relevance of the program and enable modifications to be made, it can be argued that the evidence for the basic interventions that improve oral health is sufficiently validated and robust that where necessary quantitative measures at the level of DMFT are not always warranted in a school-based program.

5. Conclusions

Poor oral health is an example of a worldwide public health issue of central importance for children, with caries being both the commonest childhood infectious disease and the most common preventable cause of chronic inflammation. As a consequence of caries, gingivitis, periodontal disease, and tooth loss millions of children worldwide experience significant morbidity and impairment of their quality of life. However, the majority of the poor oral health they experience can be prevented altogether or significantly improved through changes in behaviour achieved by teaching them a combination of simple factual knowledge and inexpensive healthy practices. And these two basic elements of health promotion are known to be provided through use of the WHO HPS model. In the context of oral health HPS programs have been shown to increase knowledge, reduce the self-reported incidence of halitosis, improve oral hygiene practices, change dietary preferences and increase healthy eating, decrease independently documented rates of caries, and result in improved DMFT scores [11, 15, 27–30, 39, 46].

Health care providers, those involved in public health research, and governments have a significant role to play in the ongoing transformation of health knowledge and behaviours [55, 56], and the WHO HPS model is a validated method for them to initiate collaborative community-based intervention to address a locally relevant health issue. As recent innovative approaches show, where such individuals enter into partnership with policy makers and engage in knowledge exchange with advocacy groups and professionals such as teachers, mutual benefits result that lead to more effective interventions to address the health needs prevalent in communities. Such benefits accrue because collaboration brings together different perspectives and competencies that optimize use of available expertise and elevate understanding of innovative approaches [57]. For those looking to initiate health promotion in schools poor oral health is an ideal starting point as it is a topic with no stigma or cultural or religious overtones, which has relevance to almost every population [40]. A possible exception would be communities where naturally high fluoride levels in the water result in a much lower incidence of caries than usual.

HPS programs initiated to address a variety of issues have been documented to result in children acquiring knowledge and practical skills that enable them to positively impact key determents of health [12, 39]. Such children are more likely to choose health behaviours and a lifestyle that reduces their susceptibility to preventable diseases. And, importantly, these positive attitudes and behaviours established in childhood and youth are known to contribute beneficially to their behaviours as adults, because the habits of living established in these early years, be they beneficial or negative, significantly impact their choices and how they behave in later life [58]. Today the WHO HPS model is relevant as a means of health promotion as very large numbers of children worldwide experience deficiencies that negatively impact a broad range of health indicators, yet many of these can be addressed through HPS initiatives [55, 59, 60]. Importantly, there is growing evidence of positive benefits evident amongst children in HPS schools and also in the broader community. Also, such improvement can be achieved with modest investment and in developing countries and amongst disadvantaged populations, as initiating HPS activities requires a change in mindset and small additions to the curriculum rather than major investment in resources, training of additional health care professionals, or new infrastructure.

It is relevant in the context of promotion of oral health that HPS initiatives that address prevention of caries and periodontal disease, increase knowledge of healthy dietary choices, and promote healthy practices are some of the simplest and least expensive to initiate. Also that oral health promotion is more affordable than the cost of traditional restorative treatments, a fact with particular relevance in the financial climate of current times [55]. And, as with all HPS programs, children who benefit from effective program delivery can be expected to have less dependence on government funded health care delivery because of the reduction in their predisposition to preventable illness because of the lifestyle changes, knowledge, and practices that they acquire. It is also recognized that improved health in turn promotes more successful learning, probably through both a reduction in school absence due to illness and improved academic performance. And, arguably, because of what is known about the association of poor oral health with predisposition to adult diseases, there is also a health and potential cost benefit, as pregnancy outcomes, the consequences of heart disease and stroke, and growing burden of diabetes are of growing relevance even in the developing world [61, 62]. Thus HPS programs contribute to the best possible use being made of available human, financial, and community resources and hence are of particular relevance as a health intervention in schools in low and middle income countries. And it is for such reasons that the WHO sees HPS programs as a particularly sound investment in global child health.

Conflict of Interests

The author declares that there is no conflict of interests regarding the publication of this paper.

References

[1] P. E. Petersen, D. Bourgeois, D. Bratthall, and H. Ogawa, "Oral health information systems—towards measuring progress in oral health promotion and disease prevention," *Bulletin of the World Health Organization*, vol. 83, no. 9, pp. 686–693, 2005.

[2] B. Christian and A. S. Blinkhorn, "A review of dental caries in Australian aboriginal children: the health inequalities perspective," *Rural and Remote Health*, vol. 12, no. 4, article 2032, 2012.

[3] C. McGrath, H. Broder, and M. Wilson-Genderson, "Assessing the impact of oral health on the life quality of children: implications for research and practice," *Community Dentistry and Oral Epidemiology*, vol. 32, no. 2, pp. 81–85, 2004.

[4] A. J. Grau, H. Becher, C. M. Ziegler et al., "Periodontal disease as a risk factor for ischemic stroke," *Stroke*, vol. 35, no. 2, pp. 496–501, 2004.

[5] M. Ide and P. N. Papapanou, "Epidemiology of association between maternal periodontal disease and adverse pregnancy outcomes - Systematic review," *Journal of Clinical Periodontology*, vol. 40, no. 14, supplement, pp. S181–S194, 2013.

[6] J. J. Taylor, P. M. Preshaw, and E. Lalla, "A review of the evidence for pathogenic mechanisms that may link periodontitis and diabetes," *Journal of Periodontology*, vol. 40, supplement 14, pp. S113–S134, 2013.

[7] L. L. Humphrey, R. Fu, D. I. Buckley, M. Freeman, and M. Helfand, "Periodontal disease and coronary heart disease incidence: a systematic review and meta-analysis," *Journal of General Internal Medicine*, vol. 23, no. 12, pp. 2079–2086, 2008.

[8] B. L. Pihlstrom, B. S. Michalowicz, and N. W. Johnson, "Periodontal diseases," *The Lancet*, vol. 366, no. 9499, pp. 1809–1820, 2005.

[9] P. B. Lockhart, A. F. Bolger, P. N. Papapanou et al., "Periodontal disease and atherosclerotic vascular disease: does the evidence support an independent association?: a scientific statement from the American heart association," *Circulation*, vol. 125, no. 20, pp. 2520–2544, 2012.

[10] O. Ibiyemi, J. O. Taiwo, and G. A. Oke, "Dental education in the rural community: a Nigerian experience," *Rural and Remote Health*, vol. 13, no. 2, p. 2241, 2013.

[11] S. Y. L. Kwan, P. E. Petersen, C. M. Pine, and A. Borutta, "Health-promoting schools: an opportunity for oral health promotion," *Bulletin of the World Health Organization*, vol. 83, no. 9, pp. 677–685, 2005.

[12] K.-C. Tang, D. Nutbeam, C. Aldinger et al., "Schools for health, education and development: a call for action," *Health Promotion International*, vol. 24, no. 1, pp. 68–77, 2009.

[13] A. Macnab, "The stellenbosch consensus statement on health promoting schools," *Global Health Promotion*, vol. 20, no. 1, pp. 78–81, 2013.

[14] World Health Organization, "What is a Health Promoting School?" 2013, http://who.int/school_youth_health/gshi/hps/en/.

[15] A. Kizito, C. Meredith, Y. Wang, A. Kasangaki, and A. J. Macnab, "Oral health promotion in schools: rationale and evaluation," *Health Education*, vol. 114, no. 4, pp. 293–303, 2014.

[16] R. C. Page and H. E. Schroeder, "Pathogenesis of inflammatory periodontal disease: a summary of current work," *Laboratory Investigation*, vol. 34, no. 3, pp. 235–249, 1976.

[17] M. Anderson, "Risk assessment and epidemiology of dental caries: review of the literature," *Pediatric Dentistry*, vol. 24, no. 5, pp. 377–385, 2002.

[18] R. H. Selwitz, A. I. Ismail, and N. B. Pitts, "Dental caries," *The Lancet*, vol. 369, no. 9555, pp. 51–59, 2007.

[19] G. C. Armitage, "Periodontal diagnoses and classification of periodontal diseases," *Periodontology 2000*, vol. 34, pp. 9–21, 2004.

[20] P. J. Moynihan, "The role of diet and nutrition in the etiology and prevention of oral diseases," *Bulletin of the World Health Organization*, vol. 83, no. 9, pp. 694–699, 2005.

[21] A. Pau, S. S. Khan, M. G. Babar, and R. Croucher, "Dental pain and care-seeking in 11–14-yr-old adolescents in a low-income country," *European Journal of Oral Sciences*, vol. 116, no. 5, pp. 451–457, 2008.

[22] P. E. Petersen, "Global policy for improvement of oral health in the 21st century—implications to oral health research of World Health Assembly 2007, World Health Organization," *Community Dentistry and Oral Epidemiology*, vol. 37, no. 1, pp. 1–8, 2009.

[23] A. Rowan-Legg, "Oral health care for children—a call for action," *Paediatrics and Child Health*, vol. 18, no. 1, pp. 37–43, 2013.

[24] G. Tsakos and C. Quiñonez, "A sober look at the links between oral and general health," *Journal of Epidemiology & Community Health*, vol. 67, no. 5, pp. 381–382, 2013.

[25] H. Löe, "Oral hygiene in the prevention of caries and periodontal disease," *International Dental Journal*, vol. 50, no. 3, pp. 129–139, 2000.

[26] C. D. Wu, I. A. Darout, and N. Skaug, "Chewing sticks: timeless natural toothbrushes for oral cleansing," *Journal of Periodontal Research*, vol. 36, no. 5, pp. 275–284, 2001.

[27] R. Harrison, D. Duffy, D. Benton, and A. J. Macnab, "Brighter smiles: service learning, inter-professional collaboration and health promotion in a first nations community," *Canadian Journal of Public Health*, vol. 97, no. 3, pp. 237–240, 2006.

[28] A. J. Macnab, J. Rozmus, D. Benton, and F. A. Gagnon, "3-year results of a collaborative school-based oral health program in a remote First Nations community," *Rural and Remote Health*, vol. 8, no. 2, p. 882, 2008.

[29] H. V. Worthington, K. B. Hill, J. Mooney, F. A. Hamilton, and A. S. Blinkhorn, "A cluster randomized controlled trial of a dental health education program for 10-year-old children," *Journal of Public Health Dentistry*, vol. 61, no. 1, pp. 22–27, 2001.

[30] W. H. van Palenstein Helderman, L. Munck, S. Mushendwa, M. A. van't Hof, and F. G. Mrema, "Effect evaluation of an oral health education programme in primary schools in Tanzania," *Community Dentistry and Oral Epidemiology*, vol. 25, no. 4, pp. 296–300, 1997.

[31] G. Bos, "The miswāk, an aspect of dental care in Islam," *Medical History*, vol. 37, no. 1, pp. 68–79, 1993.

[32] World Health Organization Expert Committee on Comprehensive School Health Education and Promotion, "Promoting health through schools," WHO Technical Report Series 870, 1997.

[33] D. Lister-Sharp, S. Chapman, S. Stewart-Brown, and A. Sowden, "Health promoting schools and health promotion in schools: two systematic reviews," *Health Technology Assessment*, vol. 3, no. 22, pp. 1–207, 1999.

[34] A. M. Moon, M. A. Mullee, L. Rogers, R. L. Thompson, V. Speller, and P. Roderick, "Helping schools to become health-promoting environments—an evaluation of the Wessex Healthy Schools Award," *Health Promotion International*, vol. 14, no. 2, pp. 111–122, 1999.

[35] I. Young, "Health promotion in schools—a historical perspective," *Promotion & Education*, vol. 12, no. 3-4, pp. 112–117, 2005.

[36] S. Stewart-Brown, "What is the evidence on school health promotion in improving health or preventing disease and, specifically, what is the effectiveness of the health promoting schools approach?" WHO Regional Office for Europe, Copenhagen, Denmark (Health Evidence Network Report) 2006, http://www.euro.who.int/document/e88185.pdf.

[37] L. St Leger, I. Young, C. Blanchard, and M. Perry, "Promoting health in schools from evidence to action," http://www.dhhs.tas.gov.au/__data/assets/pdf_file/0007/117385/PHiSFromEvidence-ToAction_WEB1.pdf.

[38] World Health Organization, "Nairobi Call to Action for Closing the Implementation Gap in Health Promotion," WHO, Geneva, Switzerland, 2009, http://javeriana.edu.co/redcups/Nairobi_Call_for_Action.pdf.

[39] R. Langford, C. P. Bonnell, H. E. Jones et al., "The WHO health promoting school framework for improving the health and well-being of students and their academic achievement," *The Cochrane Database of Systematic Reviews*, no. 4, Article ID CD008958, 2014.

[40] M. Bardi, A. Burbank, W. Choi et al., "Activities for engaging schools in health promotion," *Health Education*, vol. 114, no. 4, pp. 271–280, 2014.

[41] J. Inchley, J. Muldoon, and C. Currie, "Becoming a health promoting school: evaluating the process of effective implementation in Scotland," *Health Promotion International*, vol. 22, no. 1, pp. 65–71, 2007.

[42] A. J. Macnab, F. A. Gagnon, and D. Stewart, "Health promoting schools: consensus, strategies, and potential," *Health Education*, vol. 114, no. 3, pp. 170–185, 2014.

[43] O. Samdal and L. Rowling, "Theoretical and empirical base for implementation components of health-promoting schools," *Health Education*, vol. 111, no. 5, pp. 367–390, 2011.

[44] A. J. Macnab, D. Stewart, and F. Gagnon, "Health promoting schools: initiatives in Africa," *Health Education*, vol. 114, no. 4, pp. 246–259, 2014.

[45] S. Dharamsi, R. Woollard, P. Kendal, I. Okullo, and A. J. Macnab, "Health promoting schools as learning sites for physicians in-training," *Health Education*, vol. 114, no. 3, pp. 186–196, 2014.

[46] A. MacNab and A. Kasangaki, ""Many voices, one song": a model for an oral health programme as a first step in establishing a health promoting school," *Health Promotion International*, vol. 27, no. 1, pp. 63–73, 2012.

[47] S. Nörmark and H. J. Mosha, "Relationship between habits and dental health among rural Tanzanian children," *Community Dentistry and Oral Epidemiology*, vol. 17, no. 6, pp. 317–321, 1989.

[48] E. O. Sote, "The relative effectiveness of chewing sticks and toothbrush on plaque removal," *African Dental Journal*, vol. 1, no. 2, pp. 48–53, 1987.

[49] V. O. Rotimi and H. A. Mosadomi, "The effect of crude extracts of nine African chewing sticks on oral anaerobes," *Journal of Medical Microbiology*, vol. 23, no. 1, pp. 55–60, 1987.

[50] A. G. Jagtap and S. G. Karkera, "Extract of *Juglandaceae regia* inhibits growth, in-vitro adherence, acid production and aggregation of *Streptococcus mutans*," *Journal of Pharmacy and Pharmacology*, vol. 52, no. 2, pp. 235–242, 2000.

[51] J. J. Dietrich, J. Coetzee, K. Otwombe et al., "Adolescent-friendly technologies as potential adjuncts for health promotion," *Health Education*, vol. 114, no. 4, pp. 304–318, 2014.

[52] M. Quirynen, J. Dadamio, S. van den Velde et al., "Characteristics of 2000 patients who visited a halitosis clinic," *Journal of Clinical Periodontology*, vol. 36, no. 11, pp. 970–975, 2009.

[53] World Health Organization, *Oral Health Surveys. Basic Methods*, World Health Organization, Geneva, Switzerland, 3rd edition, 1987.

[54] L. M. Muwazi, C. M. Rwenyonyi, F. J. Tirwomwe et al., "Prevalence of oral diseases/conditions in Uganda," *African Health Sciences*, vol. 5, no. 3, pp. 227–233, 2005.

[55] M. Sparks, "The changing contexts of health promotion," *Health Promotion International*, vol. 28, no. 2, pp. 153–156, 2013.

[56] B. Hutchison, J.-F. Levesque, E. Strumpf, and N. Coyle, "Primary health care in Canada: systems in motion," *Milbank Quarterly*, vol. 89, no. 2, pp. 256–288, 2011.

[57] J. G. Kosteniuk, D. G. Morgan, J. Bracken, and P. Kessler, "Adventures in rural and remote health services innovation: the role of researcher as collaborator," *Rural and Remote Health*, vol. 14, article 2898, 2014.

[58] P. R. W. Kendall, C. Mangham, and D. W. Young, "An ounce of prevention," *Paediatrics and Child Health*, vol. 9, no. 3, pp. 151–152, 2004.

[59] R. G. Davidson, S. Rustein, K. Johnson, E. Suliman, A. Wagstaff, and A. Amouzou, *Socioeconomic Differences in Health, Nutrition, and Population within Developing Countries: An Overview*, The World Bank, Washington, DC, USA, 2007.

[60] A. Wagstaff, "Poverty and health sector inequalities," *Bulletin of the World Health Organization*, vol. 80, no. 2, pp. 97–105, 2002.

[61] Y.-L. Lee, H.-Y. Hu, N. Huang, D.-K. Hwang, P. Chou, and D. Chu, "Dental prophylaxis and periodontal treatment are protective factors to ischemic stroke," *Stroke*, vol. 44, no. 4, pp. 1026–1030, 2013.

[62] J. C. N. Mbanya, A. A. Motala, E. Sobngwi, F. K. Assah, and S. T. Enoru, "Diabetes in sub-Saharan Africa," *The Lancet*, vol. 375, no. 9733, pp. 2254–2266, 2010.

6

Neighborhood Social Environment and Health Communication at Prepregnancy and Maternal Stages among Caucasian and Asian Women: Findings from the Los Angeles Mommy and Baby Survey

Lu Shi[1] and Yuping Mao[2]

[1]*Department of Public Health Sciences, Clemson University, Clemson, SC 29634-0745, USA*
[2]*Department of Media & Communication, Erasmus University Rotterdam, 3000 DR, Netherlands*

Correspondence should be addressed to Lu Shi; lushi.pku@gmail.com

Academic Editor: Apostolos Vantarakis

Introduction. We study whether the relationship between neighborhood social environment and maternal communication with healthcare providers differs between Asians and Caucasians. *Method and Materials.* Using the 2007 Los Angeles Mommy and Baby (LAMB) survey, we measure new mother's neighborhood social environment by four key variables: (1) instrumental/emotional support during pregnancy, (2) neighborhood social cohesion, (3) neighborhood social exchange, and (4) neighborhood services. Logistic regressions were applied for data analysis. Neighborhood social exchange predicts less chance of lacking communication about sensitive issues in preconception visits among Caucasians (logged odds: −0.045; $P < 0.01$) and Asians (L.O.: −0.081; $P < 0.001$) and predicts less chance of lacking communication during preconception visits among Asians (L.O.: −0.092; $P < 0.05$). Neighborhood social cohesion predicts more chance for lacking communication about preparation for pregnancy only among Asians (L.O.: 0.065; $P < 0.05$). Neighborhood services predict less chance of lacking communication about stigmatized issues in the prenatal visit among Asians (L.O.: −0.036; $P < 0.05$). *Discussion.* Caucasians and Asians with more neighborhood social exchange are more likely to discuss sensitive issues during preconception visits. Neighborhood service significantly predicts maternal discussion of stigmatized issues with health care providers, but only among Asians.

1. Introduction

In developed nations, racial/ethnic disparities persist in receipt of a wide range of health services such as specialty care, pain assessment and treatment, and mental health services [1]. Asian women above 35 years are at higher risk of giving birth to a child with Down syndrome in comparison with Caucasian women in the same age group [2]. This risk could be effectively reduced by seeing an obstetrician prior to the pregnancy and obtaining recommended nutritional supplements such as folic acid, as well as by taking a prenatal screening to monitor the fetal growth. However, a study from the United Kingdom shows that South Asian women with positive attitudes toward taking prenatal screening for Down syndrome are less likely to take the test than

Caucasian women with positive attitudes toward the test [3]. The racial difference in receiving maternal health services is an important topic in racial/ethnic health disparities, since maternal health affects both women and their children's health. It is also a health service the majority of women will receive at least once in their lives. Thus, the disparity of receiving maternal health services between Asian pregnant women and non-Hispanic Caucasian (to be referred to as "Caucasian" hereafter) pregnant women requires more research attention, given the severity of this disparity.

Some of the racial disparities between Asian women and Caucasian women in receiving healthcare services may be attributed to challenges associated with the former's intercultural communication with their healthcare providers, the economic difficulties during the immigration process, and the psychological challenges during the acculturation process. Female immigrants encounter various challenges such as economic strain, acculturation stress, and language barriers, which may negatively affect health [4]. As an additional challenge, sometimes the acculturation process seems to have a negative rather than positive health impact on maternal health, as is the case for many Southeast Asian immigrant women in Canada [5]. Some evidence from the United States even indicates that the general health status of certain Asian and Pacific Islander immigrants could deteriorate when their length of residency in the US increases [6]. These findings contradict the stereotype of "the model minority" and suggest that challenges to Asian immigrants' health might be underestimated and understudied.

Communication between healthcare providers and recipients is a potential contributing factor of disparities in health outcomes [7]. During women's prepregnancy and prenatal visits with healthcare providers, it is especially challenging for women and their healthcare providers to discuss socially stigmatized health topics that are important to the health of both mother and baby. Many barriers exist for Asian and Latino women in the US who seek help from healthcare providers when experiencing intimate partner abuse including social isolation, language barriers, discrimination and fears of deportation, dedication to the children and family unity, shame related to the abuse, and the cultural stigma of divorce [8]. HIV/AIDS positive status disclosure is one sensitive issue investigated in this study. One of few research papers on Asian population's HIV/AIDS disclosure found the communication barriers among the Asian population on this topic include fear of stigma, concerns of disappointing, burdening others, fear of discrimination, protection of family from shame, protection of family from obligation to help, and avoidance of communication regarding highly personal information [9, 10]. Thus it is worthwhile to explore what might facilitate or hinder Asian women's communication about these sensitive issues with health care providers in the host country.

One possible factor that may have a dubious impact on women's communication with health care providers is the kind of social support they receive. Social support is a complex process involving "transactions between individuals and their social networks, for example, providing and receiving tangible (material) or intangible (emotional, informational, or cognitive guidance) support, and developing and maintaining support network resources" [11]. A lot of research has focused on the relationship between social support and particular medical maternal outcomes such as birth weight [12] and fetal growth [13]. It is also evident that, among women experiencing intimate partner violence, the more social support these women receive, the lower their risk of perceived poor mental health, physical health, anxiety, current depression, and suicide attempts [13]. During their interactions with healthcare providers, prospective mothers choose to share or not to share some important health information that might be considered as sensitive or private in their own cultures. This decision on communication with their healthcare providers and their health decision-making might be influenced by information and support that they receive from different sources such as neighbors and friends. For immigrant women who stay among fellow immigrants from one sending country, folk belief and folk medicine could displace health care utilization such as physician visits and thus serve as a roadblock to health outcome maximization [14]. As low social support has been shown to be associated with more health care utilization [15], it is reasonable to suspect that heightened social support for a mother could lower the likelihood of her prepregnancy and prenatal visits.

This study examines the relationship between social support and women's health communication with healthcare providers such as whether women make prepregnancy and maternal visits with their healthcare providers and to what extent women communicate sensitive issues (e.g., abuse and illegal drug use) as well as mental health issues (e.g., anxiety and depression) with their healthcare providers. In particular, our study examines the association of neighborhood social support with prospective mothers' health communication since neighborhood is an important and convenient source of social support for many people. Neighborhood characters and social support are related to various health issues. For instance, neighborhood cohesion has been found to positively correlate to youth participation in physical activity [16]. Buka et al. [17] reported that neighborhood-level factors are significantly associated with infant birth weight. In the existing literature on maternal and child health in relation to neighborhood context, the following categories of neighborhood characteristics have been addressed: income/wealth, employment, family structure, population composition, housing, mobility, education, occupation, social resources, violence and crime, deviant behavior, and physical conditions [18]. Only in more recent years, research has been conducted on neighborhood social support in relation to maternal health. Nkansah-Amankra et al.'s [19] research shows low neighborhood social support is an independent risk for low birth weight or preterm births. Mothers with more supportive social networks are found to experience better mental health outcomes [20]. While the association between neighborhood social support and maternal health outcomes has been examined by these studies, researchers have not examined the role of patient-physician communication as a possible intervening variable between social support and health outcome.

Our study explores the racial difference in prospective mothers' communication with healthcare providers, as quality communication between a physician and a patient positively influences the health outcomes and thus constitutes an integral part of health care [21]. To the best of our knowledge, our study is the first to explore social support's influence on health communication among Asian immigrant women in the US. The rising number of Asian immigrants in the US makes studies on Asian American women's maternal health even more important.

2. Method

We use the 2007 Los Angeles Mommy and Baby (LAMB) survey to study overall health disparities in maternal and child health before and during pregnancy. The 2007 LAMB survey was conducted to new mothers who had a live birth in the Los Angeles County four to seven months before. The survey contains items examining maternal and child health indicators such as prenatal care, health behaviour during pregnancy, and postnatal recovery. Participating mothers were recruited through multilevel sampling and were asked to fill out the sections of the survey that were relevant to their experience. For the purpose of this research, we analyzed survey items related to participating mothers' prepregnancy and prenatal visits to health providers and social environment. We use four sets of questionnaire items to construct four scales that measure different aspects of social environment, adapted from the Project on Human Development in Chicago Neighborhoods (PHDCN) [16] and the LAMB project team. In this study, we measure Asian women's and Caucasian women's neighborhood social environment by four related key variables: (1) instrumental and emotional support during pregnancy, (2) neighborhood social cohesion, (3) neighborhood social exchange, and (4) neighborhood services characterized by safety, friendliness, quietness, cleanliness, and public service.

2.1. Instrumental and Emotional Support during Pregnancy.
The 2007 LAMB survey asked each respondent "During your last pregnancy, how often would you get these kinds of support, if you needed them?" and the respondent would choose from "Never," "Rarely," "Sometimes," "Most of the time," and "All of the time" for each of the following seven items:

> (a) Someone to loan me $50; (b) Someone to help me if I were sick and needed to be in bed; (c) Someone to take me to the clinic or doctor if I needed a ride; (d) Someone to give me a place to live; (e) Someone to help me with babysitting or child care; (f) Someone to help me with household chores; (g) Someone to talk to about my problems.

For each of the seven items, we coded this Likert scale as 1 through 5 with "Never" being 1 and "All of the time" being 5 and summed up the seven items to create a scale of prenatal social network support.

2.2. Neighborhood Social Cohesion.
The 2007 LAMB survey asked each respondent "Do you agree that people in your neighborhood...

> (a) Are willing to help their neighbors? (b) This is a close-knit (tight) neighborhood? (c) Can be trusted? (d) Generally do not get along with each other? (e) Do not share the same values?"

The respondent would choose from "Strongly disagree," "Disagree," "Neutral," "Agree," and "Strongly agree" for each of the above five items. For each of the first three items we coded this Likert scale as 1 through 5 with "Strongly disagree" being 1 and "Strongly agree" being 5, while coding the remaining two items in the reverse order as conceptually Item D and Item

E measure the antonymous construct of neighborhood social cohesion. We summed up the five items to create a scale for neighborhood social cohesion.

2.3. Neighborhood Social Exchange.
The 2007 LAMB survey asked each respondent "And how often do your neighbors...

> (a) Do favors for each other? (b) Ask each other advice about personal things such as child rearing or job openings? (c) Have parties or other get-togethers where other people in the neighborhood are invited? (d) Visit in each other's homes or on the street? (e) Watch over each other's property?"

and the respondent would choose from "Never," "Almost never," "Sometimes," "Fairly often," and "Very often" for each of the above five items. For each of the five items, we coded this Likert scale as 1 through 5 with "Never" being 1 and "Very often" being 5 and summed up the five items to create a scale of neighborhood social exchange.

2.4. Neighborhood Services.
The 2007 LAMB survey asked each respondent "How would you rate this neighborhood in terms of its...

> (a) Police protection; (b) Protection of property; (c) Safety from violence; (d) Friendliness; (e) Cleanliness; (f) Quietness; (g) Quality of schools; (h) Availability of parks, playgrounds, or sidewalks; (i) Municipal services (e.g., trash pickup, road repair, libraries, water)"

and the respondent would choose from "Very poor," "Poor," "Sometimes," "Good," and "Very good" for each of the above nine items. For each of the nine items, we coded this Likert scale as 1 through 5 with "Very poor" being 1 and "Very good" being 5 and summed up the nine items to create a scale of neighborhood services.

2.5. Dependent Variables.
We use the following three dummy variables to measure the communication between White/Asian women and health care providers: whether the respondent had talked to provider to prepare for pregnancy (women who did not do so were coded as 1 and women who did so were coded as 0); whether she talked about sensitive issues in preparatory visit prior to pregnancy (women who talked about domestic violence, anxiety/depression, or birth control during her prepregnancy visit were coded as 0, and women who did not do so were coded as 1); whether she talked about stigmatized issues in prenatal visits (women who talked about domestic abuse, illicit drug, and HIV during her prenatal visits were coded as 0 while women who did not do so were coded as 1).

2.6. Logistic Regressions with Geographic Fixed Effects.
We use six logistic regressions to examine the association between the social environment and women's communication with

TABLE 1: Logistic regressions of neighborhood factors in predicting communication during prepregnancy and prenatal visit to health care providers.

	Not talking to a health care provider to get prepared for pregnancy (prepregnancy visits)		Not talking about sensitive issues (prepregnancy visits)		Not talking about stigmatized issues (prenatal visits)	
	Asian	Caucasian	Asian	Caucasian	Asian	Caucasian
Instrumental and emotional support	No data was collected				−0.023	−0.017
Neighbor social cohesion	0.065*	−0.007	0.010	0.049	0.056	0.022
Neighbor social exchange	−0.092***	−0.027	−0.081**	−0.045*	−0.042	−0.012
Neighbor services	−0.010	−0.001	0.006	0.010	−0.036*	−0.012

Notes:
(1) *if $P < 0.05$, **if $P < 0.01$, ***if $P < 0.001$;
(2) controlled for the following covariates: age, education, income, and geographic units (operationalized as seven dummy variables accounting for the eight service planning areas in Los Angeles County).

health care providers (operationalized as the three above-mentioned dependent variables), stratified by race (Caucasians versus Asians). To control for confounding factors, we use the respondent's age, education (dummy-coded by level of educational attainment), household income (dummy-coded by 5 levels of household income), and geographic units (operationalized as seven dummy variables accounting for the eight service planning areas in Los Angeles County) as covariates in our logistic models.

3. Results

Table 1 summarizes the results of the six regressions. Neighborhood social exchange is negatively associated with not talking about sensitive issues in prepregnancy visits among Caucasian women (logged odds: −0.045; $P < 0.01$) and Asian women (logged odds: −0.081; $P < 0.001$), which indicates both Caucasian and Asian women living in a neighborhood with a higher level of social exchange tend to talk about sensitive issues in prepregnancy medical visits. However, the negative association between neighborhood social exchange and not talking to a health care provider to prepare for pregnancy is only significant among Asian women (logged odds: −0.092; $P < 0.05$), meaning Asian women living in a neighborhood with higher level of social exchange tend to talk to their health care provider about preparing for pregnancy. Neighborhood social cohesion has a significant positive association with not talking to provider to prepare for pregnancy among Asians (logged odds: 0.065; $P < 0.05$), which is a pattern that is not seen among Caucasian women (logged odds: −0.007; $P > 0.05$). During prenatal visits to health care providers, the only significant association exists between neighborhood services and not talking about stigmatized issues among Asian women (logged odds: −.036; $P < 0.05$), a pattern that is not statistically significant among Caucasian women (logged odds: −.012; $P > 0.05$).

4. Discussion

As social support is significantly correlated with a woman's "maternal confidence" to provide infant care [22], it might be plausible to infer that such confidence could trigger the mother to skip physician visits before, during, and after her pregnancy. According to our study, Asian women with higher neighborhood social exchange are more likely to visit health care providers to prepare for pregnancy while Asian women from a more cohesive neighborhood sharing similar values are less likely to visit healthcare providers to prepare for pregnancy. This might indicate the feared "displacement effect" (word-of-mouth experience sharing in a more cohesive community displaces the resident's physician visits) could be happening in immigrant or minority neighborhoods, yet the reciprocal help among neighbors is unlikely to displace a woman's visit to health care providers in preparation for her pregnancy. This "displacement effect," however, is not evident among Caucasian women when it comes to their visit to health care providers. Future research could further examine ethnic differences in social support and maternal confidence in relation to women's possibility of making prepregnancy visits.

It is worth noting that Caucasian women and Asian women do share an important similarity in discussing sensitive issues such as domestic violence, anxiety, and depression during their prepregnancy visits to health care providers: those who enjoy more neighborhood social exchange are more likely to discuss these issues during their visit to healthcare providers to prepare for their pregnancy. While our study of associations cannot be used as causal evidence, this significant pattern shared by both Caucasian women and Asian women might give us a hypothesis for future experimental studies: living in an environment of friendliness and trust helps people open up about sensitive topics in their conversation with health care providers.

Caucasian and Asian women differ in their likelihood of discussing stigmatized issues (such as drinking, abuse, illegal drug use, and HIV/AIDS) during their prenatal visit. Better neighborhood services (characterized by safety, cleanness, and public services) are positively associated with Asian women's likelihood of discussing stigmatized issues with their healthcare providers during prenatal visits, while this association is much weaker and statistically insignificant among Caucasian women, albeit with the same sign of the logistic coefficient. Exactly why the pattern differs between Asians and Caucasians is unknown to us, but we do notice in our data that Caucasian women on average reported having significantly higher instrumental and emotional support level from their personal networks than Asian women. This might mean that Asian women with their lower level of instrumental and emotional support from their personal networks actually need neighborhood services more than their Caucasian counterparts to have a sense of trust and security for opening a conversation about stigmatized issues during pregnancy.

On average, Asian women in this study lived in neighborhoods with lower service quality than Caucasians. As our study shows that neighborhood service is a significant predictor of Asian women's discussion of stigmatized issues with health care providers (usually considered as a good sign in health communication), it could be critical to improve the safety, cleanness, and public service in neighborhoods with higher proportions of Asian population, as the improvement of the public service quality of those neighborhoods could be an indirect way to reduce the racial disparities in benefiting from maternal health services. From the perspective of planning interventions, initiatives like improving neighborhood services could be easier to implement than improving neighborhood social support or enhancing one's personal network, as the latter two tend to be individual choices and community culture rather than policy makers' actionable targets.

Conflict of Interests

The authors declare that there is no conflict of interests regarding the publication of this paper.

References

[1] M. van Ryn and S. S. Fu, "Paved with good intentions: do public health and human service providers contribute to racial/ethnic disparities in health?" *American Journal of Public Health*, vol. 93, no. 2, pp. 248–255, 2003.

[2] M. Kuppermann, E. Gates, and A. E. Washington, "Racial-ethnic differences in prenatal diagnostic test use and outcomes: preferences, socioeconomics, or patient knowledge?" *Obstetrics & Gynecology*, vol. 87, no. 5 I, pp. 675–682, 1996.

[3] M. H. Davis, M. M. Morris, and L. A. Kraus, "Relationship-specific and global perception of social support: associations with well-being and attachments," *Journal of Personality and Social Psychology*, vol. 74, no. 2, pp. 468–481, 1998.

[4] J. S. Ali, S. McDermott, and R. G. Gravel, "Recent research on immigrant health from statistics Canada's population surveys," *Canadian Journal of Public Health*, vol. 95, no. 3, pp. I9–I13, 2004.

[5] I. Hyman, "Negative consequences of acculturation on health behavior, social support and stress among pregnant Southeast Asian immigrant women in Montreal: an exploratory study," *Canadian Journal of Public Health*, vol. 91, no. 5, pp. 357–360, 2000.

[6] W. P. Frisbie, Y. Cho, and R. A. Hummer, "Immigration and the health of Asian and pacific islander adults in the United States," *American Journal of Epidemiology*, vol. 153, no. 4, pp. 372–380, 2001.

[7] R. M. Perloff, B. Bonder, G. B. Ray, E. B. Ray, and L. A. Siminoff, "Doctor-patient communication, cultural competence, and minority health: theoretical and empirical perspectives," *American Behavioral Scientist*, vol. 49, no. 6, pp. 835–852, 2006.

[8] H. M. Bauer, M. A. Rodriguez, S. S. Quiroga, and Y. G. Flores-Ortiz, "Barriers to health care for abused Latina and Asian immigrant women," *Journal of Health Care for the Poor and Underserved*, vol. 11, no. 1, pp. 33–44, 2000.

[9] M. R. Yoshioka and A. Schustack, "Disclosure of HIV status: cultural issues of asian patients," *AIDS Patient Care and STDs*, vol. 15, no. 2, pp. 77–82, 2001.

[10] D. Chin and K. W. Kroesen, "Disclosure of HIV infection among Asian/Pacific Islander American women: cultural stigma and support," *Cultural Diversity & Ethnic Minority Psychology*, vol. 5, no. 3, pp. 222–235, 1999.

[11] G. Choi, "Acculturative stress, social support, and depression in Korean American families," *Journal of Family Social Work*, vol. 2, no. 1, pp. 81–97, 2013.

[12] S. Cohen and T. A. Wills, "Stress, social support, and the buffering hypothesis," *Psychological Bulletin*, vol. 98, no. 2, pp. 310–357, 1985.

[13] A. L. Coker, P. H. Smith, M. P. Thompson, R. E. McKeown, L. Bethea, and K. E. Davis, "Social support protects against the negative effects of partner violence on mental health," *Journal of Women's Health & Gender-based Medicine*, vol. 11, no. 5, pp. 465–476, 2002.

[14] D. J. Bearison, N. Minian, and L. Granowetter, "Medical management of asthma and folk medicine in a hispanic community," *Journal of Pediatric Psychology*, vol. 27, no. 4, pp. 385–392, 2002.

[15] A. C. Kouzis and W. W. Eaton, "Absence of social networks, social support and health services utilization," *Psychological Medicine*, vol. 28, no. 6, pp. 1301–1310, 1998.

[16] A. L. Cradock, I. Kawachi, G. A. Colditz, S. L. Gortmaker, and S. L. Buka, "Neighborhood social cohesion and youth participation in physical activity in Chicago," *Social Science & Medicine*, vol. 68, no. 3, pp. 427–435, 2009.

[17] S. L. Buka, R. T. Brennan, J. W. Rich-Edwards, S. W. Raudenbush, and F. Earls, "Neighborhood support and the birth weight of urban infants," *American Journal of Epidemiology*, vol. 157, no. 1, pp. 1–8, 2003.

[18] J. K. Rajaratnam, J. G. Burke, and P. O'Campo, "Maternal and child health and neighborhood context: the selection and construction of area-level variables," *Health and Place*, vol. 12, no. 4, pp. 547–556, 2006.

[19] S. Nkansah-Amankra, A. Dhawain, J. R. Hussey, and K. J. Luchok, "Maternal social support and neighborhood income inequality as predictors of low birth weight and preterm birth outcome disparities: analysis of South Carolina pregnancy risk assessment and monitoring system survey, 2000–2003," *Maternal and Child Health Journal*, vol. 14, no. 5, pp. 774–785, 2010.

[20] A. B. Balaji, A. H. Claussen, D. C. Smith, S. N. Visser, M. J. Morales, and R. Perou, "Social support networks and maternal mental health and well-being," *Journal of Women's Health*, vol. 16, no. 10, pp. 1386–1396, 2007.

[21] L. M. L. Ong, J. C. J. M. De Haes, A. M. Hoos, and F. B. Lammes, "Doctor-patient communication: a review of the literature," *Social Science and Medicine*, vol. 40, no. 7, pp. 903–918, 1995.

[22] P. L. Ruchala and D. C. James, "Social support, knowledge of infant development, and maternal confidence among adolescent and adult mothers," *Journal of Obstetric, Gynecologic, and Neonatal Nursing*, vol. 26, no. 6, pp. 685–689, 1997.

7

Factors Associated with Men's Awareness of Danger Signs of Obstetric Complications and Its Effect on Men's Involvement in Birth Preparedness Practice in Southern Ethiopia, 2014

Alemu Tamiso Debiso,[1] Behailu Merdekios Gello,[1] and Marelign Tilahun Malaju[2]

[1]*Department of Public Health, College of Medicine and Health Science, Arba Minch University, Arba Minch, Ethiopia*
[2]*Department of Public Health, College of Health Sciences, Debre Tabor University, Debre Tabor, Ethiopia*

Correspondence should be addressed to Alemu Tamiso Debiso; tamisodebiso@gmail.com

Academic Editor: Guang-Hui Dong

Background. Compared to average maternal mortality ratio of 8 per 100,000 live births in industrialized countries, Ethiopia has an estimated maternal mortality ratio of 676 per 100,000 live births. Maternal deaths can be prevented partially through increasing awareness of danger signs of obstetric complications and involving husbands (male) in birth preparedness practice. *Methods*. Community based cross-sectional study was done. All adult males with a wife or partner who lives in the selected kebeles were our study population. Data was collected by pretested and structured questionnaires and two-stage cluster sampling procedure was used in order to collect study samples. Data was cleaned and entered into Epi Info 7 and exported to SPSS (IBM-21) for further analysis. Ordinary and hierarchical logistic regression model were used and AOR with 95% CI were used to show factors and the effect of men's awareness of danger sign on men's involvement in birth preparedness practice. *Results*. Total numbers of men interviewed were 836 making a response rate of 98.9%. 42% of men had awareness of danger sign and 9.4% (95% CI: (7.42, 11.4) of men were involved in birth preparedness practice. Respondents who live in the rural area [(AOR: 8.41; (95% CI: (4.99, 14.2)], governments employee [(AOR: 3.75; (95% CI: (1.38, 10.2)], those who belong to the highest wealth quintile [(AOR: 3.09; (95% CI: (1.51, 6.34)], and husbands whose wives gave birth in the hospital [(AOR: 2.09; (95% CI: (1.29, 3.37)], health center [(AOR: 1.99; (95% CI: (1.21, 3.28)], and health post [(AOR: 2.2; (95% CI: 2.16 (1.06, 404)] were positively associated and those who had no role in the health development army [(AOR: 0.43; (95% CI: (0.26, 0.72)] were negatively associated with men's awareness of danger signs of obstetric complications. *Conclusion*. The prevalence of men awareness of danger sign was low and male involvement in birth preparedness practice was very low. Since there is a low level of awareness (17.1%) particularly in the urban area and men act as gatekeepers to women's health, the respective organization needs to review urban health extension program and give due emphasis to husband education in order that they are able to recognize danger signs of obstetric complications in a way to increase their involvement in birth preparedness practice.

1. Introduction

Compared to the average MMR of 8 per 100,000 live births in industrialized countries, Ethiopia has an estimated MMR of 676 per 100,000 live births, which is the greatest contribution for maternal mortality that occurs worldwide [1, 2].

Globally there are five obstetric causes that lead to four-fifths of maternal deaths; those are divided into direct causes (severe bleeding, sepsis, unsafe abortion, hypertensive disorder of pregnancy, obstructed labor, and other causes like ectopic pregnancy, embolism) and indirect causes (malaria, anemia, and heart diseases) [3]. The preventable ones are prevented and controlled partially by increasing awareness of the signs and symptoms of obstetric complications and timely access to appropriate emergency obstetric care, even in the poorest communities [4].

The birth plan is also a very important strategy in developing countries where obstetric services are weak and thus contribute significantly to maternal and neonatal morbidity and mortality [5]. The key elements of the birth plan include a plan for skilled birth attendants, place of delivery, and arrangement of money for transport or other costs [6]. In Ethiopia, a husband at an antenatal clinic is rare in many communities and it is unthinkable to find men accompanying their partners during antenatal care and delivery [7].

In Ethiopia the top four causes of maternal mortality in the last decade were obstructed labor/uterine rupture (36%), hemorrhage (22%), hypertensive disorders of pregnancy (19%), and sepsis/infection (13%) [8, 9]. With understanding of unacceptable death due to common obstetric complications, the Ethiopian government has expressed its commitment to improving maternal health and reducing maternal mortality by three-quarters (MDG5), by launching innovative health extension program (HEP) [10]. Since the government's introduction of this new health program in 2003, individual counseling about danger signs of obstetric complications and birth preparedness have been emphasized. Furthermore, those women identified as being "at risk" of a complicated birth can be advised to give birth at a healthcare facility or government hospital, having a health worker with midwifery skills, and this is now seen as one of the most critical interventions for making motherhood safer [11–13].

However, the majority of women in Ethiopia have poor status in society and lack decision-making power, a factor that can contribute significantly to adverse pregnancy outcomes [14]. Studies in Africa, particularly in Ethiopia, have found that husbands and other family members often make the decision about where a woman will deliver [15, 16], and although it is unlikely that men are actively ignoring the signs of complications during pregnancy and labor, it is possible that they lack awareness of what to look for, thereby hindering their ability to judge when emergency actions must be taken. If men are acting as gatekeepers to women's health, it is of paramount importance if they are able to recognize the danger signs of obstetric complications and be involved in birth preparedness practices [17]. The aim of this study therefore was to determine factors associated with men's awareness of danger signs of obstetric complications and its effect on men's involvement in birth preparedness practice at Chencha district of Gamo Gofa Zone, southern Ethiopia, 2014.

2. Method and Materials

2.1. Study Area and Period. The study was conducted in Chencha district of Gamo Gofa Zone of southern Ethiopia. It is located 562 Km southwest of the capital city of Ethiopia, Addis Ababa, and 295 Km southwest of the regional capital, Hawassa, with a total population of 137,196 and estimated women with child bearing age of 31,966. The district has 50 kebeles, five urban and 45 rural, with 27,999 households until the end of 2013. The district has one primary hospital, six health centers, and 50 health posts. The study was conducted from April to May 2014.

2.2. Study Design. Community based cross-sectional study was implemented.

2.3. Study Population. All adult males with a wife or partner who live in the selected kebeles and participants with a wife or partner who had been through childbirth in the preceding 36 months were study population and included in the study, respectively.

2.4. Sample Size and Sampling Procedures

2.4.1. Sample Size Determination. The required sample size was determined by using StatCalc program of the Epi Info version 7; five percent desired precision, 95% confidence level, 50% men awareness of danger signs of obstetric complications (due to absence of previous finding on men in Ethiopia), ten percent of nonresponse rate, and design effect of two were considered which resulted in 845 study participants.

2.4.2. Sampling Procedures. Two-stage cluster sampling technique was used to reach household level. The district was stratified into urban and rural area; then nine kebeles from urban and one kebele from rural area were selected by simple random sampling considering 20% minimum sample. Proportional to size allocation technique was used to allocate the sample, and kebeles were divided into different clusters based on "*Got*" (small-villages) and number of participants in each cluster was calculated. Based on the allocated sample size, K clusters were selected from each kebele and total participants in each cluster were asked until we reached the adequate sample from each kebele.

2.5. Data Collection. Data was collected by using face-to-face interview technique using pretested and structured questionnaires, and it includes sociodemographic characteristics, household characteristics, reproductive characteristics, men's awareness of danger signs of obstetric complications at three stages, and questions related with birth preparedness practices.

After three days of extensive training on basic skills of interview, ways of obtaining verbal consent, and objective of the study, nine B.S. nurses conducted home to home visit for data collection also supervised by four public health professionals.

2.6. Data Quality Assurances. To maintain the quality of data, data collectors were trained. Pretest was done on 43 individuals (5% of the study participants) out of the study area with similar population in order to assess the validity of the instrument. Definition of concepts and terms was made so that they harmonize with a local language of the district to avoid ambiguity. Supervisors underwent onsite supervision during data collection period and reviewed all filled questionnaires before the next morning of each data collection, so as to identify incomplete and incoherent responses. Data was cleaned by performing frequencies for all variables to check for incorrectly coded data.

2.7. Definition of Terms

> After childbirth: this is the period from expulsion of placenta to 6 weeks.
>
> Danger signs of obstetric complications: these are signs and symptoms of obstetric complications which occur during pregnancy and childbirth and immediately after delivery and are measured by the total number of correct spontaneous answers to 15 items on knowledge of danger signs during pregnancy, labor, and childbirth.
>
> Men involved in birth preparedness practice: they are the men involved at least in two BPP (a plan for skilled birth attendants, place of delivery, and arrangement of money for transport or other costs).
>
> Pregnancy: it is the period from conception to onset of labor.
>
> Vaginal bleeding: this is any vaginal bleeding irrespective of the amount during pregnancy and excessive vaginal bleeding or not the same as previous deliveries during labor and delivery.
>
> Knowledgeable/had awareness: this is a man who knew danger signs of obstetric complications more than mean average score during any of the three phases (pregnancy, childbirth, or postpartum period).
>
> Not knowledgeable/had no awareness: this is a man who knew danger signs of obstetric complications less than mean average score during the three phases.

2.8. Data Processing and Analysis. Each completed questionnaire was checked manually for completeness before data entry. The data was coded and entered into EPI Info version 7 and cleanup was made to check accuracy and consistency, and any error identified was corrected. Final data was exported to SPSS version 21 for further cleanup and analysis. Descriptive and summary statistics were carried out. Hosmer-Lemeshow goodness of fit test was used to check the assumption (P value = 0.71) of logistic regression model. Bivariable logistic regression analysis was used to identify the crude effect and variables that have P value of less than or equal to 0.2 were fitted to multiple logistic regression model to identify the presence and strength of association. Adjusted odds ratio with 95% CI was calculated to determine the presence and strength of association between the independent variables and men's awareness of danger signs. Hierarchical logistic regression model was fitted to know association between explanatory and outcome variables. Crude odds ratio and adjusted odds ratio with 95% CI were used to determine the presence and strength of association between men's awareness of danger signs and men's involvement in birth preparedness practices.

3. Results

3.1. Sociodemographic and Economic Characteristics. Total numbers of husbands/partners interviewed were 836 (98.9%). Among them, two hundred thirty-five (28.1%) of them had completed primary education, the majority of them were married (97.8%), almost all (97.8%) of them were Gamo by ethnicity, and five hundred eight (60.8%) were orthodox by religion. Regarding economic status, 20.3% (170) were found in the second wealth quintile and median and range of age of husbands were 35 and 48, respectively. The majorities (74.2%) of the wives were housewives by occupation and had not received any education (54.1%) (Table 1).

3.2. Reproductive Characteristics. The mean time taken to reach health facility for delivery services was 40.5 ± 34.9 min. More than three-fourths (93.1%) of the study households have two or more children. More than half (60.6%) of the households use local transportation/Kareza to take pregnant women in labor to health facility and almost all (96.3%) of the husbands knew where to go if labor occurs to their wives. Wives of four hundred ninety-seven (59.6%) husbands gave birth at home and 41.6% delivered at different public health facilities such as public hospitals (16.5%), public health centers (16.4%), and health posts (7.7%) in the past three years.

3.3. Men's Awareness of Obstetric Danger Signs during Pregnancy and Labor and after Childbirth. Three hundred thirty-six (42.2%), 95% CI (39%, 46%), men knew danger signs of obstetric complications which was measured by mean score at three stages (Figure 1).

The percentage of men who knew vaginal bleeding related to pregnancy was (34%), in relation to delivery (60.4%) and in relation to postpartum period (32.2%). Severe abdominal pain (87%) was the most recognized danger sign and water breaking/leaking before labor (1.2%) was the least mentioned danger sign during pregnancy. Severe vaginal bleeding was the most recognized danger sign during labor and childbirth and after delivery by 32.2% and 60.4%, respectively. Loss of consciousness was the least recognized danger sign during labor (13%) and after childbirth (2.8%).

Prolonged labor was known only by 21.4% of the husbands, while retained placenta was recognized by 19.7%.

3.4. Bivariable Logistic Regression Analysis

3.4.1. Sociodemographic and Economic Characteristics. Except marital status and religion, all other sociodemographic and economic characteristics were significantly associated with men's awareness of danger signs of obstetric complications on bivariable logistic regression analysis.

3.4.2. Association between Reproductive Characteristics and Men's Awareness of Obstetric Danger Signs. Good knowledge about place of delivery, time taken to reach health facility, and place of delivery such as public hospital, public health center, and health post were significant factors of men's awareness of danger signs of obstetric complications, but all other reproductive characteristics were not significant.

3.5. Multiple Logistic Regression Analysis. The independent variables, residence, paternal and maternal occupation,

TABLE 1: Sociodemographic and socioeconomic characteristics of household, husband, and wives at Chencha district, southern Ethiopia, 2014.

Variables	Frequency	%
Household characteristics		
Residence (place of living)		
Rural	610	73
Urban	226	27
Marital status		
Married	818	97.8
Widowed	7	0.8
Separated	11	1.3
Religion		
Protestant	326	39.0
Orthodox	508	60.8
Catholic	2	0.2
Wealth index quintile (economic status)		
Lowest	167	20.1
Second	170	20.3
Middle	164	19.6
Fourth	167	20.0
Highest	168	20.0
Involvements status in HDA (health development army)		
Leader	284	34.0
Member	351	42.0
Neither of the two	201	24.0
Husband/partner characteristics		
Age of husband		
≤19	5	0.6
20–29	192	22.9
30–39	370	44.2
40–49	231	27.6
50–59	39	4.7
Educational status of husbands		
No education	330	39.5
Primary education	235	28.1
Secondary education	151	18.1
Above secondary education	120	14.4
Occupational status of husband		
Farmer	355	42.5
Weaver	229	27.4
Merchant	64	7.7
Government employee	108	12.9
Private gainful work	49	5.9
Others (no specified job)	31	3.7

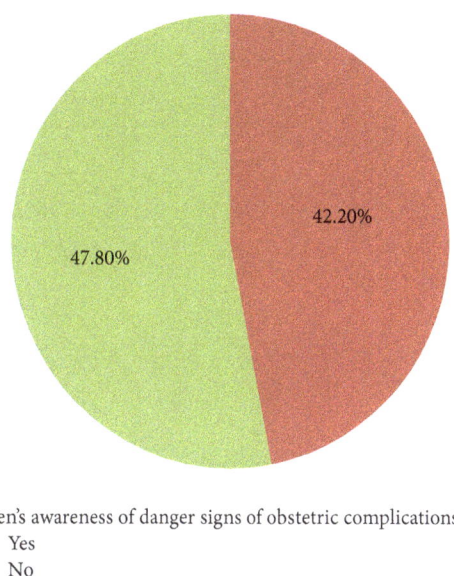

FIGURE 1: Men's awareness of danger signs of obstetric complications at Chencha district, southern Ethiopia, 2014.

associated with men awareness of danger signs of obstetric complications.

Accordingly, husbands who live in the rural area were 8.4 times [(AOR: 8.41; (95% CI: (4.99, 14.2)] more knowledgeable than urban husbands. Compared to wives whose occupation was housewife, women whose occupation was weaver had 6 times [(AOR: 5.94; (95% CI: (1.07, 33.0)] higher odd of being aware of danger sign. Husbands whose occupation is weaver also and government employee were 2 times [(AOR: 1.95; (95% CI: (1.24, 3.06)] and 4 times [(AOR: 3.75; (95% CI: (1.38, 10.2)] more knowledgeable than their farmer counterparts, respectively. Economic status was also significantly associated with men's awareness of danger signs of obstetric complications. Husbands in the highest wealth quintile (wealthiest) were 3 times [(AOR: 3.09; (95% CI: (1.51, 6.34)] more knowledgeable compared to the lowest wealth index quintile (poorest). Final household factor which has association with men's awareness of danger signs of obstetric complications was role in the health development army; thus husbands who did not involve themselves in the health development army were by 57% less [(AOR: 0.43; (95% CI: (0.26, 0.72)] knowledgeable than leaders of health development army.

Husbands whose wives gave birth in the hospital [(AOR: 2.09; (95% CI: (1.29, 3.37)], health center [(AOR: 1.99; (95% CI: (1.21, 3.28)], and health post [(AOR: 2.16; (95% CI: (1.06, 404)] were 2 times more aware than husbands whose wives gave birth at home.

Finally, households with one child were by 50% [(AOR: 0.50; (95% CI: (0.27, 0.93)] less aware of the danger signs than those who had two or more alive children (Table 2).

3.6. Male Involvements in Birth Preparedness Practices. The prevalence of men's involvements in birth preparedness practice was 9.4% (95% CI: 7.42, 11.4) (Figure 2).

wealth index, participation in the health development army, number of children, and place of delivery were factors

TABLE 2: Factors associated with men's awareness of danger signs of obstetric complications at Chencha district of southern Ethiopia, 2014.

Variables	Male awareness N (%)		COR (95% CI)	AOR (95% CI)
	Yes	No		
Household characteristics				
Residences				
Rural	296 (48.5)	314 (51.5)	4.38 (3.01, 6.39)	8.41 (4.99, 14.2)**
Urban	40 (17.7)	186 (82.3)	1	1
Wealth index quintile				
Lowest	106 (63.1)	62 (36.9)	1	1
Second	80 (47.1)	90 (52.9)	4.23 (2.56, 698)	1.83 (0.94, 3.57)
Middle	67 (40.9)	97 (59.1)	3.29 (1.98, 5.46)	1.53 (0.82, 2.86)
Fourth	54 (32.3)	113 (67.7)	2.27 (1.36, 3.81)	1.23 (0.67, 2.25)
Highest	29 (17.4)	138 (82.6)	8.14 (4.89, 13.5)	3.09 (1.51, 6.34)**
Role in health development army				
Leader	90 (31.7)	194 (68.3)	1	1
Member	151 (43.0)	200 (57.0)	1.63 (1.17, 2.26)	0.80 (0.52, 1.24)
Neither of the two	95 (47.7)	106 (53.3)	1.93 (1.33, 2.81)	0.43 (0.26, 0.72)
Husband characteristics				
Age of husband				
≤19	2 (40.0)	3 (60.0)	1.69 (0.25, 11.6)	—
20–29	67 (35.1)	124 (64.9)	1.38 (0.64, 2.94)	
30–39	176 (47.6)	194 (52.4)	2.31 (1.12, 4.78)	
40–49	80 (34.6)	151 (65.4)	1.35 (0.64–2.85)	
50–59	11 (28.2)	28 (71.8)	1	
Partner/wife characteristics				
Occupation status of wife				
Housewife	236 (38.0)	385 (62.0)	1	1
Farmer	13 (18.8)	56 (81.2)	0.38 (0.23, 0.71)	0.52 (0.24, 1.15)
Weaver	8 (80.0)	2 (20.0)	6.53 (1.37, 30.9)	5.94 (1.07, 33.0)*
Government employee	34 (66.7)	17 (33.3)	3.26 (1.78, 5.97)	1.11 (0.51, 2.43)
Others (private work)	45 (52.9)	40 (47.1)	1.85 (1.16, 2.89)	0.77 (0.41, 1.42)
Reproductive characteristics				
Number of alive children in the family				
≤1	29 (50.0)	29 (50.0)	1.54 (0.89, 2.62)	0.50 (0.27, 0.93)*
2 or more	307 (39.5)	471 (60.5)	1	1
Place of delivery				
Home	171 (34.4)	326 (65.6)	1	1
Public hospital	83 (60.1)	55 (39.9)	2.88 (1.95, 4.24)	2.09 (1.29, 3.37)*
Public health center	57 (41.6)	80 (58.4)	1.39 (0.92, 2.00)	1.99 (1.21, 3.28)*
Health post	25 (39.1)	39 (60.9)	1.22 (0.72, 2.09)	2.16 (1.06, 404)*

Note: *P* value: *<0.05; **<0.001.

3.7. Effect of Men's Awareness of Danger Signs of Obstetric Complications on Involvement in Birth Preparedness Practice. The results showed a clear association of men's awareness of danger signs of obstetric complications with male involvement in birth preparedness practice in the district. The effect remained statistically significant even after controlling for possible confounding of residence, wealth index, educational status, and occupational status of women. Thus husbands who had awareness of danger signs of obstetric complications were two times [(AOR: 1.91; (95% CI: (1.06, 3.41)] more likely involved in birth preparedness practice than respondents

who had no awareness of danger signs of obstetric complications (Table 3).

4. Discussion

Although researches have not previously assessed men's awareness of danger signs of obstetric complications and associated factors in Ethiopia, this study assumes that men potentially would have an equal understanding compared to women and based on this assumption, it utilized the study done in women to compare the findings. On top of this, we

TABLE 3: Association (odds ratio, 95% CI) between men's awareness of danger signs of obstetric complications and birth preparedness: hierarchical logistic regression analysis.

Male involvements in birth preparedness practice	Crude odds ratio	Model 1 (adjusted for residence)	Model 2 (adjusted for residence and wealth index)	Model 3 (adjusted for residence, wealth index, education, and occupational status)
Men's awareness				
Has awareness	1.79 (1.12, 2.8)	2.58 (1.54, 4.30)	2.26 (1.30, 3.92)	1.91 (1.07, 3.41)*
Has no awareness	1	1	1	1
Residences	—			
Rural		0.31 (0.19, 0.54)	0.31 (0.18, 0.54)	0.27 (0.15, 0.49)**
Urban		1	1	1
Wealth index quintile	—	—		
Lowest			0.12 (0.02, 0.99)	0.19 (0.23, 1.64)
Second			3.37 (1.55, 7.32)	4.38 (1.93, 9.92)**
Middle			5.29 (2.44, 11.5)	7.04 (3.01, 16.5)**
Fourth			0.86 (0.29, 2.49)	1.21 (0.39, 3.77)
Highest			1	1
Paternal education	—	—	—	
No education				0.77 (0.28, 2.13)
Primary education				1.71 (0.68, 4.28)
Secondary education				4.61 (1.91, 11.1)**
Above secondary education				1
Maternal occupation	—	—	—	
Housewife				1
Farmer				0.23 (0.061, 0.88)
Weaver				1.06 (0.10, 10.3)
Government employee				0.54 (0.14, 2.02)
Others (merchant)				0.79 (0.35, 1.78)

Note: P value: *<0.05; **<0.001.

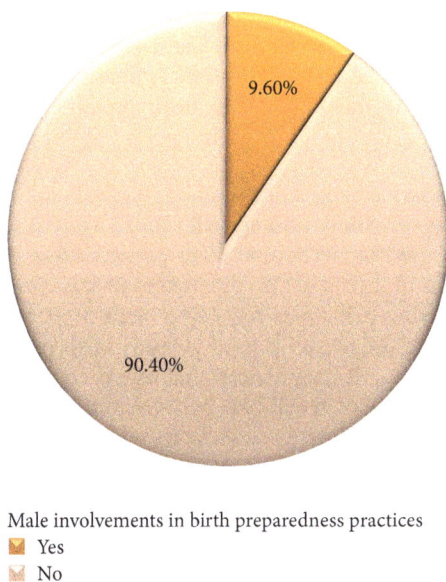

Male involvements in birth preparedness practices
- Yes
- No

FIGURE 2: Prevalence of male involvement in birth preparedness practices at Chencha district, southern Ethiopia, 2014.

used the study done among men in sub-Saharan Africa and other parts of the world.

The finding of this study revealed that the prevalence of men's awareness of danger signs of obstetric complications was 42.2% (95% CI (39%, 46%) which was assessed by mean score and this was lower than findings in the study done among men in rural area of Kenya and women in Tanzania [18, 19] and lower than the study conducted in Egypt, Alexandria, and the study done in Uganda among women [20, 21]. The lower awareness could be explained by poor counseling of danger signs among men and less involvement in health development army in urban area, since the majority of the study subjects in urban area lack good awareness. The higher awareness in rural area might be due to the Ethiopian government's emphasis on health extension program that made the majority of men aware of danger signs of obstetric complications [13, 22].

Residences, wealth index, number of children/parity, occupational status, role in health development army, and place of delivery were significantly associated with men's awareness of danger signs of obstetric complications.

Being a rural resident increased men's awareness of danger signs of obstetric complications; this was contradictory with the study done in Aleta-Wondo district of southern Ethiopia among women, where urban residents were more knowledgeable than rural ones [23]. The finding surprises investigators but this might be explained by standard health education offered by rural health extension worker and more involvement of rural men in maternal and child health packages in rural area by enrolling them in the health development army.

Economic statuses of households were significantly associated with men's awareness of danger signs. This was shown in the study done in Uganda [21], but the study done in Tigray region of Ethiopia [24] and Tanzania [19] showed that economic status was not associated with knowledge on danger signs of obstetric complications. This might be due to the fact that men with the highest economic status buy radio and other media to get more information about maternal health. In addition men with the highest economic status seek delivery service from health facility and are exposed to health education that is given in the health institution.

Moreover, wives occupation seems to influence the level of men's awareness about danger signs of obstetric complications. This could be explained by the fact that working women have better opportunity to share experiences with others and transfer those to husbands than housewives [20].

Place of delivery was significantly associated with men's awareness of danger signs of obstetric complications. Husbands whose wives gave birth in the health institutions (health center, hospital, and health post) were more knowledgeable than husbands whose wives gave birth at home. This is consistent with the study done in Tanzania [19], in which wives/partners who gave birth in the health institution have had more knowledge when compared with wives who gave birth at home. This may be explained by standard health education offered by healthcare professionals and health extension workers to women and they also transfer information to their husbands at home; in addition health extension workers in rural side involve more men during ANC forum and disseminate maternal and child health related packages which initiate men's involvement in the delivery services from health institution, which in turn open the way to get information from health facility [25].

Parity which was measured by number of children in this study was a significant factor associated with men's awareness. The finding was consistent with the study done in Egypt and Tanzania [19, 20]. This might be due to high antenatal coverage and relatively high frequency of visits among women of high parity which provides an excellent opportunity for information, education, and communication, and they in turn transfer it to their husbands [19, 26].

Husbands who did participate in health development army (HDA) had more awareness of danger signs, compared to husbands who did not participate in HDA; this might be due to the fact that the former ones are exposed to health education which is provided in different meeting with health professional and health extension worker; in addition, health development army members gather together

and discuss the reproductive issue with each other and health professionals, which in turn increases their awareness [25]. Finally educational status has no significant association with that of men's awareness; this might be due to masking of the effect of education due to rural health extension program achievements.

The magnitude of men's involvement in birth preparedness practices of 9.4% estimated in our study appears to be higher than what was reported from Kenya (7%) [27] but lower than ((20%–22%), 44.3%, and 48%) studies done in Ethiopia, Uganda, and India, respectively [28–31]. Low level of involvement in birth preparedness might be due to low level of economic status, in the district, which in turn hampers husbands' involvement in the birth preparedness practices, particularly involving themselves in saving money. In addition this study showed that males give due emphasis to food and cloth preparation for upcoming baby and mother than preparing for transportation and saving money; this might also be due to one-way ambulance service that has been provided freely for the laboring mother and delivery services in the health center [25].

The study also showed significant association between men's awareness of danger signs of obstetric complications and involvement in birth preparedness practice. Accordingly husbands who were aware of danger signs of obstetric complications were two times more likely involved in birth preparedness practice than husbands who had no awareness of danger signs. This was evidenced by the study done in Uganda in which women's awareness of danger signs predicts the level of birth preparedness practices [32]. This might be due to the assumption that knowledge of danger signs leads to greater anticipation and preparation to mitigate effects of pregnancy and childbirth complications by reducing the first two delays and the third delay if health facilities are prepared to address obstetric complications.

Furthermore educational status, economic status which was measured by wealth index quintile, and place of residence had significant effect on male involvements in birth preparedness practices, but occupational status has no significant effect on male involvement in birth preparedness practices.

Limitation and Strength of the Study. It is difficult, however, to compare our study findings with those from others as the measures used to determine birth preparedness had some variations and there are also differences in sex. Nevertheless, the underlying principles regarding birth preparedness are the same and the methods used to study birth preparedness were the same. It is possible that there may have been different degrees of recall bias between men who did have wife who gave birth before two years and within two years. This may introduce misclassification bias, resulting in positive/negative association. Confounding was controlled in the analysis by stepwise hierarchical logistic regression model. Possible confounders were introduced into the level and they did not have significant effect on the association between men's awareness of danger signs and involvement in birth preparedness practices.

5. Conclusion

Our study showed low levels of awareness of obstetric danger signs among men in Chencha district of southern Ethiopia. Since men are acting as gatekeepers to women's health, it is of paramount importance if they are able to recognize the danger signs of obstetric complications which in turn decrease one of the three delays. Residences, wealth index, number of children, occupational status, role in health development army, and place of delivery were important factors associated with men's awareness of danger signs. So the government and stakeholders should start innovative maternal health intervention to encourage institutional delivery and to discourage home delivery, and the Ministry of Health needs to review urban health extension program, to review the focus and include men in health education regarding danger signs of obstetric complications. The government and stakeholders should emphasize boosting household economic status and providing work opportunity that brings income for respondents. Health extension program especially urban HEP should focus on men health education to boost men's awareness of danger signs through involving them in the health development army.

Our study showed very low involvement in birth preparedness practice among men in Chencha district. The study also demonstrated strong association between men's awareness of dangers signs of obstetric complications and men's involvements in birth preparedness. It is of paramount importance if husbands are able to recognize the danger signs of obstetric complications which are an indication that urgent emergency care needs to be sought from skilled attendants and which in turn increase their involvement in birth preparedness practice.

Ethical Approval

Ethical clearance for the study was obtained from the Institutional Ethical Review Board (IRB) of the College of Medicine and Health Sciences, Arba Minch University, and a permission letter was taken from Chencha district health offices.

Consent

Informed oral consent was taken from individual participants. No form of identifiers was included in the questionnaires to maintain confidentiality. Participation was voluntary and participants were informed that they could withdraw from the study at any stage if they wanted, without any penalty.

Conflict of Interests

The authors declare that there is no conflict of interests.

Authors' Contribution

Alemu Tamiso Debiso was the primary researcher, envisioned the study, designed, participated in supervision and

quality assurances, conducted data analysis, and drafted and finalized the paper for publication. Behailu Merdekios Gello and Marelign Tilahun Malaju assisted in data collection and reviewed the initial and final drafts of the paper. Behailu Merdekios Gello and Marelign Tilahun Malaju read and approved the final paper.

Acknowledgments

The authors are very grateful to Chencha district health office, for its administrative and technical assistance. Arba Minch University deserves special acknowledgement for funding opportunity and data collectors and supervisors are acknowledged for their support in data collection and supervision.

References

[1] G. J. Hofmeyr, R. A. Haws, S. Bergström et al., "Obstetric care in low-resource settings: what, who, and how to overcome challenges to scale up?" *International Journal of Gynecology & Obstetrics*, vol. 107, supplement 1, pp. S21–S45, 2009.

[2] Central Statistical Agency [Ethiopia] and ICF International, *Ethiopia Demographic and Health Survey 2011*, ICF International, Calverton, Md, USA; Central Statistical Agency, Addis Ababa, Ethiopia, 2012.

[3] N. Gupta, "Maternal Mortality: magnitude causes and concerns," *Journal of Obstetrics and Gynaecology*, vol. 9, pp. 555–558, 2004.

[4] O. M. Campbell and W. J. Graham, "Strategies for reducing maternal mortality: getting on with what works," *The Lancet*, vol. 368, no. 9543, pp. 1284–1299, 2006.

[5] M. Drennan, *Reproductive Health: New Perspectives on Men's Participation*, vol. 46 of *Population Reports Series J*, Johns Hopkins University, Population Information Programme, Baltimore, Md, USA, 1998.

[6] R. C. Del Barco, *Monitoring Birth Preparedness and Complication Readiness. Tools and Indicators for Maternal and Newborn Health*, JHPIEGO, Baltimore, Md, USA, 2004.

[7] S. Babalola and A. Fatusi, "Determinants of use of maternal health services in Nigeria—looking beyond individual and household factors," *BMC Pregnancy and Childbirth*, vol. 9, article 43, 2009.

[8] Y. Berhan and A. Berhan, "Causes of maternal mortality in Ethiopia: a significant decline in abortion related death," *Ethiopian Journal of Health Sciences*, vol. 24, pp. 15–28, 2014.

[9] A. Abdella, "Maternal mortality trend in Ethiopia," *Ethiopian Journal of Health Development*, vol. 24, no. 1, pp. 115–122, 2010.

[10] A. Sebhatu, "The implementation of Ethiopia's Health Extension Program: an overview," 2012.

[11] A. Starrs, *The Safe Motherhood Action Agenda: Priorities for the Next Decade. Report on the Safe Motherhood Technical Consultation 18–23 October 1997 Colombo Sri Lanka*, Family Care International, New York, NY, USA, 1997.

[12] E. B. Keyes, A. Haile-Mariam, N. T. Belayneh et al., "Ethiopia's assessment of emergency obstetric and newborn care: setting the gold standard for national facility-based assessments," *International Journal of Gynecology & Obstetrics*, vol. 115, no. 1, pp. 94–100, 2011.

[13] J. Wilder, *Ethiopias Health Extension Program: Pathfinder Internationals Support 2003–2007*, Pathfinder International, Watertown, Mass, USA, 2008.

[14] B. Alemu and M. Asnake, *Women's Empowerment in Ethiopia: New Solutions to Ancient Problems*, Pathfinder International, 2007.

[15] A. Starrs, *The Safe Motherhood Action Agenda: Priorities for the Next Decade. Report on the Safe Motherhood Technical Consultation, 18–23 October 1997, Colombo, Sri Lanka*, Family Care International, New York, NY, USA, 1998.

[16] B. Evjen-Olsen, S. G. Hinderaker, R. T. Lie, P. Bergsjø, P. Gasheka, and G. Kvåle, "Risk factors for maternal death in the highlands of rural northern Tanzania: a case-control study," *BMC Public Health*, vol. 8, no. 1, article 52, 2008.

[17] M. N. Wegner, J. Ruminjo, E. Sinclair, L. Pesso, and M. Mehta, "Improving community knowledge of obstetric fistula prevention and treatment," *International Journal of Gynecology and Obstetrics*, vol. 99, supplement 1, pp. S108–S111, 2007.

[18] A. Dunn, S. Haque, and M. Innes, "Rural Kenyan Men's awareness of danger signs of obstetric complications," *Pan African Medical Journal*, vol. 10, no. 39, 2011.

[19] A. B. Pembe, D. P. Urassa, A. Carlstedt, G. Lindmark, L. Nyström, and E. Darj, "Rural Tanzanian women's awareness of danger signs of obstetric complications," *BMC Pregnancy and Childbirth*, vol. 9, no. 1, article 12, 2009.

[20] W. A. Rashad and R. M. Essa, "Women's awareness of danger signs of obstetrics complications," *Journal of American Science*, vol. 6, no. 10, pp. 1299–1306, 2010.

[21] J. K. Kabakyenga, P.-O. Östergren, E. Turyakira, and K. O. Pettersson, "Knowledge of obstetric danger signs and birth preparedness practices among women in rural Uganda," *Reproductive Health*, vol. 8, no. 1, article 33, 2011.

[22] A. Medhanyie, M. Spigt, Y. Kifle et al., "The role of health extension workers in improving utilization of maternal health services in rural areas in Ethiopia: a cross sectional study," *BMC Health Services Research*, vol. 12, no. 1, article 352, 2012.

[23] M. Hailu, A. Gebremariam, and F. Alemseged, "Knowledge about obstetric danger signs among pregnant women in Aleta Wondo district, Sidama Zone, Southern Ethiopia," *Ethiopian Journal of Health Sciences*, vol. 20, no. 1, 2011.

[24] D. Hailu and H. Berhe, "Knowledge about obstetric danger signs and associated factors among mothers in Tsegedie district, Tigray region, Ethiopia 2013: community based cross-sectional study," *PLoS ONE*, vol. 9, no. 2, Article ID e83459, 2014.

[25] FMOH, "Ethiopia five year Health Sector Development Program IV (2010/11–2014/15)," in *Maternal Health Services*, Federal Ministry of Health, Addis Ababa, Ethiopia, 2010.

[26] N. Regassa, "Antenatal and postnatal care service utilization in southern Ethiopia: a population-based study," *African Health Sciences*, vol. 11, no. 3, pp. 390–397, 2011.

[27] S. M. Mutiso, Z. Qureshi, and J. Kinuthia, "Birth preparedness among antenatal clients," *East African Medical Journal*, vol. 85, no. 6, pp. 275–283, 2008.

[28] M. Hailu, A. Gebremariam, F. Alemseged, and K. Deribe, "Birth preparedness and complication readiness among pregnant women in Southern Ethiopia," *PLoS ONE*, vol. 6, no. 6, Article ID e21432, 2011.

[29] M. Hiluf and M. Fantahun, "Birth preparedness and complication readiness among women in Adigrat town, north Ethiopia," *Ethiopian Journal of Health Development*, vol. 22, no. 1, pp. 14–20, 2008.

[30] S. Agarwal, V. Sethi, K. Srivastava, P. K. Jha, and A. H. Baqui, "Birth preparedness and complication readiness among slum women in Indore city, India," *Journal of Health, Population and Nutrition*, vol. 28, no. 4, pp. 383–391, 2010.

[31] O. Kakaire, D. K. Kaye, and M. O. Osinde, "Male involvement in birth preparedness and complication readiness for emergency obstetric referrals in rural Uganda," *Reproductive Health*, vol. 8, article 12, 7 pages, 2011.

[32] S. N. Mbalinda, A. Nakimuli, O. Kakaire, M. O. Osinde, N. Kakande, and D. K. Kaye, "Does knowledge of danger signs of pregnancy predict birth preparedness? A critique of the evidence from women admitted with pregnancy complications," *Health Research Policy and Systems*, vol. 12, no. 1, article 60, 2014.

8

Effect of Physical Activity on Blood Pressure Distribution among School Children

Anisa M. Durrani and Waseem Fatima

Department of Home Science, Aligarh Muslim University, India

Correspondence should be addressed to Anisa M. Durrani; anisamd@gmail.com

Academic Editor: Jennifer L. Freeman

The present study analyzed the relationship between physical activity and blood pressure in 701 school children aged 12–16 years (girls = 338, boys = 363). During the baseline examination, systolic blood pressure (SBP) and diastolic blood pressure (DBP), height, weight, and 24-hour recall of the working day activity with duration were recorded. Total activity score and type of activity were calculated by weighing the activity level. Mean, standard deviation, and correlation coefficient were calculated by using SPSS 12.0 version. The results revealed that rise in blood pressure was directly proportional to the increase in age. The range of systolic blood pressure was found to be high in low risk blood pressure (LBP) group than in elevated blood pressure (EBP) group showing direct association of activity level and systolic blood pressure. Physical activity score was found to be more in LBP group than in EBP group. Our results support the hypothesis that SBP is independently related to the level of habitual physical activity in children.

1. Introduction

There is a strong, continuous, and independent relationship between blood pressure and cardiovascular disease and all-cause mortality. Physical inactivity is strongly positively associated with hypertension, and intervention studies have demonstrated that increased physical activity is effective in the treatment of high blood pressure in a variety of populations [1]. Several studies have provided ample evidence that hypertension in adults has its onset in childhood which has caused growing concern with monitoring arterial BP in children in the last few decades [2]. Therefore, the trend in blood pressure in children with respect to increase in age may be important predictors of subsequent trend in adult hypertension. A number of physical activities and intervention studied performed in children and adolescents described the influence of physical activity pattern and blood pressure [3, 4]. Several studies have reported useful data on the benefits of exercise, health, and nutritional program in children [5, 6]. However, to the best of our knowledge, relationships between physical activity and hypertension have not been studied in Indian context.

Physical activity and health behavior are tracked into adulthood; thus, it is important to study blood pressure distribution among children in school and community setting for designing and implementing effective policy and program to promote physical activity in the young people. In the present study, the relationship of blood pressure and physical activity of school children has been studied.

2. Material and Methods

This cross-sectional study was conducted in city of Aligarh among school children aged 12–16 years. The total population of Aligarh in this age group was found to be 46.850 (Municipal Corporation of Aligarh, 2004-2005).

Considering 11.7% prevalence of hypertension among adolescence [7] and with 20% possible error, the sample size was calculated to be 755 by using the formula $N = 4pq/L^2$. A sample of 701 school children ranging in age 12–16 years participated in the study, with response rate of 92.84%. Four schools were selected based on the consent and active cooperation of the school authorities, by stratified random sampling by dividing the city into four specific zones on the geographical layout to ensure that the study was representative of whole city. Consent was obtained from parents of all the selected samples of school children.

The age was determined to the nearest birth date from the school registration record. Blood pressure measurements (BP) were taken with a mercury sphygmomanometer and stethoscope. The cuff used was adapted to the arm circumferences and was inflated to a level at which the distal arterial pulse was not palpable. Three consecutive readings of blood pressure after 5 minutes of rest at two minutes of interval were taken for both systolic blood pressure (SBP) and diastolic blood pressure (DBP) and their mean values were used in subsequent analysis. The measurements were taken by the researcher during the school hours, mostly in the morning in sitting position with the arm at the level of the heart, in a quiet isolated setting.

On the basis of these readings, 5th and 95th percentile were computed for each age group, genderwise for both systolic and diastolic blood pressure. Blood pressure ranging from 60 to 75 mmHg (DBP) and 76 to 100 mmHg (SBP), equal to or below 25th percentile, is considered for the low risk pressure group (LBP), and pressure range from 85 to 100 mmHg (DBP) and 120 to 140 mmHg (SBP), equal to or greater than 95th percentile, is considered for the high risk or elevated pressure group (EBP).

In the LBP group 81 (11.6%) adolescents were identified and in EBP group 66 (9.4%) adolescents were identified. From these adolescent populations an equal number of boys and girls from LBP and EBP group were selected from each age group. While comparing the EBP and LBP groups according to age and sex, the least number of five students was observed at the age of 12 years in girls. In order to reduce the influence of confounding variables in the two groups, the children were also matched with age, sex, and number for the purpose of comparing and evaluating the results between two pressure groups. A total number of 100 students were selected through purposive sampling method, comprising 50 boys and 50 girls. As only five girls were identified in the low mean pressure group (LBP) in 12-year age group, equal number of 5 boys and 5 girls from 12 to 16 years of age comprising 50 adolescents (25 boys and 25 girls) were selected in LBP group. The equal numbers of 50 adolescents (25 boys and 25 girls) constituted the elevated blood pressure (EBP) group, thereby matching the two pressure groups (LBP and EBP) with age, sex, and number. In the final sample of 100 adolescents, an in-depth study was carried out. The comprehensive data was collected through a validated questionnaire to find out physical activity pattern.

The 24-hour recall of the previous working day activities and their duration was recorded. Total activity score and the type of activity for the two groups (LBP and EBP) were also calculated by weighing the activity level in the following manner. Time spent in sleeping and in the very light activity categories was multiplied by a factor one, light activity by a factor two, moderate activity by three, and strenuous activity by a factor four. Physical activity score for total activity was calculated by summation of these scores. The collected data were stored in a database (Microsoft Excel 2003) and mean, standard deviation (SD), and correlation coefficient were calculated by using SPSS 12 to establish significance between the LBP and EBP adolescent. The results were seen at 5% level of significance and P value < 0.05 was considered to be statistically significant.

3. Results

A total of 701 school children between 12 and 16 years constituting 363 (51.78%) boys and 338 (48.21%) girls were included for the study. Table 1 presents the range of blood pressure (mmHg) in LBP and EBP groups. The range was more or less the same for diastolic blood pressure in both the LBP and EBP groups. In case of systolic blood pressure, the range was found to be more in LBP group than in EBP group without any significance. The percentile value of both systolic blood pressure (Figure 1) and diastolic blood pressure (Figure 2) revealed that the rise in blood pressure was directly proportional to the increase in the age and was found to be highly significant ($P < 0.05$).

The mean and standard deviation of one-day physical activity (hrs/day) and energy expenditure in LBP and EBP group are presented in Table 2. The total activity score of LBP and EBP group was 37.67 ± 4.4 and 35.41 ± 6.05, respectively, $P < 0.05$ level. Children of LBP did more moderate activity than EBP children and highly significant difference at $P < 0.001$ level was observed in the two pressure groups. However, no significant difference was found in time spent in sleeping, very light activity, and light and strenuous activity.

The physical activity correlate of blood pressure seen in Table 3 indicates a positive association of moderate activity and energy expenditure with diastolic blood pressure of boys in EBP group at $P < 0.05$ level. In LBP group, no association between physical activity and blood pressure was found in boys.

In EBP group, no association was found between physical activity and blood pressure among girls. But LBP group showed direct association of strenuous activity with diastolic blood pressure and it was found to be significant at ($P < 0.05$) level.

4. Discussion

The pathological processes associated with development of cardiovascular disease begin early in life. For example, elevated blood pressure (BP) can be seen in childhood and is tracked into adulthood. The relationship between physical activity (PA) and BP in adults is well established, but findings in children have been inconsistent with few studies.

Thakor et al., 2004, found that both SBP and DBP were significantly associated with outdoor playing taking the whole sample as one, but not in different sex or age group, except that the SBP was significantly correlated with outdoor playing in 10–13 years of age group in boys [8]. Hansen and Hyidebebrendt 1989 found an inverse correlation between blood pressure and physical fitness [9]. Klesges et al., 1990, found no consistent relationship between various childhood activity factors and cardiovascular risk factors, weight and blood pressure [10]. Jenner et al., 1992, reported that the

Table 1: Range of blood pressure (mmHg) in LBP and EBP groups.

Group	Diastolic blood pressure	Systolic blood pressure
LBP	60–75	76–100
EBP	85–100	120–140

Table 2: Mean and standard deviation of one-day physical activity (hrs/day) and energy expenditure in both boys and girls of LBP and EBP groups.

Physical activity (hrs)	LBP ($n = 50$)	EBP ($n = 50$)	Z
sleep	8.21 (1.22)	8.28 (1.15)	0.60
Very light	1.58 (1.1)	1.59 (1.27)	0.50
Light	22.46 (5.3)	21.72 (4.9)	0.080
Moderate	4.2 (3.3)	2.37 (2.57)	1.9**
Strenuous	1.15 (2.3)	1.63 (2.56)	0.60
Total activity score	37.67 (4.4)	35.41 (6.05)	1.4*

Figures in parenthesis indicate standard deviation.
*$P < 0.05$.
**$P < 0.001$.

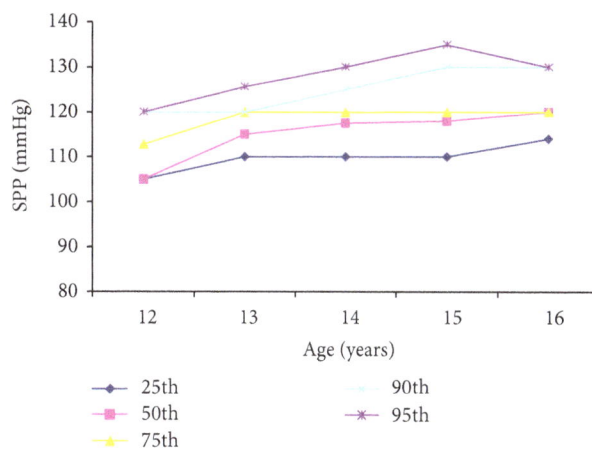

Figure 1: Percentile distribution of systolic blood pressure.

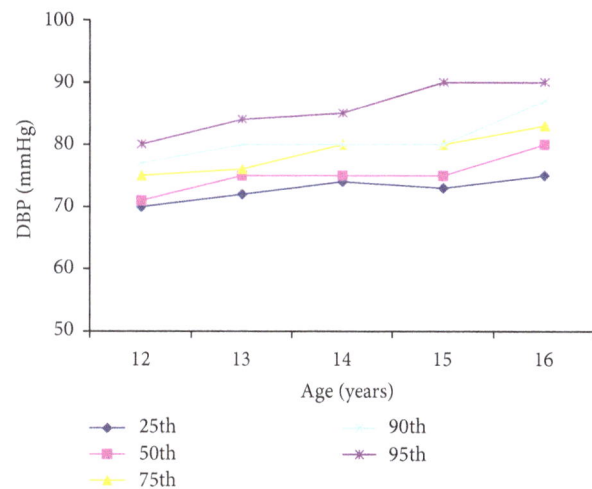

Figure 2: Percentile distribution of diastolic blood pressure.

number of physical active days per week was negatively correlated with DBP in girls, while relationship with SBP in girls and SBP and DBP in boys was nonsignificant [11].

Leary et al., 2008, concluded that higher levels of physical activity were associated with lower blood pressure, and results suggested that the volume of activity may be more important than the intensity [6]. In the present study also girls in LBP group showed significant association with physical activity and blood pressure.

The physical activity correlate of blood pressure indicates a positive association of moderate activity and energy expenditure with diastolic blood pressure of boys in EBP group at $P < 0.05$ level. But in comparison to girls, the boys in LBP group showed no association between physical activity and blood pressure.

A number of studies have emerged recently describing the influence of lifestyle interventions on various risk factors associated with high blood pressure in overweight and obese children and adolescence. The benefits of physical activity in the prevention and treatment of high blood pressure in adults have been very well described by Hagberg et al. and Whelton et al. [3, 12].

Regular physical activity and restriction of sedentary activity will improve efforts at weight management and may prevent an excess increase in blood pressure over time. A recent meta-analysis study of Kelley et al., which combined 12 randomized trials, for a total of 1266 children and adolescents, concluded that physical activity leads to a small but not statistically significant decrease in blood pressure. However, both regular physical activity and decreasing sedentary activities (such as watching television and playing video or electronic games) are important components of pediatric obesity treatment and prevention [13].

Public health approaches, such as reducing calories, saturated fat, and salt in processed foods and increasing community/school opportunities for physical activity, can achieve a downward shift in the distribution of a population's BP; thus potentially reducing morbidity, mortality, and the lifetime risk of an individual's becomes hypertensive.

When public health intervention strategies address the diversity of racial, ethnic, cultural, linguistic, religious, and social factors in the delivery of their services, the likelihood of their acceptance by the community increases. These public health approaches can provide an attractive opportunity to interrupt and prevent the continuing costly cycle of managing hypertension and its complications.

In conclusion, higher levels of PA were associated with lower BP, and results suggested that the volume of activity may be more important than the intensity.

Conflict of Interests

The authors declare that there is no conflict of interests regarding the publication of this paper.

TABLE 3: Correlation coefficient of blood pressure of LBP and EBP group in boys and girls by physical activity and energy expenditure.

| Physical activity | LBP ($n = 50$) | | | | EBP ($n = 50$) | | | |
| | DBP | | SBP | | DBP | | SBP | |
	Girls (25)	Boys (25)	Girls (25)	Boys (25)	Girls (25)	Boys (25)	Girls (25)	Boys (25)
Sleep	0.00	−0.17	0.21	−0.01	−0.01	−0.11	−0.30	−0.36
Very light	0.10	−0.07	−0.07	−0.39	−0.20	−0.14	−0.10	0.25
Light	−0.10	−0.02	−0.02	−0.22	−0.18	0.21	0.17	0.34
Moderate	−0.17	−0.16	0.04	−0.01	−0.01	0.42*	−0.08	0.27
Strenuous	0.48*	0.19	0.13	0.24	0.17	−0.09	−0.06	−0.30
Total activity score	−0.10	−0.05	0.09	0.30	−0.14	0.23	0.09	0.16

Figures in parenthesis indicate number of boys and girls.
*$P < 0.05$.

References

[1] J. Stamler, R. Stamler, and J. D. Neaton, "Blood pressure, systolic and diastolic, and cardiovascular risks: US population data," *Archives of Internal Medicine*, vol. 153, no. 5, pp. 598–615, 1993.

[2] N. J. Wareham, M.-Y. Wong, S. Hennings et al., "Quantifying the association between habitual energy expenditure and blood pressure," *International Journal of Epidemiology*, vol. 29, no. 4, pp. 655–660, 2000.

[3] S. P. Whelton, A. Chin, X. Xin, and J. He, "Effect of aerobic exercise on blood pressure: a meta-analysis of randomized, controlled trials," *Annals of Internal Medicine*, vol. 136, no. 7, pp. 493–503, 2002.

[4] G. A. Kelley and K. S. Kelley, "Aerobic exercise and resting blood pressure in women: a meta-analytic review of controlled clinical trials," *Journal of Women's Health and Gender-Based Medicine*, vol. 8, no. 6, pp. 787–803, 1999.

[5] G. A. Kelley, K. A. Kelley, and Z. Vu Tran, "Aerobic exercise and resting blood pressure: a meta-analytic review of randomized, controlled trials," *Preventive Cardiology*, vol. 4, no. 2, pp. 73–80, 2001.

[6] S. D. Leary, A. R. Ness, G. D. Smith et al., "Physical activity and blood pressure in childhood: findings from a population-based study," *Hypertension*, vol. 51, no. 1, pp. 92–98, 2008.

[7] S. L. Chadha, R. Tandon, S. Shekhawat, and N. Gopinath, "An epidemiological study of blood pressure in school children (5–14 years) in Delhi," *Indian Heart Journal*, vol. 51, no. 2, pp. 178–182, 1999.

[8] H. G. Thakor, P. Kumar, and V. K. Desai, "Effect of physical activity and mental activity on blood pressure," *The Indian Journal of Pediatrics*, vol. 71, no. 4, pp. 307–312, 2004.

[9] S. H. Hansen and M. Hyidebebrendt, "Familiar aggregation of BP in children," *Scandinavian Journal of Clinical and Laboratory Investigation*, vol. 49, pp. 55–57, 1989.

[10] R. C. Klesges, C. K. Haddock, and L. H. Eck, "A multimethod approach to the measurement of childhood physical activity and its relationship to blood pressure and body weight," *Journal of Pediatrics*, vol. 116, no. 6, pp. 888–893, 1990.

[11] D. A. Jenner, R. Vandongen, and L. J. Beilin, "Relationships between blood pressure and measures of dietary energy intake, physical fitness, and physical activity in Australian children aged 11-12 years," *Journal of Epidemiology and Community Health*, vol. 46, no. 2, pp. 108–113, 1992.

[12] J. M. Hagberg, J.-J. Park, and M. D. Brown, "The role of exercise training in the treatment of hypertension: an update," *Sports Medicine*, vol. 30, no. 3, pp. 193–206, 2000.

[13] G. A. Kelley, K. S. Kelley, and Z. V. Tran, "The effects of exercise on resting blood pressure in children and adolescents: a meta-analysis of randomized controlled trials," *Preventive Cardiology*, vol. 6, no. 1, pp. 8–16, 2003.

9

Assessment of Knowledge, Attitude, and Practice of Risky Sexual Behavior Leading to HIV and Sexually Transmitted Infections among Egyptian Substance Abusers: A Cross-Sectional Study

Atef Y. Bakhoum,[1] **Max O. Bachmann,**[1] **Ehab El Kharrat,**[2] **and Remon Talaat**[3]

[1] *Norwich Medical School, University of East Anglia, Norwich, UK*
[2] *Freedom Drugs and HIV Program, Cairo, Egypt*
[3] *Ipsos Healthcare, 35A Saray El Maadi Tower, Cairo, Egypt*

Correspondence should be addressed to Atef Y. Bakhoum; atefbakhoum@gmail.com

Academic Editor: Livio Pagano

Background. Rapidly growing youth population with changing sexual trend in Egypt raised HIV potential. The aim of this study is to assess knowledge, attitude, and practice regarding unsafe sexual behavior among Egyptian drug abusers. *Methods.* This cross-sectional study was conducted in 2008 in the Freedom Drugs and HIV Program on 410 drug abusers in Egypt. Included respondents were subanalyzed by gender, age, education, and intravenous drug usage. *Results.* KAP average scores on safe sexual behavior were low compared to the maximum possible denoting low awareness and action of drug addicts towards avoidance of infection. Respondents with higher education had significantly better knowledge about safe sexual behavior. Significant positive correlation was shown between age and knowledge of safe sexual behavior. Older age groups were predicted to know more about safe sex, while gender; educational level and intravenous drug usage were not. Similarly, females and intravenous drug users were predicted to have higher attitude for safe sex while age and educational level did not. *Conclusion.* KAP of safe sexual behavior were low among drug addicts in Egypt increasing potential towards infection with STDs including HIV. The more the age and education level, the better the knowledge towards safe sexual behavior.

1. Introduction

AIDS was first recognized in United States in summer of 1981, when the U.S. Centers for Disease Control and Prevention (CDC) reported the unexplained occurrence of *Pneumocystis carinii* pneumonia in five previously healthy homosexual men in Los Angeles and of kaposi sarcoma in 26 previously healthy homosexual men in New York and Los Angeles [1].

Since 2001, the number of people newly infected in the Middle East and North Africa has increased by more than 35% (from 27 000 to 37 000). Middle East and North Africa were the second most suffering region which experienced significant increases in mortality from AIDS. The limited HIV information available for the Middle East and North Africa indicates that approximately 300 000 (250 000–360 000) people were living with HIV in 2011 compared to 210 000 (170 000–270 000) in 2001 [2].

It was 1986 when the first AIDS case patient in Egypt was identified. Egypt was estimated to have 11,000 of PLWHA till the end of 2010, with adults 25–40 years being the majority, and male-female ratio of all detected cases was 4 : 1 (UNAIDS). According to the Bio-Behavioral Surveillance Survey (BBSS) in 2010 [3], Egypt had a low HIV prevalence <0.2% [4], with a concentrated epidemic among men having sex with men (MSM) and intravenous drug users in Cairo and Alexandria [5]. HIV prevalence in most-at-risk groups like MSM populations was estimated at 6.2% denoting that Egypt may be witnessing a concentrated epidemic among MSM [6].

As per the Egypt-NAP [4], by the end of 2011, there were 4,781 HIV reported cumulative cases (468 new cases detected in 2011 only). Since 1990 and to 2011, there has been a steady increase in the HIV detected cases; that is, number has increased from 1,040 cases (from 2001 to 2005) to 1,663 cases (from 2006 to 2009) yet, a population-based survey was never conducted.

Risk behaviors like unprotected sex, multipartnership, no or inconsistence use of condoms, and drug abuse are extremely determinants to health of adolescents and young adults putting them at high risk to HIV and other sexual transmitted infections (STIs) [7]. Wahdan et al. [8] had conducted a study on prevalence of condom use among people living with HIV/AIDS in Egypt that showed a prevalence of condom use of 45.0% in regular sexual relations while it was only 18.1% in casual relations. Another study in 2007 [9] conducted in the Nile delta among males aged 15–49 years also confirmed the low use of condoms where only 23.9% had ever been using condoms, and only a quarter reported knowing how to use condoms properly.

Egyptian MOHP [10, 11] reported that other factors participating in the rapid spread of HIV, for example, more liberal sexual attitude and behavior among the youth (sexual revolution), immigration, and travel, and increased intravenous drug use.

Before formulating public health policies for the prevention of HIV, it is critical to obtain information about the prevalent knowledge, attitude, and practice regarding HIV, other STIs, and sexuality in the target community. Few studies on KAP regarding HIV have been reported from Egypt to address the increased risk of HIV infection [8, 9] associated with acquisition of other STIs in addicts. Therefore, the aim of the study is to assess drug addicts' knowledge, attitudes, and practice regarding safe/unsafe sexual behavior risking their infection with HIV and other STIs. We also investigated the impact of age, gender, and educational level and intravenous drug usage on the respondents' KAP of sexual behavior.

2. Methods

2.1. Study Area and Design. A cross-sectional study was conducted back in summer and autumn, 2008, in the Freedom Drugs and HIV Program, in male and female addicts' treatment and rehabilitation facilities, which are scattered in 20 facilities all over Egypt. Estimated residents and outreached active addicts were 500–600 individuals at a cross section basis. These facilities provide peaceful place for recovery and allow for support if relapses happen.

2.2. Study Population and Sampling Procedure. There were a total of 500 drug addicts (injecting and noninjecting) in Freedom Program facilities during the study period distributed into the different recovery/treatment/rehabilitation facilities. All the program residents were invited to take part voluntarily where 90 cases were excluded from the major stage; *48 volunteers* consented to piloting of questionnaire before the major phase. The pilot phase revealed some careless approaches by the participating addicts resulting in some incomplete answers to the questions and so improvements in techniques were taken in the major phase to insure better gathering of completed answers.

Another *42 addicts* were excluded for various reasons, for example, due to uncooperativeness, inconsistency of data, or hugely missing of data.

A total of 410 addicts consented to take part in the major survey and completed the questionnaire. Study included males and females, young and old subjects, urban and rural inhabitants, different socioeconomic classes, and low and high education levels. The biggest number of participants was targeted for this study and so all the resident drug addicts in the facilities, who completed the study questionnaire to the maximum possible, were included in the study.

2.3. Data Collection. The study instrument was a self-administered questionnaire which comprised fourteen parts. Part-1 was related to respondents' personal sociodemographic background, Part-2 was on marriage and sexual partner, Part-3 was on sexual history (number and criteria of sexual partners), Part-4 was on sexual history with regular sexual partners (if any), Part-5 was on sexual history with CSWs (if any), Part-6 was on sexual history (irregular relationships), Part-7 was on condoms, Part-8 was on STIs, Part-9 was on HCV and HBV, Part-10 was on knowledge, attitude, practice, and health education to HIV, Part-11 was on knowledge, attitude, practice, and health education to hepatitis virus B and hepatitis virus C, Part-12 was on medical advice seeking-behavior, Part-13 was on sex education and gender issues, and Part-14 was on substance use/misuse and needle sharing behavior. This paper is discussing research findings of the first 7 parts of the survey.

The knowledge, attitude, and practice questionnaire was modified from the instrument used by a survey on HIV knowledge, attitude, and practice adopted from the FHI (Family Health International) questionnaire [6].

As for knowledge on sexual behavior, addicts were asked to respond to 112 statements about safe sexual (as included in the study questionnaire based on FHI questionnaire) behavior. Items were rated on a two-response options: 1: yes, 0: no in 99 statements, while in 13 statements items were rated on a 6-point rating scale (Likert): 0: not at all to 5: very much. Final scores ranged from 0 to 164, with high scores suggesting more positive knowledge or more information on safe sex.

As for attitude on sexual behavior, respondents were asked to respond to 95 statements about safe sex (as included in the study questionnaire based on FHI questionnaire). Items were rated on a two-response option: 1: yes, 0: no in 80 statements, while in 14 statements items were rated on a 6-point rating scale: 0: not at all to 5: very much, and in 1 statement items were rated on a 4-point rating scale: 0: nil to 3: severely. Final scores ranged from 0 to 153, with high scores suggesting less risky attitude to STIs infection.

As for safe sexual practice, participants were asked to respond to 20 statements about safe sex (as included in the study questionnaire based on FHI questionnaire). Items were rated on a two-response option: 1: yes, 0: no in 17 statements, while in three statements items were rated on a 4-point rating scale: 0: none to 3: each time. Final scores ranged from 0 to 26, with high scores suggesting less risky practices and protection from STIs.

Higher knowledge scores indicated correct answers to more questions about knowledge. Higher attitude and practice scores meant attitudes and practices that were more towards avoidance of infection.

The English questionnaire was translated into simple Arabic (colloquial) and back-translated into English. Questionnaire was pretested/piloted on a sample of respondents and the results were used to improve the phrasing of questions in the questionnaire.

However the lengthy study tool/questionnaire procedures were strictly taken to keep the highest quality standards in collecting the data from respondents/addicts. This is mainly was in the form of (1) logistically, offering the addicts refreshments during the survey and allowing them to smoke cigarettes to concentrate; (2) though it was a self-administered survey (except for the illiterate who needed to be interviewed and explained by a literate supervisor one-to-one), research facilitator(s), addicts' supervisors, and even the main study investigator (Dr. Atef Bakhoum) had been in the same room with the respondents while answering the questionnaire in order to keep more discipline, explain a hard question, rephrase it, complete the questionnaire with an impatient addict, or to allow an addict to withdraw and take back his signature on the consent form.

2.4. Data Management and Analysis. During data collection process, the data were checked for completeness and any incomplete or misfiled questions were checked with the respondents for correction. Data were analyzed using SPSS-17 statistical software (SPSS Inc. Chicago, 2010). Descriptive statistics were used to give a clear picture of background variables like age, sex, and other variables. The frequency distribution of both dependent and independent variables was worked out. The association between variables was measured and tested using Chi-square or Mann-Whitney test. Mann-Whitney was used in situations involving a categorical independent variable (IV) and an ordinal (rank) dependent variable (DV) while Chi-square was used in situations where both the IV and DV are categorical. t-test was used according to type of data. Spearman correlation was used to test the correlation between age and other variables while multivariate regression with odds ratio was used to get an idea on the prediction of KAP scores with age, sex, education, and intravenous drug usage status. P value < 0.05 was considered significant in all cases.

2.5. Ethical Consideration. Prior to data collection, all study participants were given complete introductory information on the nature of study (supervisors, researchers, and research facilitators). Informed consent forms for voluntary participation in the study with no intimidation or coercion and respect of withdrawal at any time or asking any query, plus proper considering of the participants' privacy, confidentiality, and anonymity, were distributed and had been signed by all participants. Introductory forms and signed informed consent forms were made in English and colloquial Arabic and are being saved in Norwich Medical School, University of East Anglia, UK.

3. Results

3.1. Demographics and Sexual History. 410 drug addicts participated voluntarily and completed the questionnaire in The Freedom Program's facilities. The mean age of respondents was 28.63 ± 6.27 years and ranged from 16 to 53 years. 361 (88%) were male. 278 (70%) had a college degree, university degree, or higher education. 203 (49.5%) were intravenous drug users.

165 (40.2%) respondents reported that they have ever been married (Table 1), with mean age at marriage of 24.81 years (range 14–38). However only 26% reported being currently married versus 64% who reported being currently unmarried but sexually active.

387 (94%) respondents reported that they have ever had sex, with mean age at first sexual experience of 17 years (range 6–31). 303 (78%) reported having sex during the past year. Their mean number of sexual partners during the past year was 2.5 of whom regular sex partners were an average of 1.4 and commercial sex workers were 0.85, that is, commercial sex workers constituting 1/3 of the sexual partners of respondents over the last year.

8.5% of those who had sex during the last year reported having sex with a person of the same sex, that is, 6.3% (26/410) of all respondents. 18 (4.3% of all respondents) reported having had anal sex during the past 12 months.

During sex with regular sexual partners in the past 12 months, 10 (3.3%) respondents reported using a condom each time, while 100 (33%) reported never using a condom (Table 2), with the commonest reasons being "because they did not like it," 57 (52.8%).

With a close focus on females compared to males, female addicts were significantly younger (mean age was 26.1 versus 28.9 years for males) and less likely to have ever been to school (less educated) (91.8% versus 97.2% of males) (P value (*chi square test*) < 0.05) where only 57% had college degree or university degree versus 71% of males. Females were statistically significant to be more likely to have been married, in general (67% versus 37% of males). Those who had been married, they married at younger ages (average of 19.02 years old) than men did (26.28 years old). (P value (t test) < 0.05).

3.2. Knowledge, Attitude, and Practice (KAP) of Safe Sexual Behavior. In order to identify the total knowledge, attitude, and practice scores of participants for safe sex, each respondent was asked to respond to number of statements about safe sex (as included in the study questionnaire based on FHI questionnaire) and then items were rated on a scoring system to get the final score, with high scores suggesting less risky practices and protection from STIs.

Respondents under the study had shown fair knowledge and attitude towards safe sex while they had poor practice as shown by the KAP scores stating higher knowledge scores than attitude and practice scores. In general, scores tended to be of low mean values (Table 3), compared to the maximum possible showing to what extent KAP of respondents towards safe sex was not up to the desirable standard. In order to better understand these scores, further analysis was done by gender (males versus females), education level (high versus

TABLE 1: Sample characteristics and sexual history.

Sex	
Male, *n* (%)	361 (88.0%)
Female, *n* (%)	49 (12.0%)
Age	
N	374
Mean (SD)	28.63 (6.27)
Min.–Max.	16–53
If ever gone to school, what is the highest qualification you have?	
Primary, *n* (%)	17 (4.3%)
Preparatory, *n* (%)	17 (4.3%)
Vocational, *n* (%)	38 (9.7%)
Secondary, *n* (%)	39 (9.9%)
College or institute, *n* (%)	48 (12.2%)
University or higher, *n* (%)	230 (58.5%)
No answer, *n* (%)	4 (1.0%)
Intravenous drug usage (IVDU)	
IVDUs, *n* (%)	203 (49.5%)
Non-IVDU, *n* (%)	207 (50.5%)
Have you ever been married?	
Yes, *n* (%)	165 (40.2%)
No, *n* (%)	239 (58.3%)
No answer, *n* (%)	6 (1.5%)
If married, how old were you when you first married?	
N	165
Mean (SD)	24.81 (5.0)
Min.–Max.	14–38
What describes your current marital/sexual activity status?	
Married and having sex with my wife/husband, *n* (%)	85 (20.7%)
Married and having sex with another woman/man, *n* (%)	14 (3.4%)
Married and not having sex with someone, *n* (%)	8 (2.0%)
Unmarried and having sex with a woman/man, *n* (%)	134 (32.7%)
Unmarried and not having sex with someone *n* (%)	129 (31.5%)
No answer, *n* (%)	40 (9.8%)
Have you ever had a sexual relationship before? (sex means vaginal or rectal sex)	
Yes, *n* (%)	387 (94.39%)
No, *n* (%)	22 (5.37%)
No answer, *n* (%)	1 (0.24%)
How old were you when you first had sex?	
N	297
Mean (SD)	16.89 (3.5)
Min.–Max.	6–31
Don't know, *n* (%)	70 (23.6%)
No answer, *n* (%)	20 (6.7%)
Have you had sex within the past 12 months?	
Yes, *n* (%)	303 (78.29%)
No, *n* (%)	67 (17.31%)
Don't know, *n* (%)	7 (1.81%)
No answer, *n* (%)	10 (2.58%)

TABLE 1: Continued.

In total, do you know how many were they in the past 12 months?	
N	202
Mean (SD)	2.5 (2.3)
Min.–Max.	0–24
Don't know, *n* (%)	65 (32.17%)
No answer	36 (17.82%)
In those past 12 months, how many of them were regular sex partners, for example, as your wife/girl friend or husband/boyfriend or anybody else without money for sex?	
N	204
Mean (SD)	1.4 (1.22)
Min.–Max.	0–9
1–3 regular partners	162 (79%)
4–6 regular partners	9 (4%)
7–9 regular partners	2 (1%)
Don't know, *n* (%)	31 (15%)
In those past 12 months how many of them were commercial sex workers?	
N	173
Mean (SD)	0.85 (1.83)
Min.–Max.	0–17
1–3 CSWs	115 (66%)
4–6 CSWs	21 (12%)
7–9 CSWs	1 (1%)
10 or more CSWs	3 (2%)
Don't know, *n* (%)	33 (19%)
In the past 12 months, how many of those irregular sex partners have you never lived with except with money for sex?	
N	171
Mean (SD)	1.22 (1.84)
Min.–Max.	0–12
Don't know, *n* (%)	47 (27.48%)
We talked about having sex with people from the other sex; now, have you ever had sex with a person of the same sex?	
Yes, *n* (%)	70 (18.08%)
No, *n* (%)	164 (42.37%)
No answer, *n* (%)	153 (39.53%)
Have you had sex with a person of your same sex, within the past 12 months?	
Yes, *n* (%)	26 (8.58%)
No, *n* (%)	91 (30.03%)
No answer, *n* (%)	186 (61.38%)
Have you had anal sex in the past 12 months?	
Yes, *n* (%)	18 (69.27%)
No, *n* (%)	5 (19.23%)
Don't know, *n* (%)	3 (11.53%)

TABLE 2: Condom usage.

In the past 12 months, how would you describe your practice for using condoms?	Each time, n (%)	10 (3.3%)
	Almost every time, n (%)	6 (2.0%)
	Sometimes, n (%)	39 (12.9%)
	Never, n (%)	100 (33.0%)
	Don't know, n (%)	2 (0.7%)
	No answer, n (%)	146 (48.2%)
Why didn't you use a condom this time?		
I don't like it	Yes, n (%)	57 (52.8%)
I didn't think of it	Yes, n (%)	38 (35.5%)
We used other contraceptive measures	Yes, n (%)	33 (31.1%)
I didn't think it was important	Yes, n (%)	28 (26.2%)
No answer	Yes, n (%)	17 (15.6%)
Other, mention	Yes, n (%)	14 (13.6%)
Partner refused	Yes, n (%)	5 (4.7%)
Don't know	Yes, n (%)	4 (3.8%)
Wasn't available	Yes, n (%)	1 (1.0%)

TABLE 3: KAP scores of sexual behavior in overall sample.

Cases	Safe sexual behavior		
	Knowledge	Attitude	Practice
Mean	70.1	54.3	3.7
Min.	0	0	0
Maximum	149	99	23
Poor	90 (22%)	64 (15.6%)	348 (84.9%)
Fair	278 (67.8%)	235 (57.3%)	55 (13.4%)
Good	42 (10.2%)	111 (27.1%)	7 (1.7%)

low education), and intravenous drug usage (injectors versus noninjectors) (Table 4).

No significant differences in the knowledge, attitude, and practice scores for sexual behavior were found between males and females or between Injectors and noninjectors; that is, gender and drug injection were not determining factors in KAP about safe sex (P value (*Mann Whitney test*) > 0.05). With regard to education, respondents with above university education had significantly higher scores for knowledge about safe sexual behavior than those with below university education (P value (*Mann Whitney test*) < 0.05). Other attitude and practice scores did not differ significantly with education level.

A significant (weak) positive correlation (*Spearman R coefficient* is 0.170) was shown between age and knowledge of safe sexual behavior (P value < 0.05); that is, the more the addicts grew older the more their proper knowledge about safe sexual behavior was. Still, getting older did not affect the attitude or practice towards safe sex (Table 5).

Trying to *associate* the KAP scores with gender, educational level, and intravenous drug usage (Table 6), females, higher education students were more likely to have higher knowledge than males, lower education students while non-injectors had higher practice scores than injectors (P value < 0.05).

Our study showed that 94–98% of respondents who participated in the survey had heard about STIs, HIV, HCV, and HBV.

4. Discussion

Generally speaking, average knowledge, attitude, and practice (KAP) scores were low denoting the low knowledge, attitude, and practice towards safe sex procedures/behavior. The total mean score of knowledge was 70.1 (range 0–149); attitude was 54.3 (range 0–99) while practice was 3.7 (range 0–23), among addicts. Our study showed no significant differences in the knowledge, attitude, and practice scores for sexual behavior between males and females; that is, the overall behavior status of participants was not statistically influenced by gender. In line with our findings there was a research in Ethiopia by Shiferaw et al. in 2011 [12], while in contrast to our findings, there was a study in India which indicated that good knowledge was observed in males compared to females [13]. This discrepancy might be due to cultural differences where females in India might have had more social restrictions than males of the same age, which was not observed in our study, leading to lower knowledge scores in females in their study compared to us.

With consideration to education, those with university degree (higher education level) had better knowledge on sexual behavior (mean rank of 229.526 versus 174.800) but their attitude and practice did not significantly differ from those with lower education level. Education might lead to better knowledge on safe sex. Our finding emphasised the need to improve the role of teachers in HIV awareness programs. This is important because educating school children about safe sex is one of the most crucial ways of postponing the onset of sexual activity among them [14]. Intervention programs providing sex education had been reported to result in a marked improvement in the knowledge of attendees about HIV and have been associated with a positive change in their attitude towards the disease [15].

This discrepancy between knowledge scores on one side and attitude and practice scores on the other side was not surprising; similar findings have been reported from developed countries [16].

Our results showed positive correlation between age and knowledge of safe sexual behavior which meant the more the addicts grew older the more their knowledge about safe sex was. Still knowledge was not translated into better attitude or practice.

Another interesting finding in our study was that 94–98% of respondents participated in the survey had heard about STIs (sexually transmitted infections), that is, HIV, HBV, and HCV. This was an encouraging finding which should further be strengthened by establishing educational seminars on HIV. It is very important to link this finding in addicts (and general population) minds with the safe sexual practices. People in Egypt should be aware that STIs including HIV, HBV, and HCV are very linked to poor sexual practices.

TABLE 4: KAP scores versus gender, education level, and IVDU (Mann-Whitney).

| | Mean rank for Mann Whitney | | Mann-Whitney test significance | | Mean rank for Mann Whitney | | Mann-Whitney test significance | | Mean rank for Mann Whitney | | Mann-Whitney test significance | |
	Male	Female	Z	P value	University and above	Below university	Z	P value	Injectors	Noninjectors	Z	P value
Knowledge	202.294	229.122	−0.64	0.522	229.526	174.800	−4.64	0.001*	209.249	201.751	−0.641	0.522
Attitude	204.130	215.592	−0.27	0.783	213.128	195.753	−1.47	0.141	203.888	207.112	−0.276	0.783
Practice	199.463	249.980	−1.15	0.248	201.678	210.383	−0.74	0.454	198.832	212.168	−1.155	0.248

*Means significant at <0.05.

TABLE 5: Correlation between age and knowledge, attitude, and practice to sexual practice scores.

	Age versus	
	Spearman R	P value
Knowledge (sexual practice)	0.170	0.001*
Attitude (sexual practice)	0.032	0.531
Practice (sexual practice)	−0.069	0.181

*Means significant at <0.05.

TABLE 6: KAP scores versus gender, education level, and IVDU.

	Average (SD) of knowledge	Average (SD) of attitude	Average (SD) of practice
Gender			
Female	74.97 (21.24)	56.16 (20.22)	5.22 (4.92)
Male	69.47 (26.46)	54.06 (20.28)	3.44 (4.22)
P value	**0.042***	**0.435**	**0.96**
Education			
Below university	63.71 (25.78)	52.64 (20.53)	3.89 (4.54)
University and above	75.15 (24.98)	55.62 (19.99)	3.47 (4.19)
P value	**0.045***	**0.301**	**0.678**
Injection			
IVDU	70.81 (25.54)	54.16 (19.73)	3.26 (3.94)
Non-IVDU	69.44 (26.37)	54.46 (20.81)	4.04 (4.69)
P value	**0.153**	**0.864**	**0.014***

*Means significant at <0.05.

Our study suggested that the education system needs to implement specific and focused educational programs for students in school prior to college admission and to promote health promotion. It is important that school students understand STIs (including HIV, HCV, and HBV) prevention, and transmission, as well as developing positive attitude and safe sex practice. The school is an appropriate place and time to have educational programs that address healthy sexual attitudes, for example, abstinence till marriage, delay onset of first sexual intercourse, and negotiate safer sexual practices.

Our study also suggested that more efforts need to be made to educate addicts in Egypt about safe sexual practices with consideration to its main correlation with HIV/AIDS and other STIs. Policy makers should be made aware that if this trend towards having more sexual partners continued, the potential for HIV to be spread through heterosexual sex will definitely increase. Condom use should be promoted, especially among the sexually active youth with multiple sexual partners, as well as studies conducted to introduce sex education to increase condom use [17, 18] as well as decrease sexual intercourse associated to alcohol or drugs [19].

Figures regarding the variety of sexual risky behaviors and the variety of factors involved in the performance of preventive sexual behaviors increase the importance of implementing programs and campaigns that aim specifically to change behaviors and promoting sexual and reproductive health [20, 21].

In order to fully understand an addict, one has to consider the individual family contexts where the addict interacts as well as the ways individuals organize sexual experiences. This means that the way addicts relate sexually to others is deeply influenced by family and social models.

5. Study Limitations

Our study was confronted by multiple limitations, for example, the sample was not random and so there might be a difficulty to generalize these results; however this can defended by the diversity of respondents included from 20 facilities nationwide in Egypt (males and females, young and old subjects, urban and rural inhabitants, different socioeconomic classes, and low and high education levels). Also among limitations is no inclusion of subjects outside rehabilitation centers and this is defended by the fact that some outreach addicts were included in the study. Also the study subjects were under rehabilitation; however these freedom facilities are for treatment as well as rehabilitation of addicts and hence some respondents were actually under treatment. Time and budget constraints were among the most important limitations in this study; in addition it is very difficult in a Muslim conservative country like Egypt to reach such a high number of addicts, MSMs (men having sex with men) and CSWs (commercial sex workers) unless you can reach them via specialized centers like the freedom facilities.

6. Conclusion and Recommendations

In our cross-sectional survey of drug addicts in the Freedom Drugs and Rehabilitation Program's facilities in Egypt, awareness/knowledge of STIs and HIV in relation to sexual behavior was better than attitude and practice. Older age groups and those with higher education tended to have better awareness/knowledge about these STIs.

Therefore, our study urges continued and strengthened drug rehabilitation and health education to bring a positive change in knowledge and hence attitude and practice, for safer sex to protect from threat of infection by STIs and HIV in Egypt.

Education might have played a major role in lowering the dissemination of HIV and other STIs.

Ethical Approval

This paper receives an ethical approval from the Freedom Program Prevention, Treatment and Rehabilitation of Drugs and AIDS Research Ethics Committee, Egypt.

Disclosure

Max O. Bachmann and Ehab El Kharrat are coauthors.

Conflict of Interests

The authors declare that there is no conflict of interests regarding the publication of this paper.

Acknowledgments

The authors acknowledge the Founder and President, Programs Heads, Sector Managers, Hostel Managers, and Supervisors in the Freedom Drugs and HIV Program for their kind efforts in facilitating a safe, organized, and quite environment to conduct this study. They also acknowledge the research facilitators for their efforts with observing and note-taking. They are also so grateful to the individuals who kindly volunteered to participate in this study and give their time, effort, and trust.

References

[1] A. S. Fauci, "The AIDS epidemic—considerations for the 21st century," *The New England Journal of Medicine*, vol. 341, no. 14, pp. 1046–1050, 1999.

[2] UNAIDS, *Report on the Global AIDS Epidemic*, UNAIDS, Geneva, Switzerland, 2012.

[3] Ministry of Health Egypt, *HIV/AIDS Biological and Behavioral Surveillance Survey: Summary Report*, National AIDS Programme, Cairo, Egypt, 2010.

[4] Egypt-NAP data, 2010 and 2011.

[5] UNGASS, GLOBAL AIDS Response Progress Report, 2012.

[6] HIV/AIDS Biological & Behavioral Surveillance Survey, Summary, National AIDS Program Egypt, 2006.

[7] G. Abebe and A. Fekadu, "A health concerns and challenges among high school adolescents," *Ethiopian Journal of Health Development*, vol. 10, no. 1, pp. 37–40, 2000.

[8] I. Wahdan, A. Wahdan, M. El Gueneidy, and I. Abd El Rahman, "Prevalence and determinants of condom utilization among people living with HIV/AIDS in Egypt," *Eastern Mediterranean Health Journal*, vol. 19, no. 12, 2013.

[9] I. A. Kabbash, N. M. El-Sayed, A. N. Al-Nawawy, I. K. Shady, and M. S. Abou Zeid, "Condom use among males (15–49 years) in lower Egypt: knowledge, attitudes and patterns of use," *Eastern Mediterranean Health Journal*, vol. 13, no. 6, pp. 1405–1416, 2007.

[10] "Ministry of Health and Population takes to the rails to promote awareness for HIV/AIDS," The Daily Star-Egypt Edition, December 2006.

[11] Egyptian Ministry of Health and Population, Bio-Behavioral Serveillance Surveys, 2007.

[12] Y. Shiferaw, A. Alemu, A. Girma et al., "Assessment of knowledge, attitude and risk behaviors towards HIV/AIDS and other sexual transmitted infection among preparatory students of Gondar town, north west Ethiopia," *BMC Research Notes*, vol. 4, article 505, 2011.

[13] S. S. Lal, R. S. Vasan, P. S. Sarma, and K. R. Thankappan, "Knowledge and attitude of college students in Kerala towards HIV/AIDS, sexually transmitted diseases and sexuality," *National Medical Journal of India*, vol. 13, no. 5, pp. 231–236, 2000.

[14] R. Short, "Teaching safe sex in school," *International Journal of Gynecology & Obstetrics*, vol. 63, supplement 1, pp. S147–S150, 1998.

[15] H. K. Agrawal, R. S. P. Rao, S. Chandrashekar, and J. B. S. Coulter, "Knowledge of and attitudes to HIV/AIDS of senior secondary school pupils and trainee teachers in Udupi District, Karnataka, India," *Annals of Tropical Paediatrics*, vol. 19, no. 2, pp. 143–149, 1999.

[16] N. E. MacDonald, G. A. Wells, W. A. Fisher et al., "High-risk STD/HIV behavior among college students," *The Journal of the American Medical Association*, vol. 263, no. 23, pp. 3155–3159, 1990.

[17] D. B. Kirby, B. A. Laris, and L. A. Rolleri, "Sex and HIV education programs: their impact on sexual behaviors of young people throughout the world," *Journal of Adolescent Health*, vol. 40, no. 3, pp. 206–217, 2007.

[18] T. E. Mueller, L. E. Gavin, and A. Kulkarni, "The association between sex education and youth's engagement in sexual intercourse, age at first intercourse, and birth control use at first sexual intercourse," *Journal of Adolescent Health*, vol. 42, no. 1, pp. 89–96, 2008.

[19] A. S. Madkour, T. Farhat, C. T. Halpern, E. Godeau, and S. N. Gabhainn, "Early adolescent sexual initiation as a problem behavior: a comparative study of five nations," *Journal of Adolescent Health*, vol. 47, no. 4, pp. 389–398, 2010.

[20] M. G. Matos, Ed., *Sexualidade, Segurança e SIDA*, Sexuality, Safetiness and AIDS, IHMT/FMH/FCT, Lisbon, Portugal, 2008.

[21] M. G. Matos, C. Simões, G. Tomé et al., "A Saúde dos Adolescentes Portugueses—Relatório do Estudo HBSC 2010," The Health of Portuguese Adolescents—HBSC Study Report, 2011, ACS/FMH/UTL/CMDT-UNL.

10

Sociodemographic Correlates of Choice of Health Care Services in Six Rural Communities in North Central Nigeria

Onyemocho Audu,[1] Ishaku Bako Ara,[1] Abdujalil Abdullahi Umar,[2] Victoria Nanben Omole,[3] and Solomon Avidime[4]

[1]Department of Epidemiology & Community Health, Benue State University, PMB 10 2119, Makurdi, Benue, Nigeria
[2]Department of Public Health, Ministry of Health, Katsina, Katsina State, Nigeria
[3]Department of Community Medicine, Kaduna State University, Kaduna, Nigeria
[4]Department of Obstetrics/Gynaecology, Ahmadu Bello University Teaching Hospital, Zaria, Kaduna State, Nigeria

Correspondence should be addressed to Onyemocho Audu; audeeony@yahoo.com

Academic Editor: Guang-Hui Dong

Household expenditure on health has increasingly remained a major source of health care financing in Nigeria despite the introduction of several social health scheme policies provided by the government for meeting the health care costs of patients. Recognizing these limitations, this study assessed the type of health care services people commonly use in various illnesses and the sociodemographic correlates of the preferred health care services by household heads in six rural communities of North Central Nigeria. A cross-sectional community-based descriptive study design was used to study 154 household heads in the settlements using a multistage sampling method. Multiple logistic regressions were performed to investigate independent predictors that had significant chi-square at $P < 0.05$. The leading causes of illness experienced by respondents were medical conditions (42.0%) and 41.7% of them sought treatment from patent medicine vendors. The dominant reasons for health-seeking preferences were financial access (53.7%) and proximity (48.6%). Age had a higher impact (Beta = 0.892) on the health-seeking preferences of the respondents as compared to their occupation and religion (Beta = 0.368 and −0.746, resp.). Therefore, in order to meet the health care of patients, it is pertinent that the unmet needs of patients are properly addressed by appropriate agencies.

1. Introduction

Health care embraces all the goods and services designed to promote health, including preventive, curative, and palliative interventions whether directed to individuals or populations [1]. It is, therefore, a necessity and a basic human need. Based on that recognition, the Alma-Ata declaration of the 1978 Primary Health Care (PHC) conference, endorsed by practically all governments, called for social and economic guarantees that would ensure that the basic health needs for all citizens of the world will be achieved by or before the year 2000 [2]. When the goal post of the Alma-Ata declaration was almost approaching, representatives from 189 countries met at the Millennium Summit in New York to adopt the Millennium Development Goals (MDGs). The MDGs just like the PHC declaration also place health at the heart of development

and represent commitment by governments throughout the world to reduce poverty and hunger, lack of education, and gender inequality and to tackle ill-health conditions [3]. Unfortunately, for most developing countries, the prospects of achieving even a minimal level of adequacy in health services and health remains a mirage. While health care needs are increasing, governments' expenditure on health in developing countries is declining [4].

Health care providers in Nigeria in the precolonial period were predominantly made up of traditional healers and diviners. In the colonial era there was a paradigm shift from the traditional health practice to orthodox and traditional medical services running concurrently. In these cases, orthodox medical services that were initially meant for the British Army were later extended to members of the colonial government and local populations living close to them. Various religious bodies later further established hospitals to supplement the efforts of the government and that continued until the postindependence era [5]. Now it is a concurrent responsibility of the three tiers of government (local, state, and national) in the country to provide orthodox medical care to the citizenry. However, because Nigeria operates a mixed economy, private providers of health care and tradomedical health practitioners still have a visible role to play in health care delivery as well [6]. Despite the existence of these public and private health services, Nigeria as a country has never been able to meet up with the international standards that have been set for the advancement of health over the years. Nigeria's poor health care system has been described as alarming by many authorities, and that calls for urgent attention from the government at all levels as well as medical practitioners [6, 7]. In 2011, Nigeria's health care system was ranked 51st out of 53 countries in Africa, as against the case in the 60s and 70s, when Nigeria was ranked 4th in the Commonwealth [8].

Various contributory factors have been identified at the individual level, communities, and societal levels. For instance, due to poor leadership and poor political commitment, the federal government still has a low health expenditure of about 1.5% to over 150 million Nigerians [9]. These coupled with the skewed distribution of public health facilities in the country left the rural areas with high disease morbidity and mortality. About 70% of the health facilities are situated in the urban areas, while 30% are in the rural areas. However, 70% of health-related conditions are found in the rural areas where poverty also abounds [6, 9]. At the individual level, poverty and ignorance remain as the most important determinants of ill-health as they contribute significantly to increasing exposure to disease-causing agents and also prevent access to health care services. Over 20 percent of foreign patients seeking medical attention in most developed countries are from Nigeria, but the majority of these patients are, of course, the well-to-do individuals in the society. The poor ones who are in the rural areas, who have issues of poverty to contend with, cannot afford medical bills outside the shores of Nigeria. Within the country, most hospital expenditures incurred by these same poor patients are made out of pocket [6–8, 10]. Other determinant factors reported by some scholars include the age of the patient, their occupation, the nature of illness they experienced, and the functional status of the health facilities which the patients visit (i.e., in terms of the attitude and skill of staff) [7, 9, 10].

Just like any other part of the country, Benue State is not exempted. Benue State Ministry of Health (BSMoH) Report of 2009 shows that Benue State with a projected population of 4,497,988 in 2008 had 368 registered medical doctors giving doctor-patient ratio of 1 : 12,222, while the number of registered nurses/midwives is 2,172 representing nurse-patient ratio of 1 : 2,071 [11]. This study, therefore, focused on the utilization of health care services in rural areas in Benue State, based on four conceptual predictions. The first is that the patient's utilization of health services largely depends on their socioeconomic status. The second factor is based on the assumption that the income of people greatly affects their choice of health care services [12]. Another dimension is the perception of illness and the availability of health facilities,

which may determine the use of health facilities [13]. Finally, the fourth dimension is the establishment of the association between the socioeconomic status of the household heads and their belief system which may influence their health-seeking preference for themselves, other adults, and young members of their families [14].

2. Materials and Methods

2.1. Study Location. The study was community-based, conducted in Apa Local Government Area (LGA) of Benue State from January through February 2012. Apa is one of the twenty-three LGAs in Benue State, North Central Nigeria. The Local Government Area was created in August 1991 by the then Military Head of State of Nigeria, General Ibrahim Badamosi Babangida, covering what was the old Ochekwu District of Otukpo LGA. The LGA is made up of 84 villages (settlements) divided into 11 political districts/wards. The major big villages in the LGA include Ugboko (the headquarters), Oiji, Ojantele, Akpete, Iga-Okpaya, Ikobi, Odugbo, Ofoke, Oba Alifeti, Idada, Edikwu-Icho, Ugbobi, Ebugodo, and Opaha. The LGA has an estimated population of 996,000 (2006 population census). The Local Government Area shares boundary with Agatu, Otukpo, and Gwer-West Local Government Areas of Benue State to its north, south, and east, respectively, while to its west, it is bordered by Ankpa and Omala Local Government Areas of Kogi State. The Local Government Area is blessed with abundant forest resources and is one of the main sources of timber to big towns like Otukpo. The Local Government Area is also known for its agricultural products with cassava, maize, yam, melon, and guinea-corn being the main farm produce. The people of the Local Government Area predominantly speak a dialect of Idoma language. There is a Comprehensive Health Care Centre located at Ugbokpo which serves as a referral health centre for the people of the LGA. In addition, there is a Primary Health Care (PHC) facility in each of the district headquarters providing health care services to the people. Other health care providers include formal private providers, informal private providers, patent medicine vendors, traditional healers, and faith healers [15].

2.2. Study Population and Design. A cross-sectional, community-based, descriptive study design was employed for the study. The study population was the household heads in all the settlements of the 11 districts/wards. The household heads who had experienced any disease episode in the three months prior to the survey were included while those who were not around at the time of the study and those who had never experienced any disease episode 3 months prior to the survey were excluded from the study. Those who did not consent were also excluded.

2.3. Sample Size Estimation. A minimum sample size of 138 households was arrived at using the formula (see [16])

$$n = \frac{Z^2 p (1 - p)}{d^2},$$ (1)

with assumption of 90% of the household heads in the community utilizing standard health care services from a previous study [17] and 5% tolerable margin of error at 95% confidence interval. Considering attrition rate of 10%, the calculated sample size was adjusted to 154.

2.4. Sampling Technique. The World Health Organization (WHO) multistage sampling techniques used for Lot Quality Assurance Sampling (LQAS) to assess Oral Polio Vaccine (OPV) coverage in Nigeria in 2011 were adopted for the survey. In the first stage, six wards (including the LGA headquarters) out of the 11 in the LGA were selected by convenience. The selection was based on the estimated population statistics obtained from the LGA head office before the commencement of the survey. The selected wards were more populated and had more households. Six villages from the selected wards were selected later using the probability proportionate to the population size (PPS) methodology. The selected settlements were then mapped and numbered. Twenty-nine (29) households were selected from Ugbokpo and twenty-five from each of the remaining settlements to arrive at the total minimum sample size of 154. A household is defined as people eating from a common pot. A compound may include many households. The first household was selected using a table of random numbers and the subsequent households were selected by systematic method. To ensure that the sample is spread across the settlement, once a household is selected, three households next to the surveyed one were excluded and the movement was maintained continuously to the right side. In situations where the research assistants arrived at the same house again, they turn to the left and continue sampling until the maximum for each of the settlements was obtained. Where there is more than one household in a compound, only one was selected by simple random sampling using a table of random numbers [18]. In situations where an eligible household head was absent, a repeat visit was conducted by research assistants for three consecutive times before a replacement would be considered. Such households were revisited at specified periods when they were probably assumed to be present.

2.5. Data Collection. The research was conducted through the administration of structured questionnaires to household heads in the settlement. The questionnaire was first prepared in English and then translated into the local language (Idoma) and then translated back to English to check for consistency and phrasing of difficult concepts. Trained research assistants were used to collect the data. Pretesting was conducted with 16 household heads (10% of estimated sample), at Akpete ward, about 20 km away from Ugboko (the headquarters). Questions causing difficulty in the pretest were rephrased and corrected. Information obtained was the type of health-related events experienced in the three months preceding the study, type of health services sought for, and the factors influencing their choice.

2.6. Measurement. The main outcome used in the study was the common disease conditions the household heads experienced in 3 months before the survey and the health-seeking preference. Any disease condition experienced is considered as an episode and an individual can have several morbid conditions simultaneously. Where two or more episodes occur simultaneously, the primary condition is considered as the disease condition experienced. Any disease in which no form of medical attention was sought for was not considered; thus, the relative frequency of occurrence of a disease experienced by a respondent was expressed per 154 (total). The disease conditions considered were grouped into medical, surgical, and psychiatric conditions.

2.7. Data Analysis. All analyses were conducted using the Statistical Package for Social Sciences (SPSS) version 20. The analysis deals with responses to four issues, the sociodemographic characteristics, the type of disease condition experienced, where health care was sought, and reasons for health-seeking preference. Data sorted were categorized, summarized, and presented in exploratory formats as frequency tables. Chi-square (χ^2) test was used for test of association between the sociodemographic variables and the main outcome of the study, with statistical significance set at P value of 0.05. Linear relationship between the predictor variable and the outcome (criterion variable) was further performed for selected independent predictors that have significant chi-square, using multiple logistic regression models by controlling for possible confounders.

3. Results

3.1. Sociodemographic Characteristics. The sociodemographic characteristics of the respondents as shown in Table 1 show that the respondents' ages ranged from 17 to 68 years with the mean age of 34.6 years (SD = 2.9). The majority of the household heads were male ($n = 133$, 86.4%). The predominant highest educational level attained is secondary (37.7%), while the occupation and the monthly income were farming (62.3%) and 1000–5000 naira (46.1%), respectively.

Tables 2 and 3 provide information on the types of disease conditions experienced in the three months before the survey and the reported choice of health-seeking preference. The table reveals that a very small proportion of the respondents (5.8%) experienced psychiatric disease conditions, while the majority (77.9%) experienced medical disease conditions, followed by surgical conditions (16.2%). Among the medical conditions, malaria predominates (20.0%) and the least was hemorrhoids (0.8%) which was described as pile. The majority of the cases in surgery categories were abnormal growths/tumors (28.0%), while in the psychiatry category depression predominates (44.4%). The overall picture across all the disease conditions shows a strong preference for modern health care except in psychiatric disease conditions, where traditional/spiritual healers health care (55.5%) is more preferred (Likelihood Ratio = 29.039; P value = 0.000). Of the total of 120 (77.9%) respondents who had medical conditions, the majority of them (41.7%) sought patent medicine vendors when they experienced illness, while 24 (20.0%) sought private health facilities. Twenty-one (17.55%) sought self-medication, 15 (12.5%) sought public health facilities, and less

TABLE 1: Sociodemographic characteristics of respondents (n = 154).

Characteristic	Frequency	Percent
Age group (years)		
<20	12	7.8
20–30	50	32.5
31–40	35	22.7
41–50	25	16.2
51–60	20	13.0
>60	12	7.8
Sex		
Male	133	86.4
Female	21	13.6
Religion		
Christian	119	77.3
Muslim	20	13.6
Traditionalist	15	9.7
Educational status		
None	25	16.2
Quranic	8	5.2
Primary	41	26.6
Secondary	58	37.7
Tertiary	22	14.3
Occupation		
Farming	96	62.3
Business	33	21.4
Civil service	25	16.2
Monthly income (in numbers)		
<1000	40	26.0
1000–5000	71	46.1
6000–10000	28	18.1
>10000	15	9.7

TABLE 2: Respondents' major causes of disease.

Disease conditions	Frequency	Percent
Medical		
Malaria	24	20.0
Typhoid	15	12.5
Respiratory tract infection	13	10.8
Genitourinary tract (UTI)	12	10.0
Hypertension	8	6.7
Skin rashes	8	6.7
Dysentery	6	5.0
Jaundice	6	5.0
HIV/AIDS	5	4.2
Tuberculosis	5	4.2
Peptic ulcer	4	3.3
Arthritis	4	3.3
Conjunctivitis	3	5.0
Cholera	3	2.5
Diabetes mellitus	3	2.5
Hemorrhoids (piles)	1	0.8
Total	**120**	**100.0**
Surgery		
Tumors	7	28.0
Abscess	5	20.0
Lacerations/cuts	4	16.0
Hernia	2	8.0
Caesarean section	2	8.0
Fibroid	2	8.0
Appendix	2	8.0
Ectopic	1	4.0
Total	**25**	**100.0**
Psychiatry		
Depression	4	44.4
Epilepsy	3	33.3
Irrational behaviour	1	11.1
Madness	1	11.1
Total	**9**	**100.0**

than one-third (8.3%) sought traditional medications. The majority of those that had surgical conditions sought private hospitals as their first point of contact (40.0%), while a small proportion (14.3%) of the respondents resorted to self-medication. The approximate median out-of-pocket expenditure on treatment per illness episode in medical, surgical, and psychiatric conditions was two hundred and twenty-five naira (₦225.00), five thousand naira (₦5000.00), and three hundred and fifty-five naira only (₦355.00), respectively.

Table 4 explores the reasons for health care seeking preference and it reveals that there is a statistical relationship between the health-seeking preference and the reasons for choosing a particular health care service (Likelihood Ratio = 76.720; df = 12; P value = 0.000). Amongst the reasons provided by the respondents, the cost of medication (42.2%) from the preferred health care service predominates, followed by the presumed skills of the staff (21.4%) and the proximity to the health facility (20.8%). The attitude of the staff (15.6%) constitutes the least reason.

Table 5 is a multivariate analysis of sociodemographic variables (predictors) to health-seeking preference (criterion variable). Using the enter method, a significant model emerged (F6, 147 = 52.677, P < 0.0005, and Adjusted R Square = 0.826). Significant variables are age, religion, and occupation. Age has higher impact (Beta = 0.892) on the health-seeking preference of the respondents as compared to their occupation and religion (Beta = 0.368 and −0.746, resp.). Monthly income, sex, and the educational level of the respondents do not have a significant impact on their health-seeking preference (P > 0.0005).

4. Discussion

In our study, the sociodemographic correlates of choice of health care facility visited by patients vary from one disease condition to the other. The sociodemographic characteristics of the respondents in this study resemble those of a typical agrarian community as the majority of the household heads are farmers with a monthly income structure of about 5,000

TABLE 3: Health-seeking preference by disease condition of respondents.

| Health-seeking preference | Disease condition | | | Total |
	Medical freq. (%)	Surgery freq. (%)	Psychiatry freq. (%)	
Self-medication	21 (17.5)	1 (4.0)	0 (0.0)	22 (14.3)
Patent medical store	50 (41.7)	5 (20.0)	0 (0.0)	55 (35.7)
Traditional/spiritual	10 (8.3)	4 (16.0)	5 (55.6)	19 (12.3)
Private	24 (20.0)	10 (40.0)	3 (33.3)	37 (24.0)
Public	15 (12.5)	5 (20.0)	1 (11.1)	21 (13.6)
Total	**120 (100.0)**	**25 (100.0)**	**9 (100.0)**	**154 (100.0)**
Median out-of-pocket expenditure per illness episode (₦)	**225 (3.90)**	**5200 (89.97)**	**355 (6.14)**	**5780 (100.0)**

Likelihood Ratio = 29.039; df = 8; P value = 0.000.

TABLE 4: Reasons by choice of type of health care services.

| Health-seeking preference | Reasons for health-seeking preference | | | | Total |
	Cost of medication	Proximity	Attitude of staff	Skill of staff	
Self-medication	15 (68.2)	0 (0.0)	0 (0.0)	7 (31.8)	22
Patent medical store	20 (36.4)	24 (43.6)	6 (10.9)	5 (9.1)	55
Traditional	5 (26.3)	0 (0.0)	10 (52.6)	4 (21.1)	19
Private	20 (54.1)	7 (18.9)	6 (16.2)	4 (10.8)	37
Public	5 (23.8)	1 (4.8)	2 (9.5)	13 (61.9)	21
Total	65 (42.2)	32 (20.8)	24 (15.6)	33 (21.4)	154

Likelihood Ratio = 76.720; df = 12; P value = 0.000.

TABLE 5: Multiple linear regression.

| Predictor variable | Dependent variable: health-seeking preference | |
	Beta	P value
Age (years)	0.892	$P < 0.0005$
Sex	0.106	$P = 0.033$
Religion	−0.746	$P < 0.0005$
Education level	0.099	$P = 0.091$
Monthly income	−0.003	$P = 0.979$
Occupation	0.368	$P = 0.003$

naira or less. When translated to international standards of living cost, it is less than one US dollar per day. By implication, the entire family's access to appropriate health care services can be impeded since the level of income of the household head greatly affects their choice of health care services [6–8, 11].

On health-seeking preferences among patients, this study displayed nonuniformity for the different disease conditions experienced by the respondents. While there is overwhelming reliance on patent medicine vendors by patients with medical conditions, those with surgical conditions had a relatively higher preference for private health practitioners. On the other hand, a patient that primarily presents with psychiatric health challenges had preference for traditional or spiritual homes as against other options of health care services (Table 3). There is consistency between the hypothetical reasons reported in literatures [12–14] and actual behaviours reported in this study. All these is suggesting that

information on health education and the appropriate course of action for the most common diseases, which is the focus of the health intervention, seems to have been influenced mainly by the socioeconomic status of individuals. A potential explanation may lie in the source of income of the household heads [6], low doctor to patient ratio [11], and recent spread of health posts and health extension workers in Nigeria [5, 6]. By implication, since there is a skewed distribution of health facilities and professional staff across the country [6, 11], the majority of out-of-pocket expenditure by patients in North Central Nigeria will commonly be wasted on ineffective or unnecessary products and services. Hence, going by the WHO standard of health care [19], there is a lot of improvement desired in this area of the health sector and even the health-seeking preferences of patients.

In terms of access to health service as a determining factor to the quality of care that patients may seek [12, 14], our study identifies cost of medication, proximity to health facility, and attitude of staff as being among the major determinants of patients' preference for the different types of health care options available in the rural areas of North Central Nigeria (Table 4). In this study, there is a significant statistical relationship between the costs of medication and the health-seeking preference displayed in all the disease conditions examined (Likelihood Ratio = 76.720; df = 12; P value = 0.000). The direct implication is that increasing user charges decreases the likelihood of seeking health care from the formal health provider relative to self-treatment and patent medicine vendor. Our findings are consistent with those reported in other studies where user fees were reported to be a key factor determining health-seeking behavior of sick individuals [20, 21]. However, this contradicts the findings by Schwartz et al. and Akin et al. who found user fees to be insignificant determinants of choice of health care providers in the Philippines [22] and Nigeria [23], respectively.

This study also demonstrates the influence of distance on health-seeking preference. Increasing the distance would increase the likelihood of a patient opting for informal health care providers rather than any of the formal health care providers. This negative impact of proximity of patient to health facility is higher at the patent medicine vendor (43.6%), followed by private health facility. These findings are comparable to findings in a research carried out in Kenya [20, 24] and the Philippines [22]. The effect of the distance in this study can be explained by the extra monetary cost which distance adds to the total cost of treatment. Looking at the average out-of-pocket expenditure on treatment per illness episode in this study (Table 3), if those who visit private or public health facilities have already made a decision to spend extra money on treatment, the impact of distance on the choice probability for their health-seeking preference should not affect their choice substantially. However, assuming that visiting private or public facility is driven by low user fees, holding other factors constant, an increase in distance is synonymous with increasing price (i.e., through travel cost) and has the effect of lowering the probability of visiting such a facility. In the final analysis, the patient may seek options like the patent medicine vendors which may even carry the drugs to the patient's door post. However, the findings in this study differ from those reported in Benin Republic by Bolduc et al. who used travel time as an indicator of access to medical care and found it to be implausibly positively correlated with the probability of seeking health care at both public and private facilities [25].

Regarding the attitude and skill of the health providers, our study shows that the attitude of the staff (52.6%) increases the likelihood of patients opting for traditional health care providers, while the presumptive negative perception of the skill of the practitioner by the patient made most of the patients settle for self-medication (31.8%). The implication of this is that the patients may build more trust in traditional health providers and themselves in the event of any illness or injury relative to going for modern treatment. This could be explained by the sociodemographic characteristics of the respondents. Being from an agrarian community, the patients' perspectives on the services they receive could be shaped by their cultural values, previous experiences, perceptions of the role of the health system, and interactions with providers; and all these in many ways affect how clients view the risks and benefits of care.

In the multivariate analysis carried out in our study, the effect of age and religion on the demand for health care is significant and positive across all the health facilities indicating that the probability of using professional health care service relative to self-treatment increases with age ($P < 0.0005$) and the type of religion practiced by the individual ($P < 0.0005$). This finding could be confounded by other variables such as educational level ($P = 0.091$) and monthly income ($P = 0.979$) which are likely to increase with age. The result is in line with the fact that the households headed by older people have a higher propensity of seeking professional health care rather than self-medicate. This to a large extent implies that the head of the household still controls economic resources even in a rural area [6, 26].

5. Conclusion

The leading causes of illness experienced by respondents were medical conditions and the majority of them sought treatment from patent medicine vendors while those who experienced surgical cases predominantly sought private health facilities and those who had psychiatric cases often sought traditional medications. The overall median out-of-pocket expenditure on treatment per illness episode was one thousand nine hundred and twenty-six naira and sixty-seven kobo (₦1926.67) only. The dominant determining sociodemographic variables were age and religion of the patients and the financial access and proximity of the health facility. Hence, in order to meet the health care needs of patients, it is pertinent that the unmet needs of patients are properly addressed by appropriate agencies.

Limitations of the Study

Since the inclusion was based on past experience of disease episodes 3 months prior to the survey, there could be recall bias which must have missed some important subjects which could have provided very useful information. Courtesy bias may be a significant limitation to this study. The interviewed subjects may have been reluctant to disclose use of traditional healers and traditional medicine as they may tend to be in hospitalized cohorts.

Ethical Approval

Ethical approval for the study was obtained from the ethical committee of Benue University Teaching Hospital, Makurdi, before the study was conducted. An informed written consent was also obtained from Apa LGA Council Chairman and the entire selected village heads. Verbal consent of the respondents was also sought.

Conflict of Interests

The authors declare that there is no conflict of interests regarding the publication of this paper.

References

[1] K. Park, "Concept of health and disease," in *Parks Textbook of Preventive and Social Medicine*, pp. 12–46, M/s Banarsidas, 18th edition, 2005.

[2] "Primary health care: Report of the International Conference No1. Primary Health Care, Alma-Ata, USSR, September, 1978," jointly sponsored by the World Health Organization and the United Nations Children's Fund. Geneva, World Health Organization, 1978 (Health for All Series No. 1).

[3] United Nations Development Group, "The Millennium Declaration and the MDGs," 2001, http://www.un.org/millenniumgoals/bkgd.shtml.

[4] WHO, *Progress in Achieving the MDGs in Africa*, 2013, http://www.uneca.org/sites/default/files/document_files/report-on-progress-in-achieving-the-mdgs-in-africa.pdf.

[5] E. O. A. Nwaha, "Concepts and constraints of health care administration in Nigeria," in *Proceedings of Seminar by Continuing Medical Education Programme Ahmadu Bello University Zaria*, pp. 5–10, 1997.

[6] O. Akin, "Health care resources," in *Nigeria: Situation and Prospects*, pp. 1–5, Com-Heal Nigeria, Lagos, Nigeria, 1st edition, 2005.

[7] WHO, African Region: Nigerian Statistics Summary, 2002–2012, http://www.who.int/country/nga/en.

[8] Vanguard news, on October 16, 2012: Mo Ibrahim 2012 Index of African Governance report, 2012, http://www.vanguardngr.com/2012/10/mo-ibrahim-2012-index-of-african-governance-repor.

[9] Y. A. Arigbede, R. O. Yusuf, and K. Lawal, "Population growth, access to health-care services and health-seeking behaviours in zaria , kaduna state," in *Proceedings of the 54th Annual Conference of the Association of Nigerian Geographers*, Kano State University of Science and Technology, Wudil, Nigeria, September 2012.

[10] B. L. Ajibade, P. O. Amoo, M. A. Adeleke, G. O. Oyadiran, O. A. Kolade, and R. O. Olagunju, "Determinants of mothers health seeking behaviour for their children in a Nigerian teaching hospital," *Journal of Nursing and Health Science*, vol. 1, no. 6, pp. 9–16, 2013.

[11] BENUE State Ministry of Health (BSMoH), *Benue State Strategic Health Development Plan, 2010–2015*, 2012.

[12] O. Otit and W. Ogiomwo, *An Introduction to Sociological Studies*, Heinemann Educational Books, Ibadan, Nigeria, 1996.

[13] W. S. Tile, *Medical Sociology and Social Works: Evolving Professions for a Human Society*, Enugu Vougasen, 1999.

[14] T. Ruijter, *Cultural Dynamics in Developing Process*, UNESCO Publishing/Netherlands Commission for UNESCO, Paris, France, 1995.

[15] Wikipedia, "The free encyclopedia. Apa Nigeria," 2011, http://en.wikipedia.org/wiki/APA#Apa_.28without_caps.29.

[16] I. Taofeek, *Research Methodology and Dissertation Writing for Health and Allied Health Professionals*, Cress Global Link limited Publishers, Abuja, Nigeria, 1st edition, 2009.

[17] M. Kamatenesi-Mugisha and H. Oryem-Origa, "Traditional herbal remedies used in the management of sexual impotence and erectile dysfunction in Western Uganda," *African Health Sciences*, vol. 5, no. 1, pp. 40–49, 2005.

[18] WHO, *Lot Quality Assurance Sampling (LQAS) to Asses OPV Coverage Nigeria, Operational Manual*, 2012.

[19] A. L. Fitzpatrick, N. R. Powe, L. S. Cooper, D. G. Ives, J. A. Robbins, and E. Enright, "Barriers to health care access among the elderly and who perceives them," *American Journal of Public Health*, vol. 94, no. 10, pp. 1788–1794, 2004.

[20] G. Mwabu, M. Ainsworth, and A. Nyamete, "Quality of medical care and choice of medical treatment in Kenya: an empirical analysis," *Journal of Human Resources*, vol. 28, no. 4, pp. 838–862, 1993.

[21] A. Cisse, "Analysis of health care utilization in Cote d'Ivoire," Final Report, AERC, 2006.

[22] J. B. Schwartz, J. S. Akin, and B. M. Popkin, "Price and income elasticities of demand for modern health care: the case of infant delivery in the philippines," *World Bank Economic Review*, vol. 2, no. 1, pp. 49–76, 1988.

[23] J. S. Akin, D. K. Guilkey, and E. H. Denton, "Quality of services and demand for health care in Nigeria: a multinomial probit estimation," *Social Science and Medicine*, vol. 40, no. 11, pp. 1527–1537, 1995.

[24] K. M. Moses, "The determinants of health-seeking behavior in a Nairobi Slum, Kenya," *European Scientific Journal*, vol. 9, no. 8, pp. 151–164, 2013.

[25] D. Bolduc, G. Lacroix, and C. Muller, "The choice of medical providers in rural Benin: a comparison of discrete choice models," *Journal of Health Economics*, vol. 15, no. 4, pp. 477–498, 1996.

[26] D. E. Sahn, S. D. Younger, and G. Genicot, "The demand for health care services in rural Tanzania," *Oxford Bulletin of Economics and Statistics*, vol. 65, no. 2, pp. 241–259, 2003.

11

Changing Smoking Behavior of Staff at Dr. Zainoel Abidin Provincial General Hospital, Banda Aceh

Said Usman,[1] **Soekidjo Notoadmodjo,**[2] **Kintoko Rochadi,**[1] **and Fikarwin Zuska**[1]

[1]*Faculty of Public Health, University of North Sumatra, Medan 20155, Indonesia*
[2]*Indonesia Respati University, Jakarta 13890, Indonesia*

Correspondence should be addressed to Said Usman; saidusmanmkes@yahoo.co.id

Academic Editor: Jennifer L. Freeman

Smoking tobacco is a habit of individuals. Determinants of smoking behavior are multiple factors both within the individual and in the social environment around the individual. Staff smoking has been an undesirable phenomenon at Dr. Zainoel Abidin Provincial General Hospital in Banda Aceh. Health promotion efforts are a strategy that has resulted in behavioral changes with reductions in smoking by staff. This action research was designed to analyze changes in smoking behavior of hospital staff. The sample for this research was all 152 male staff who were smokers. The results of this research showed that Health Promotion Interventions (HPI) consisting of personal empowerment plus social support and advocacy to improve employee knowledge and attitudes influenced staff to stop or to significantly. HPI employed included counseling programs, distribution of antismoking leaflets, putting up antismoking posters, and installation of no smoking signs. These HPI proved effective to increase knowledge and create a positive attitude to nonsmoking that resulted in major reductions in smoking by staff when offsite and complete cessation of smoking whilst in the hospital. Continuous evaluation, monitoring, and strengthening of policies banning smoking should be maintained in all hospitals.

1. Introduction

1.1. Background. Human behavior is a reflection of various psychological tendencies that are based on stimuli from outside, both intentional and unintentional, having either positive responses or negative responses. Behavior has three domains that can be measured, namely, knowledge, attitudes, and practices. Knowledge and attitudes are passive responses, whereas practice is an active response.

Health behavior is a form of stimulus that is related to health and sickness. One form of unhealthy behavior is smoking tobacco or cigarettes. As described in Act number 36 of 2009, health is a state of health, including physical, mental, spiritual, and social health which allows everyone to live productively in a social and economic way. Smoking is an individual and/or group behavior which is injurious to the health of the smoker and also to the health of others through secondary smoking so that the individual who smokes can be categorized as unhealthy.

Cigarette smoking is a form of behavior that is a manifestation of specific needs that can be satisfied when a person smokes. Smoking behavior is the action of a person who sucks tobacco smoke into their own mouth and lungs. Smoking behaviour can be observed or measured by looking at the volume or frequency of smoking of that person [1].

In epidemiology, smoking tobacco, especially from cigarettes, is a worldwide health problem. The World Health Organization (WHO) predicts that by 2020 tobacco-related disease will be one of the world's major health problems and will cause approximately 8.4 million deaths every year. The incidence of men smoking in countries with low to middle incomes is very high, that is, 39% as compared to 35% for men in countries with middle to high incomes. Another health fact is that on average smokers die 13 to 14 years sooner than nonsmokers. Smoking results in macroeconomic losses. In Indonesia smokers smoke 230 billion cigarettes per year costing US$14 billion per year; moreover, the medical costs or losses due to smoking, in Indonesia alone, amounted to

US$185 million per year (WHO, 2011) which is 12 (twelve) times greater than the cost of the cigarettes themselves.

Smoking can cause harm to health because smoke from a tobacco cigarette contains over 7,000 chemicals, many of which are very dangerous to health, including many which can cause cancer especially the three main components of the smoke, namely, nicotine, tar, and carbon monoxide. In 2012, the WHO stated that smoking is a cause of cancer, heart disease, strokes, and lung diseases (including bronchitis, emphysema, and chronic pulmonary obstruction [CPO]).

Various studies have proven that smoking is extremely harmful to health. According to McEwen et al. [2], the leading causes of death associated with smoking are cancer, cardiovascular disease, and pulmonary diseases like bronchitis, emphysema, that is, CPOD and pneumonia. Research at Sanglah General Hospital in Denpasar, Bali, showed that, amongst patients who sought treatment for pulmonary diseases, 71% of the patients who sought treatment for lung disease had been exposed to cigarette smoke. Of these 14% were active smokers, 42% were former smokers, and the rest, 15%, were passive smokers, that is, people who lived with smokers.

Some health workers in clinics, health centers, hospitals, and other health related institutions also smoke. Research by Cofta and Staszewski [3] at the Hospital of the Lord's Transfiguration in Poland found that 27% of health care personnel were smokers, 35% of these were nurses; what is more, 82% of them smoked at work. The research of Moneer et al. [4] at the National Cancer Institute, Cairo, Egypt, found 20% of health workers were active smokers, 5% were occasional smokers, and the rest, 75%, were nonsmokers.

Research by Nagle et al. [5] with nurses at six hospitals in New South Wales, Australia, found that knowledge amongst nurses about the damage to health caused by smoking significantly lowered the habit of smoking, whilst working and such knowledge tended to be influenced by information about smoking bans and awareness to change. This indicates that the continuous delivery of information to hospital employees both medical personnel and others can influence the health behavior of the employees concerned; in particular, it can result in the employees concerned changing, that is, reducing their smoking behavior.

The reasons a person smokes vary a lot. A person learns about smoking from their environment. Initially they observe people smoking. After they try smoking for the first time, some individuals may feel a desire to smoke again for a variety of reasons, for example, to reduce anxiety, to lose the feeling of overload and stress from work, to feel accepted within a particular group, and, for some, to relax especially because of stress from family or other problems.

When the smoking habit is already formed, social factors play an important role to keep the smoking behavior going. According to Kaplan and James [6], the tendency of individuals to continue to smoke is a phase to sustain the smoking behavior stage, that is, a stage in behavior due to a combination of psychological factors and biological mechanisms.

Smoking behavior is one type of behavior that can be changed. According to Notoatmodjo [7], change in behavior can be categorized into three types: namely, (1) natural changes, mainly due to changes in the physical environment or to changes in social, cultural, or economic activities with respect to the individual; (2) planned change, that is, change in behavior due to planning by the individual concerned; and (3) change due to the willingness for change (readiness for change), that is, changes due to innovations and new programs that allow individuals to change. Changes can be rapid or slow depending on each individual's willingness. According to various experts behavior can be changed if it is based on strong intentions and a belief that such changes in behavior will be good plus there is strong motivation to change.

Behavior change according to Green [8] is influenced by three main factors, namely, (1) predisposing factors, that is, factors which more easily affect someone's behavior, amongst other things knowledge, beliefs, values, traditions, and so forth; (2) enabling factors, that is, factors that facilitate behavior or that enable action, and they include tools and infrastructure or facilities for the behaviors to be done; and (3) reinforcing factors (amplifier factors), that is, factors that encourage or strengthen the occurrence of the behavior concerned. Even if someone knows and is able to adopt healthy behavior, they sometimes do not do so for various reasons.

Smoking behavior can be changed; however, stopping smoking behavior is not an easy thing. Results from surveys conducted by the LMMM (*Lembaga Menanggulangi Masalah Merokok* or Foundation for Overcoming Smoking Problems) show that 66% of smokers have tried to quit smoking but have failed. Some failed because they did not know how to stop smoking and some failed because they said they found it too hard to concentrate when not smoking. Of the respondents who successfully quit smoking, 76% did so because of awareness itself, 16% because of illness, and 8% because of the demands of their profession according to Helman [9].

Changing the behavior of smoking of health workers or staff at a hospital is not an easy thing to do. Efforts to stop the smoking habits of staff in hospitals can be done with a health education approach. In general, hospital employees are individuals with a background of health who already understand and know about the impact of smoking tobacco and cigarettes and the effects of the smoke itself on others; nevertheless, it is a fact that many health workers smoke; thus, it can be assumed that the approach to change the behavior of hospital employees to get them to quit their smoking habit will not be easy. But one thing that can be done is to stop the staff who smoke from smoking in the hospital and its grounds.

This is supported by Public Health Act number 36 of 2009 that makes public places, in particular public hospitals, *No Smoking Areas* (*KTR or Kawasan Tanpa Rokok*). A hospital is an institution that provides complete health services to individuals including in-patient, out-patient, and emergency services. One function of a hospital is (health) maintenance and improvement of individual health through complete health services according to medical needs. That is, a hospital is a place to get treatment that hopefully does not cause other health issues such as health problems caused by cigarette smoke. A hospital is one place that must be a nonsmoking area or KTR. All areas in a hospital should always be clean and healthy to support all the efforts to heal the patients.

Restrictions on smoking in hospitals can be an initiation to smoking behavior changes, especially for hospital staff themselves. This is important to do considering health professionals are supposed to stay away from smoking and become role models for the community in the fight against the problems of smoking. But, in fact, many health workers at RSUDZA were not following the rules and policies to enforce the application of no smoking in the hospital and its grounds.

Health education efforts can teach hospital staff to stop smoking in the hospital and its grounds, especially with the commitment and support of the Director of the Hospital accompanied by supervision and enforcement of sanctions. This form of health education can be done through health promotion approaches. Health promotion interventions (HPI) to change smoking behavior in hospitals can include health education including information about the dangers of smoking, the chemicals contained in cigarettes, and the impact of smoking in general on smokers and others. Changes expected from HPI are an increase in knowledge, improved attitudes, and behavioral changes, by persons exposed to the HPI, to not smoke, especially in public places such as hospitals.

The concept of health promotion applications varies with the purpose of the public health behavior change concerned; one of them is through the learning process using stimulus and response. According to Notoatmodjo [7] the process of behavior change in fact is similar to the learning process, which consists of stimuli which are accepted or rejected, and if they are noted, understood, and accepted by the individual, they result in a change of attitude whence in the end an open reaction occurs with the change action occurring as expected. This concept in principle is relevant to the stimulus information which is conveyed about smoking, the dangers of smoking, and ways of stopping smoking through media used in HPI, so that gradually an attitude is born and grows to change, that is, to quit or reduce smoking behavior.

Smoking in the Dr. Zainoel Abidin Provincial General Hospital (RSUDZA) in Banda Aceh and in the hospital grounds was still a health problem. Numerous attempts had been made by the management of the RSUDZA strengthened by policies implemented by the Director of the RSUDZA with oversight conducted by the hospital's Peoples Health Promotion Unit (PKMRS). These had also been strengthened by new regulations with the issue of a city-wide Regulation (Perda) number 6 of 2011, to make all public areas in the City of Banda Aceh nonsmoking areas. However, all these efforts had yet to bear fruit and many visitors and even hospital staff and sometimes even patients could still be found smoking in the hospital and its grounds.

All the data and facts above indicated that the phenomenon of smoking in the hospital and its grounds still remained a health problem and a social problem for a variety of reasons. Although smoking had been banned by regulations and supervision was also being carried out, the habit was still there, so some more effective methods were still needed so that staff and also patients and visitors would no longer smoke in the hospital and its grounds.

One method that can be done is to use HPI approaches to empower hospital staff to adopt healthy behavior with outreach, that is, use of media with social support approaches including seminars, counseling, and partnerships with advocacy. The HPI can build on the commitment of the hospital Director as well as the support of regulatory oversight to stop smoking in the hospital and its grounds. HPI approaches are effective for raising awareness amongst staff to quit smoking even though only in the hospital and its grounds.

Based on the above background, this research effort has been directed at finding effective HPI methods that can be applied to modify the behavior of employees who smoke to (a) stop smoking in the hospital and its grounds and (b) to quit or reduce smoking altogether.

1.2. Problems. The phenomenon of smoking by staff of the RSUDZA in Banda Aceh has had implications for the health functions of the organization and for the human resource functions for health because, as the premier hospital in Aceh, it should play an active role and set a leading example in the health recovery efforts for all the patients that come to the hospital.

Stopping smoking by staff is not an easy goal. Ways that can be used to try to achieve this goal include HPI, that is, health education and health promotion approaches, empowering staff, providing social support and advocacy plus the wholehearted commitment of the Director, and the implementation and enforcement of no smoking regulations. In summary, the research problem formulated is how can the use of HPI, that is, health promotion activities, empowerment, advocacy, and social support, influence all the staff of RSUZA to (a) quit smoking in the hospital and its grounds and (b) quit or reduce smoking altogether.

1.3. Research Question. The problems posed above are summarized in the following research question: can health promotion interventions (HPI) including increasing knowledge about the dangers of smoking plus building positive attitudes for behavioral change amongst smokers result in all the medical staff of RSUZA (a) quitting smoking in the hospital and its grounds and (b) quitting or reducing smoking altogether?

1.4. Research Objective. The purpose of this study was to analyze the influence of various HPI to get each and every member of the RSUZA medical staff who smokes to change their smoking behavior and henceforth (a) to quit smoking in the hospital and its grounds and (b) to quit or reduce their individual smoking habits altogether.

1.5. Hypothesis. The hypothesis for this study is "There are Health Promotion Interventions (HPI) that can influence the behavior of employees at RSUZA to (a) quit smoking in the hospital and it's grounds and (b) to quit or reduce the smoking habit altogether".

1.6. Benefits of This Research. The benefits of this research are that it can be an input or reference that is useful for improving the effectiveness of HPI in order to get all the staff and workers at RSUZA (a) to stop smoking in the hospital and its grounds and (b) to quit or reduce their smoking habit altogether. It is also expected that this research can contribute to improvements in the effectiveness of HPI to stop and/or to reduce the smoking habit throughout Aceh Province, especially in other hospitals, health centers, and public facilities.

2. Research Methods

2.1. Type of Research. This research is action research that aims to find and analyze the influence of various HPI, in particular, employee empowerment and also social support and advocacy to change the behavior of hospital staff (a) to quit smoking in the RSUZA Hospital and its grounds and (b) to quit or reduce smoking altogether. This type of research can analyze and reveal facts and phenomena that arise in the ongoing research. Interventions in the research may be changed in accordance with conditions and situations found in the field. Action research is an integrated approach that is both quantitative and qualitative.

2.2. Population and Research Samples. The population for this study, who were exposed to the HPI, were all 862 medical staff of Dr. Zainoel Abidin Provincial General Hospital {RSUZA} in Banda Aceh. The sample selected was all medical staff who admitted that they smoked, 152 individuals in all.

The control group population were from the medical staff at a different hospital in Banda Aceh where there were no HPI interventions, namely, RS Meuraxa, which is some distance from RSUZA (about 7 km to the south). The control group also had a total of 152 medical staff who were self-admitted smokers.

2.3. Antismoking Interventions. Over 50 posters, including some very graphic ones (refer Appendix), were placed at strategic locations throughout the hospital. Antismoking signs were put up throughout the hospital and were also erected in the grounds. Counseling, of smokers, was given for 45 minutes a day, between 8 and 9 am, every working day (i.e., Monday to Friday); counseling was conducted by the Director himself and by specialist doctors and others in particular by persons who had suffered major illnesses as a result of smoking. Details of the interventions and illustrations of the posters and signs are in the Appendix.

2.4. Data Analysis. Data analysis in this research included analysis of bivariate tests using Chi-square and Fisher's exact test, independent t-test, and nonparametric Mann-Whitney tests. Independent t-test was conducted at 95% confidence level and the Wilcoxon rank test was conducted at 95% confidence level. Multivariate analysis used multiple logistic regression tests.

TABLE 1: Knowledge and attitudes of the staff before and after the tests.

Stage	Knowledge				Attitude			
	Good		Poor		Positive		Negative	
	n	%	N	%	n	%	n	%
Pretest	87	57	65	42	86	57	66	42
Posttest	109	71	43	28	116	76	36	23

TABLE 2: Description of smoking behavior of smoking medical staff.

	Smoking behavior	(n)	(%)
	Pretest		
1	Light smokers (1–5 cigarettes/day)	77	51
2	Moderate smokers (6–15 cigarettes/day)	37	24
3	Heavy smokers (>15 cigarettes/day)	38	25
	Total	**152**	**100**
	Posttest		
1	Light smokers	83	54
2	Moderate smokers	17	11
3	Heavy smokers	14	9
4	No longer a smoker	38	25
	Total	**152**	**100**

3. Results and Discussion

3.1. Knowledge and Attitudes of Staff before and after the Tests. The results of this research showed that the proportion of respondents with good knowledge and attitudes before the pretest were 57%. Then, after the interventions (posttest), there was an increase in respondents' knowledge to 71%, that is, an increase of 14%, and also an increase in those with positive attitudes to 76%, that is, an increase of 19% (refer Table 1).

3.2. Change in Smoking Behavior in the RSUZA Hospital and Its Grounds. As a result of the HPI interventions including more rigorous policing against smokers, smoking has been totally stopped within the hospital and its grounds by all staff and workers plus also by all patients and visitors.

3.3. Changes in Smoking Behavior of Smoking Staff (Smoking Away from the Hospital and Its Grounds). Table 2 shows that the highest proportion of respondents in the pretest was the light smokers with 51%. After the interventions (posttest) the proportion of respondents that were light smokers increased to 54% whilst moderate smokers more than halved with a decrease from 24% to 11% and nearly two-thirds of heavy smokers reduced their smoking significantly with a decrease from 25% to 9% and most significantly 38 or 25% of respondents quit smoking, that is, stopped smoking altogether. Thus, between 44 (29%) and 82 (54%) of the intervention group completely stopped or reduced their smoking with up to 44 (29%) reducing their smoking and becoming light smokers only (the number of light smokers increased from 77 to 83) (refer Table 2).

TABLE 3: Differences in knowledge, positive attitudes, and smoking behavior of staff before and after the interventions.

Variable	Mean pretest	Mean posttest	Mean difference	Z	P
Knowledge	30	33	3	−8.719	0.001*
Attitude	83	89	6	−7.644	0.001*
Quit smoking	8	3	−5	−4.219	0.001*

*Significant $\alpha \leq 0.05$.

TABLE 4: Multiple log regression models of interventions against the behavior of quitting smoking.

Variable	B	B. (Exp.)	P
Constant	−9.103		
Knowledge	1.641	5.162	0.001*
Attitude	1.682	5.375	0.004*
Health Promotion Interventions	2.481	11.949	0.001*

*Significant $\alpha \leq 0.05$.

3.4. Differences in Knowledge, Positive Attitudes, and Smoking Behavior of Staff before and after the Interventions. Table 3 shows that there are differences in the intervention group means of 3.03. Statistical analysis of the results using t-test showed that there was a significant increase in knowledge between the pre- and the posttests with a probability value of 0.001 ($P < 0.05$).

Based on attitudes, there was a mean increase in the positive attitude of the respondents of 6%. Dependent t-test results show that there was a significant increase in staff with a positive attitude before and after the test with a difference of −7.644 and a score of $P = 0.001$.

3.5. Differences in Knowledge, Positive Attitudes, and Behavior of Staff to Quit Smoking before and after HPI. The results of the multivariate analyses used a log regression test. The final multiple regression log model results are set out in Table 4.

Table 4 shows there are two variables that predict changes in the smoking behavior of staff at RSUZA as a result of health promotion interventions ($P = 0.001$: OR = 11.949). These two variables are knowledge ($P = 0.001$: OR = 5.162) and attitude ($P = 0.004$: OR = 5.375).

This indicates that the intervention campaign conducted with guidance, lectures, discussions, leaflets, and brochures effectively increased such knowledge amongst the intervention group, that is, the staff who smoked from RSUZA. The control group, who were from a different hospital in Banda Aceh, RS Meuraxa, also increased their average score, but only by 0.05; that is, the score was stable; thus, statistically there was no difference in knowledge from the start to the end of the program amongst the control group where there was no intervention campaign.

The formula used for calculating the multiple log regressions is as follows:

$$\text{Logit}(Y) = a + b_1 X_1$$

$$\text{Logit (quit smoking behavior)} = a + b_1 X_1 + b_2 X_2$$

$$X_1 = \text{Health Promotion Intervention}$$

$$X_2 = \text{Attitude}.$$

(1)

Thus, the calculations are as follows:

$$Y = a + 2.317 X_1 + 1.528$$

$$Y = -6.214 + 2.317\,(\text{Health Promotion Intervention})$$

$$+ 1.528\,(\text{Attitude})$$

(2)

$$P_1(x) = \frac{1}{1 + e^{1(-6,214+2,317+1,528*1)}} = \frac{1}{1 + e^{1(-2,369)}}$$

$$P_1(x) = 0.916 \longrightarrow 91.6\%.$$

The proportion of those smokers amongst RSUZA staff who reduced their smoking behavior as a result of the health promotion intervention plus information (about the dangers of smoking) and who had a positive attitude was 91.6%.

The most important variables that influenced the quitting smoking behavior change were the health promotion intervention and the employee's attitude variables; thus, the staff who were exposed to the health promotion intervention were 11.949 times more likely to reduce smoking behavior than staff who were not exposed to it. Similarly staff with a positive attitude to quit smoking were 5.375 times more likely to reduce smoking behavior than staff with a negative attitude to it.

3.6. The Influence of Increasing Knowledge (about the Dangers of Smoking) from HPI Interventions amongst Staff Who Smoke. Results of the independent t-test indicated that there was a significant difference in knowledge (about the dangers of smoking) between the pretest and the posttest. This indicates that the intervention campaign conducted with guidance, lectures, discussions, leaflets, and brochures effectively increased such knowledge amongst the intervention group who were staff from RSUZA. The control group, who were from a different hospital in Banda Aceh, RS Meuraxa, also increased their average score but only by 0.05; that is, the score was stable; thus, statistically there was no difference in knowledge before and after the tests/interventions (amongst the control group).

Increases in knowledge amongst the staff in the intervention group are understandable because the information contained in such health promotion interventions could be easily internalized by staff. The information was also easily made available to the employees during their routines at the hospital through banners, leaflets, and posters that were strategically placed throughout the hospital. Moreover, as the majority of the hospital employees have had higher education (mostly in health) with high-level diplomas, degrees, and postgraduate qualifications they can very easily absorb information about health. Increases in knowledge about the harm from smoking and the motivations to quit smoking varied considerably amongst the employees in the intervention group. Although employees in hospitals work in a health profession, this does not guarantee they will not smoke.

Knowledge of the dangers of smoking does not guarantee that doctors, dentists, and other health care personnel will avoid this risky behavior.

Effective media can support the delivery of the message from the facilitator because suitable media can stimulate the thoughts, feelings, concerns, objectives, and interests of the target group during the learning process.

3.7. The Influence of HPI to Increase Employees' Positive Attitudes to Stop Smoking. The attitudes in this research are the awareness and willingness of employees of RSUZA to learn about the dangers of smoking and their willingness to avoid the dangers of smoking and to adopt antismoking attitudes. There are three phases of awareness: the first phase, awareness of the dangers of smoking; the second phase, avoiding the dangers of smoking; and the third phase, adopting antismoking attitudes. Attitudes towards health can be defined as a form of reaction to feelings that can be supported or not, provoking thought and a tendency to adopt behavior that tends towards good health, free from pain or illness, not only physically but also mentally.

The results showed that 57% of the staff had a positive attitude towards nonsmoking before the pretests; this increased to 76% after the interventions, meaning that there was an increase of 19% in the positive attitude to nonsmoking. Awareness of the dangers of smoking showed little increase: from 57% strongly agreeing in the pretest to 59% in the posttests, after the interventions. However most of the respondents very much agreed when asked about the dangers of smoking to family health. Consciousness of the need to not smoke in nonsmoking areas increased from 42% in the pretest to 53% after the interventions. Whilst 35% of the sample had a positive attitude towards the will to quit smoking by removing the sense of dependence on cigarettes, 53% had a positive attitude towards antismoking programs and friends that are antismoking.

These results showed that the (hospital) staff tended to have a positive attitude towards quitting smoking. This showed that the staff of the hospital already have awareness of the desirability to quit smoking. This can be understood because generally they have a background education in health; however, factually some also had the habit of smoking. That means that the formation of consciousness or a positive attitude towards antismoking or interventions to quit smoking had not yet sparked real actions to quit smoking or at least to reduce smoking.

Independent *t*-test results showed there were significant differences in attitudes before the interventions (pretest) compared with the attitudes after the interventions (posttest). This is indicated by the value of the probability of less than 0.005 with a 95% level of certainty and a value of $t = -7.974$, meaning the difference in attitudes before and after the intervention was 9.72.

In line with the effectiveness of health promotion knowledge, the attitudes of the staff also changed after the health promotion interventions were conducted in the hospital and its grounds. This was a real change resulting from the internalization of information by the staff about the dangers of smoking, the impact of smoking, and changes in behavior needed to stop smoking. A positive or negative attitude to things concerned with cigarettes will strongly influence whether someone's smoking behavior tends to be high or not.

Interventions to promote health through health promotion media will increase knowledge and increase positive attitudes in staff towards the dangers of smoking. Results of regression tests showed that the staff with positive attitudes were 5.3 times more likely to stop smoking compared to the staff with a negative attitude. This fact shows that internalization of knowledge which the staff already have about smoking will slowly change attitudes and willingness to begin to stop smoking. Health information interventions connected to stopping smoking in public places and the dangers of smoking for personal health will form attitudes and willingness to start stopping smoking with reduction in the number of cigarettes smoked until eventually, hopefully, smoking is stopped altogether.

3.8. The Influence of HPI to Get Staff to Stop Smoking. Stopping smoking is a real-life form of individual behavior change to reduce smoking and/or not to smoke again. Results of statistical tests with Mann-Whitney tests show that the smoking behavior pretest of the intervention group with a mean value 8.38 versus 7.92 in the control group and average differences of 0.769 showed no difference because the value of the probability was 0.699 ($P > 0.05$), whilst the smoking behavior in the posttest had an average difference of 0.549 which showed significant differences in the smoking behavior between the intervention group and the control group with a value of $P = 0.002$ ($P < 0.05$), which means that with a 95% level of confidence the health promotion interventions have influenced changes in the smoking behavior of those exposed to the HPI interventions. Independent *t*-test results showed significant differences in the smoking behavior before and after the interventions which is indicated by the value of the probability being less than 0.05 ($P = 0.002$) at a 95% level of confidence with the value of $t = -3.040$.

HPI conducted in phases, starting from the stage of empowerment to counseling conducted en masse and in groups with messages about the chemicals in cigarettes, the effects of cigarettes, and ways to stop smoking were given by researchers, religious leaders, and a specialist doctor in pulmonary diseases as well as a former smoking addict who, *nota bene*, was also a specialist in radiology. This strategy provided a positive impact to decrease the number of heavy smokers (smoking more than 15 cigarettes per day) and also to increase the number of smokers who decided to stop smoking altogether. This happened because there was information directly from people who had already had serious health problems as a result of smoking and had had to undergo major treatment to regain their health.

Besides messages in media such as leaflets, flyers, and banners containing antismoking messages (refer Appendix), there were also photographs and messages from public officials in particular the Mayor and Deputy Mayor of Banda Aceh to show that efforts to combat smoking cigarettes were very strongly supported by the City of Banda Aceh.

The smoking behavior of the hospital medical staff generally started during early adulthood. The phenomenon of starting the smoking habit in early adulthood has different causes than with teenagers. According to *social stress models*, the use of addictive substances is one way for persons to overcome various stresses which they are experiencing. These stresses can arise from family (problems) or work (problems) or even from a poor environment. One response arising from such stress is the appearance of negative emotions, in particular, sadness, anger, and distress.

Such circumstances create environmental factors with the potential to influence the smoking behavior of people. Basically hospital staff understand that smoking can cause impairment of health, can affect the local environment, and can impact others as the hospital staff in general have health education background; thus, 79% of the staff in the intervention group already had an intention to stop smoking and 69% of the control group also intended to stop smoking. One of the reasons why they wanted to stop smoking was that smoking at home was not accepted by their families plus there were pressures at work to stop smoking. However, some staff who were depressed still wanted to smoke to calm themselves.

Although a lot of hospital staff already wanted to quit smoking, many still smoked. Some said *"it is very difficult to quit smoking"* because it is an addiction and they relapsed and returned to smoking if they had any stress or problems. An intention to change is a positive precedent for behavior change. According to various experts people behave based on ways that make sense considering the impact of such behavior. An action to stop smoking needs a strong intention. Any attempt to stop smoking is not easy, because we have to change previous habitual behaviors into new habits.

In accordance with the concept of behavior change expressed by Rogers and Shoemaker [10] in the theory of the *Innovation decision process*, behavior change is defined as the psychological process experienced by an individual, after receiving information or knowledge about a new concept, until such time as he accepts that new concept. If the acceptance of a new behavior through the adoption process is based on knowledge, awareness, and a positive attitude, then the behavior is likely to be long-lasting. On the contrary, if behavior change is not based on knowledge and awareness it will not last long.

Changes in the behavior of hospital staff to quit smoking can be done in various ways, for example, by HPI and/or by special therapy, as well as with stimulant health education; namely, stimulation is given to reduce internalization; that is, thinking about smoking also hypnotherapy can be used.

One strategic way to change (smoking) behavior is through health promotion interventions (HPI). This research has proven that HPI can change the behavior of people to reduce the number of cigarettes smoked per day; for example, heavy smokers can become medium or light smokers or can even quit smoking altogether.

The formation of awareness for smokers who want to quit is a must if they really want to stop. Then, after smokers really have awareness to stop smoking with actions or concrete activities, they need to get a touch of the dimension of affection. This is to reinforce the willingness to quit,

so the person and the event are really well connected and so that there will be a deep memory trace, and this memory trace will in turn give reinforcement to not start again.

If the intention to quit smoking is strong or high then the smoking behavior will be weak. Nevertheless, the intention to quit smoking will still be affected by several factors, namely, attitudes towards smoking, social support, and the ability which the smoker feels to be able to stop smoking. When his attitude towards smoking is negative (he feels unhappy to smoke and/or he wants to stop smoking) and social support (from his environment) to quit smoking is also high and the individual concerned feels highly able to effectively stop smoking, the intention and ability to stop smoking are also stronger and vice versa.

To implement a successful smoking prevention strategy it can be concluded that strategic efforts must be made by the management of the organization. These include tight supervision to totally stop smoking in the hospital and its grounds, implementing appropriate sanctions (for transgressors), banning the sale of cigarettes in the hospital and its grounds plus also increasing health promotions, and doing reevaluations every three months. Also it may be advisable to renew the HPI from time to time.

Three of the 152 individuals in the control group who did not receive the interventions also quit smoking. The reason for one person stopping smoking was that he became the Director of the hospital, so he felt ashamed to smoke in the hospital, and the reason for the others to stop was that they were in severe pain which doctors diagnosed to be due to smoking, so they also quit smoking.

The commitment of the Mayor of the City of Banda Aceh to ban smoking in public places also helped. The Mayor and Council have made bylaws and socialized them to make public places nonsmoking areas. As reported by the Serambi Daily newspaper on 31st May, 2013, the Government of Banda Aceh have made stickers for socializing smoking bans in public transport, that is, minibuses or "labi-labi," so that people are exhorted to change behavior and become "ashamed" to smoke in public. In general the nonsmoking areas where smoking is banned are public places including health facilities, schools, and places where people are teaching and learning, plus children's playing areas, places of worship, workplaces, sports facilities, public transport, and indoor public areas. People have not yet responded 100% to the bylaw, so sometimes people can still be seen smoking in public places. Quitting smoking is possible and is an absolute must, even though smoking has become almost inseparable from the everyday life of many people.

3.9. Reasons to Stop Smoking. Interventions conducted by the researchers with the health promotion approach resulted in positive impacts and positive behavior changes with all staff stopping all smoking in the hospital and its grounds. Qualitatively, the reasons to stop smoking included information from the experience of *key note speakers* for the HPI activities plus visual information in a video about the dangers of smoking in the short, medium, and long term based on personal experiences including the high cost to clean all the blood vessels in a patient's body from nicotine (a dangerous substance in cigarettes). The format of the messages was the real evidence of damage to parts of the body due to nicotine and other harmful substances in cigarettes. This was demonstrated step by step in a video. Practically, these visuals provided real stimulus for change and for the intention to quit smoking. This shows that appropriate intervention materials presented to targets by appropriate media and mechanisms can give a positive impact to change the attitudes and behavior of persons to make them want to quit smoking.

One speaker suggested that those persons who have already had experience in stopping smoking can contribute their thoughts to other staff to enable them to quit smoking. Indeed, one reason for RSUZA staff to quit smoking is the commitment of the leadership of the hospital both to support the promotion of the program to quit smoking in the hospital and to provide support for advocacy and meetings, and the Director himself even took a lead in the advocacy sessions. This resulted in smokers at RSUZA quitting out of a sense of honor and respect for the hospital leader who was so committed to get all of his employees not to smoke.

This commitment was also supported by tight supervision against smoking in the hospital and its grounds, that is, by empowering security officers to reprimand smokers caught smoking in the hospital grounds. Indeed this commitment was the highest choice selected by the participants that wanted to stop smoking and was supported by the commitment of the Director who instructed that the hospital and all its grounds must be free from cigarette smoke.

Quinn and Snyder [11] argue that people need to be empowered to realize deep change or transformation. They call their program ACT or Advanced Change Theory. Thus, changes made by the Director to consistently ensure supervision and enforcement to stop all smoking in the hospital and its grounds were able to transform the hospital and its grounds into a no smoking oasis. Leading by example and campaigning to stop smoking is one role of the hospital as a health unit to serve the community.

Results that have been achieved recently include the passing of the No Smoking Areas (NSA) Law (Qanun KTR), plus socialization of the resultant ban on smoking in public places and also celebration of Tobacco Free Day. Socializing the ban was done to all walks of life through leaflets, posters, and banners distributed throughout all Government offices and private as well as public transportation (minibuses and buses) both intraprovincially to all districts and cities in Aceh and interprovincially to provinces outside Aceh; besides, the hospital made a commitment to monitor the implementation of the NSA Law (KTR Qanun).

The fact that the hospital Director was so concerned and committed to stop smoking in the hospital and its grounds was an important factor to motivate some staff to stop smoking in the hospital and its grounds. The Director is the highest authority in the hierarchy of the hospital; he has full power to make decisions concerning human resource management in the hospital. Staff are reluctant to go against his directions and are expected to support what is requested by their leader including not to smoke in the hospital and its

grounds, even though such (conforming) behavior may only be shown in front of the leader or only in the hospital and its grounds. The hospital is a social environment that has various characteristics including hierarchical interactions. According to Giddens [12], social life is more than just individual actions but social life is also not just determined by social forces, meaning that the overall actions and activities performed in the hospital tend to also have social power, considering that all actions of the hospital staff have a social interaction too. The message from the hospital policy initiated by the Director not to smoke in the hospital and its grounds is information received by all its staff so that there is a positive interaction to mutually stop all smoking in the hospital and its grounds whether by staff, patients, or visitors. In addition, the Director in the context of the hospital structure is a free agent (who can set an example) as well as being the top figure in the structure so that he has a dual role which provides social strength to make a successful program to stop smoking in the hospital and its grounds.

In addition, another reason to stop smoking is the psychological burden each member of staff has as a health worker, meaning that there is awareness of the importance of eventually quitting all smoking in particular due to the HPI interventions of this action research program.

4. Conclusions and Suggestions

The HPI interventions implemented significantly influenced an increase in knowledge about the dangers of smoking amongst the staff and influenced positive attitudes to stop all smoking in RSUZA Banda Aceh, with the following results.

(1) Smoking within the hospital and its grounds has been completely stopped including smoking by all staff, patients, and visitors.

(2) The number of smokers in the medical staff intervention group smoking away from the hospital decreased from 100% to 75% (i.e., a decrease of 25%).

(3) As above the number of heavy smokers (>15 cigarettes/day) decreased from 25% to 9% in the intervention group.

(4) Also the number of moderate smokers (6–15 cigarettes/day) in the intervention group decreased from 24% to 12%.

(5) But the number of light smokers (1–5 cigarettes/day) in the intervention group showed a small increase from 50% to 54%.

Logistic regression tests on the results showed that the variable that most affected the behavior changes to quit smoking is the HPI (health promotion intervention) with a value OR 11.949. This means that staff provided with health promotion interventions were 11.949 times more likely to quit smoking compared to staff who were not given HPI.

HPI conducted through mass, group, and individual counseling improved employee knowledge about the dangers of smoking, so they assisted change in behavior of the RSUDZA medical staff and assisted some of them to quit smoking.

TABLE 5: Health promotion interventions strategies to change behavior of smoking staff.

Approach	Purpose	Intervention	Frequency
Empowerment	Provide and/or increase knowledge, awareness, and attitudes amongst staff towards the dangers of smoking	(i) Information campaign to staff conducted en masse and in groups	(i) 45 minutes twice weekly for 4 months
		(ii) Distributing printed leaflets	(ii) 5 types of media viz: Posters, Leaflets, Handouts, Stickers, Banners
		(iii) Putting up posters in the hospital and its grounds	(iii) For 4 months, some, e.g., banners changed often
		(iv) Putting up *no smoking* signs	(iv) Permanent signs
Social support	Provide technical support for implementing the decisions to ban smoking in the hospital and its grounds	(i) Socialization (ii) Consultations (iii) Workshop	(iv) Once every 4 months (ii) Every month for 4 months (iii) Once every 4 months
Advocacy	Provide support, direction, and written/printed decisions concerning the banning of smoking in RSUZA hospital and its grounds	(i) Audiences (ii) Consultations (iii) Meetings (iv) Reports	(i) 6 times every 4 months (i.e., about every 3 weeks) (ii) 6 times every 4 months (iii) 6 times every 4 months (iv) Every month for 4 months

Schematically, the strategy to increase knowledge, change attitudes, and change smoking behavior of the RSUZA medical staff is as shown in the figure below:

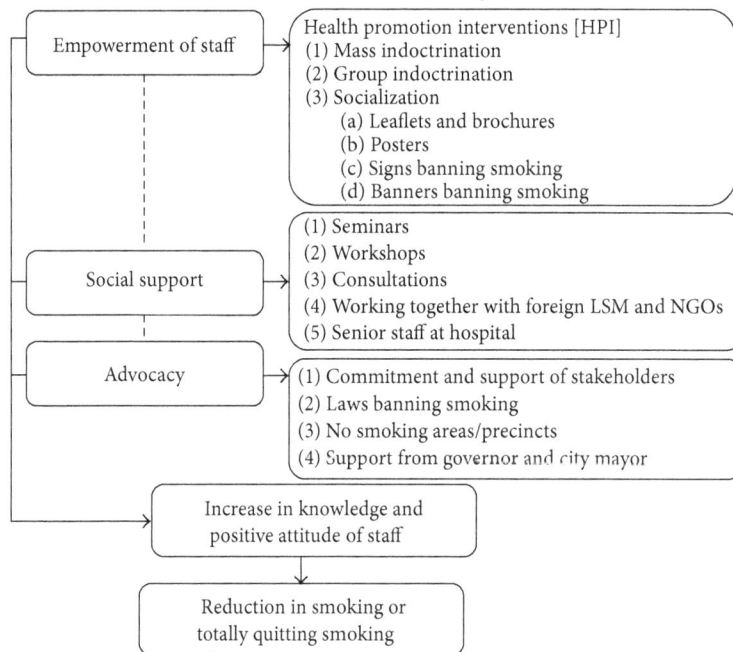

FIGURE 1: Model for change in smoking behavior of staff at RSUZA Hospital. Strategy for increasing knowledge, improving attitudes, and changing smoking behavior amongst the staff at the RSUZA Hospital.

Putting up posters about the dangers of smoking in the hospital and its grounds and installation of signs banning smoking at strategic locations throughout the hospital created a positive attitude amongst staff and a conducive environment for all staff, workers, patients, and visitors to not smoke in the RSUZA Hospital and its grounds. Strategic empowerment, social support, and advocacy carried out comprehensively and continuously can change behavior to reduce smoking and even got some staff to stop smoking away from the hospital.

It turns out that the commitment of the hospital Director can influence medical staff to change their smoking behavior. These changes can be done by making regulations for no

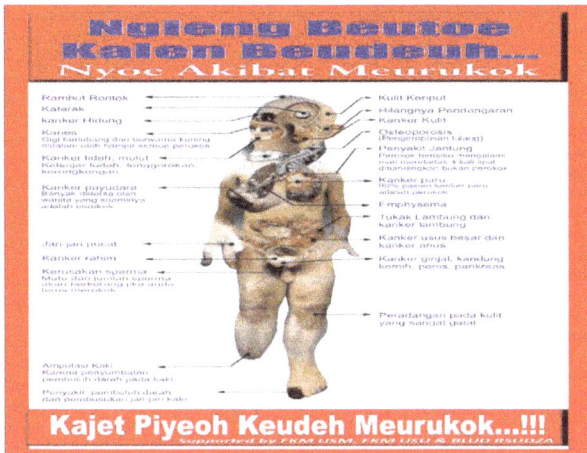

(a)

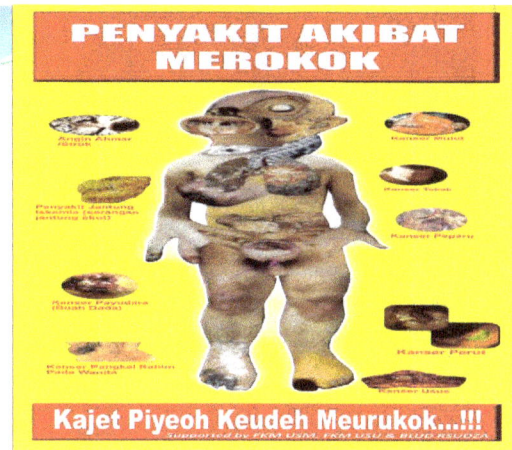

(b)

FIGURE 2: (a) Horror wall poster citing effects of smoking. (b) Another horror wall poster showing effects of smoking Both posters in both Acehnese and Indonesian languages.

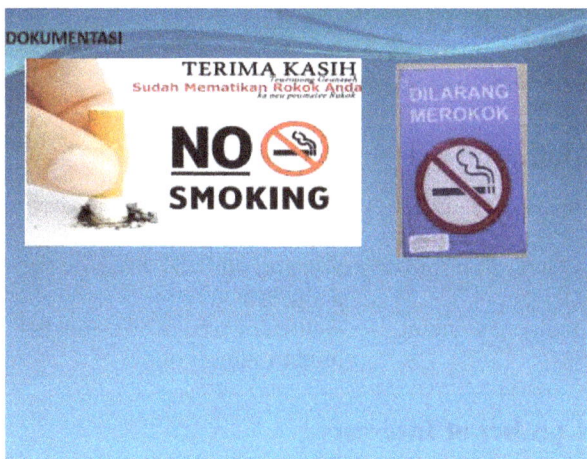

(a)

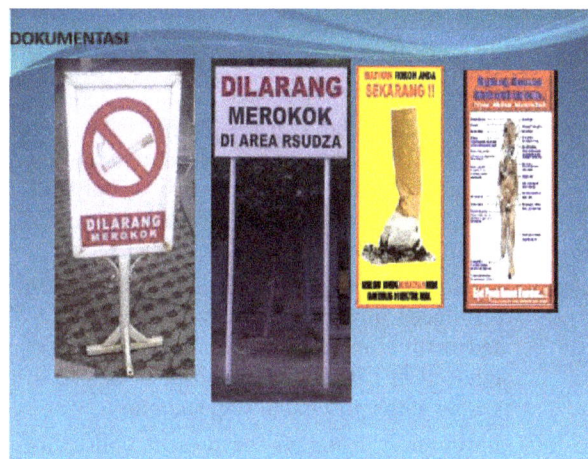

(b)

FIGURE 3: Examples of antismoking wall signs, free-standing signs, and wall posters used.

smoking in a hospital and its grounds and by close supervision of staff to ensure they do not smoke in the hospital and its grounds.

Suggestions

(1) The Government of Aceh Province, the City of Banda Aceh, and other districts in Aceh through the Aceh Provincial Health Department and City and District Health Departments need to

    (a) run routine quarterly evaluations of the implementation of the policy of nonsmoking areas in public places, particularly in hospitals;

    (b) immediately set out and pass Qanuns or local laws to implement smoke-free areas throughout the Province of Aceh, in order to reduce the number of smokers in public places in

the Province of Aceh, particularly in hospitals and other health facilities;

    (c) set policies for oversight mechanisms and technical surveillance to ensure no smoking policy in designated No Smoking Areas;

    (d) program FPI in other public institutions;

    (e) place thousands of posters, leaflets, and banners in public places providing information about the dangers of smoking.

(2) Dr. Zainoel Abidin Provincial General Hospital (RSUDZA) in Banda Aceh needs to

    (a) continue to thoroughly implement the KTR (smoke-free area) policy in the hospital and its grounds including policy of the no smoking condition and prohibiting the sale of cigarettes

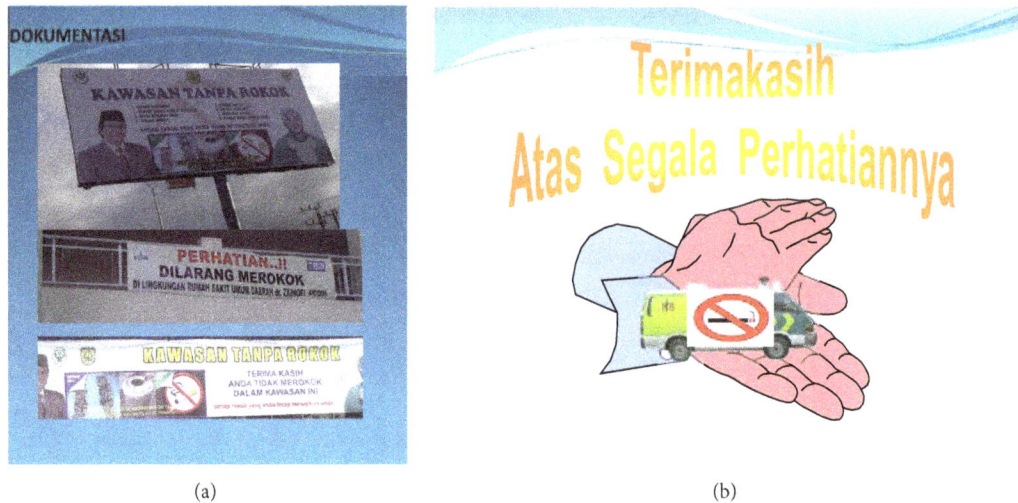

(a)   (b)

FIGURE 4: (a) Left above: example of freestanding *"No Smoking Area"* sign erected outside. Centre: example of *No Smoking* wall poster. Below: example of *"No Smoking Area"* wall sign. (b) Above: Thank You for Your Attention with no smoking sign used in slide presentations.

in the hospital and its grounds, so that the hospital areas are completely free from cigarette smoke;

(b) have systematic and structured surveillance as well as strict sanctions implemented by the Director of the hospital imposed on all staff, workers, patients and visitors who dare to try to smoke in the hospital or its grounds;

(c) sustain and continue the HPI that have been introduced in partnerships with other associated institutions to increase the awareness of staff and of patients in the hospital as well as visitors of the hospital to stop smoking;

(d) continuously maintain the present policies of the Director of RSUZA to be monitored and committed to no smoking policy in the hospital and its grounds in spite of any changes and new dynamics that may be introduced by future directors of RSUZA;

(e) have support for the commitment by the Director of RSUZA Banda Aceh to continue the policy of banning smoking in the RSUDZA hospital and its grounds in order to allow the hospital management to continuously maintain the ban in the future.

Recommendations for Academia

(1) Follow-up studies need to be done with regard to other types of health promotion interventions (HPI) using comparative analysis for different media and other variables in hospital management.

(2) There is a need for further study and analysis of policies and methods of intervention to get behavior change to stop smoking that can be a reference for implementation in other hospitals and institutions.

Appendix

See Table 5 and Figures 1, 2, 3, and 4.

Definitions

Smoking behavior:	Smoking of cigarettes, cigars, and/or pipe tobacco regularly
Quit or stop smoking:	Stopping smoking behavior altogether
Reduced smoking:	Going down from one smoking level to a lower one.

Conflict of Interests

The authors declare that there is no conflict of interests regarding the publication of this paper.

References

[1] S. Shiffman, "Assessing smoking patterns and motives," *Journal of Consulting and Clinical Psychology*, vol. 61, no. 5, pp. 732–742, 1993.

[2] A. McEwen, P. Hajek, H. McRobbie, and R. West, *Manual of Smoking Cessation a Guide for Counselors and Practitioners*, Blackwell, Oxford, UK, 2007.

[3] S. Cofta and R. Staszewski, "Hospital staff and smoking habits: do we need modification of smoking behavior in polish hospitals?" *Journal of Physiology and Pharmacology*, vol. 59, no. 6, pp. 191–199, 2008.

[4] M. N. Moneer, M. K. Noaman, and N. A. Labib, "Smoking behavior, knowledge and attitudes among medical workers in the National Cancer Institute, Cairo University," *Journal of American Sceince*, vol. 7, pp. 1059–1064, 2011.

[5] A. Nagle, M. Schofield, and S. Redman, "Australian nurses' smoking behaviour, knowledge and attitude towards providing smoking cessation care to their patients," *Health Promotion International*, vol. 14, no. 2, pp. 133–144, 1999.

[6]   R. M. Kaplan and F. S. James, *Health and Humans*, McGraw-Hill, New York, NY, USA, 1992.

[7]   S. Notoatmodjo, *Promosi Kesehatan*, PT Rineka Cipta, Jakarta, Indonesia, 2006.

[8]   L. Green, *Promotion Planning and Education: An Environmental Approach, Institute of Health Promotion Research*, University of British Colombia, British Colombia, Canada, 1980.

[9]   C. G. Helman, *Culture, Health and Illness*, Butterworth-Heineman, Oxford, UK, 1994.

[10] E. M. Rogers and F. F. Shoemaker, *Diffusion of Innovations*, Free Press, New York, NY, USA, 5th edition, 2003.

[11] R. E. Quinn and N. T. Snyder, *Advanced Change Theory in Conger J A et al. Leaders Change Handbook*, Jossey-Bass, San Francisco, Calif, USA, 1st edition, 1999.

[12] A. Giddens, *Central Problems in Social Theory*, Polity Press, London, UK, 2nd edition, 1993.

Awareness and Self-Reported Health Hazards of Electromagnetic Waves from Mobile Phone Towers in Dhaka, Bangladesh: A Pilot Study

Sheikh Mohammed Shariful Islam[1,2]

[1] Center for Control of Chronic Disease (CCCD), International Center for Diarrhoeal Disease Research, Bangladesh (ICDDR,B), 68 Shaheed Tajuddin Ahmed Sarani, Mohakhali, Dhaka 1212, Bangladesh
[2] Center for International Health (CIH), Ludwig-Maximilians-Universität (LMU), Leopoldstraße 7, 80802 Munich, Germany

Correspondence should be addressed to Sheikh Mohammed Shariful Islam; shariful.islam@icddrb.org

Academic Editor: Gudlavalleti Venkata Murthy

Background. Over the last few years there have been concerns regarding the health effects of electromagnetic waves (EMW) produced by mobile phone base transmitter stations (BTS). Data on possible health effects of EMW in developing countries are rare. This study was conducted to determine the awareness and self-reported health hazards of EMW from the mobile phone BTS in Dhaka city. *Methods*. A cross-sectional study was conducted among 220 respondents living around BTS in Dhaka city. Data was collected on sociodemographic characteristics, mobile phone use, BTS and EMW awareness, and self-reported health problems. *Results*. The majority of respondents (92.7%) reported to have seen a BTS but only 29.5% knows how it works and 74.5% had no knowledge about the EMW. 49% respondents experienced sleeping disturbances while recent episodes of headache or dizziness were reported by 47% and mood change or anxiety or depression by 41%. About 22% complained about other physical or mental symptoms. *Conclusion*. Awareness about the possible health hazards from EMW of BTS is low among the inhabitants of Dhaka city. A number of respondents mentioned recent health effects but the association with BTS could not be established.

1. Introduction

The world has witnessed rapid growth of mobile phones use over the past few decades. Worldwide in 2013, there were 6.8 billion mobile phone subscribers which are almost as many people on earth [1]. Similarly, the use of mobile phone in Bangladesh has increased over the past few years with the total number of mobile phone active subscribers reaching 114 million at the end of December 2013 from 26.66 million at the end of May 2007 [2]. With this growth in mobile phone use there has been inevitable increase in the number of mobile phone base transmitter stations (BTS), accompanied by public concern for possible health impacts associated with exposure to electromagnetic waves (EMW) emanating from BTS.

Base transmitter stations (BTS) are radio transmitters mounted on either free-standing masts or on buildings that facilitate wireless communication between user equipment and a network. The base station antennas serving macrocells are either mounted on free-standing towers, typically 10–30 m high, on short towers on top of buildings, or attached to the side of buildings. In a typical arrangement, each tower supports three antennas, each transmitting into a 120° sector. The main beam is tilted slightly downwards but does not reach ground level until the distance from the tower is at least 50 m (usually 50–200 m). Radio signals are fed through cables to the antennas and then launched as radio waves into the area or cell, around the BTS [3]. At positions where people are exposed to the radio waves from BTS, the level of exposure is much more constant over whole body than when they are exposed to a mobile phone [4].

A survey by the World Health Organization showed radio frequency (RF) exposure from BTS range from 0.002% to 0.2% of the levels of international exposure guidelines depending on the proximity to the antenna and other surrounding environmental factors [5]. This is low or comparable to RF exposure from radio or television broadcast transmitters and the temperature increase is insignificant and results in no adverse health effect. Consequently, the strength of the RF field is greatest at the source and diminishes quickly with distance [6]. Access near base station antennas is often restricted where RF signal may exceed international exposure limits. Previous studies have reported that RF exposure might be associated with several adverse health effects and complaints such as cancers in children, headache, neurological changes, loss of memory, increased blood pressure, and damage to eye cells [7–11]. However, most of these studies did not find a direct association between RF exposure and health complaints in the study population, rather a concern for the RF exposure might be responsible for the reported health effects. In addition, these symptoms are often not independent of each other and demand further evaluation.

In Bangladesh, there has been a rapid penetration of mobile phone over the past few years. Dhaka, the capital of Bangladesh, is a mega city of about 16 million people, with an area of about 1353 sq. km, and is the hub of the nation's industrial, commercial, cultural, educational, and political activities. The population is growing by an estimated 4.2% per annum, one of the highest rates amongst Asian cities. According to Far Eastern Economic Review, Dhaka will become a home of 25 million people by the year 2025. With the ever increasing number of mobile phone users, more and more BTS are being erected to support the network growth in different public areas in this city. In contrast to mobile handsets, radiation is emitted continuously from BTS and is more powerful at close quarters. Despite public concern about the safety of mobile phones and BTS, there is no published literature on the possible health effects of BTS in Bangladesh to the best of our knowledge. The objectives of this study were to determine the awareness regarding BTS and identify self-reported health problems of people living near a BTS in Dhaka city.

2. Methods

2.1. Study Population. A cross-sectional study was conducted among 220 adults from September to November 2009 in Dhaka city. The study population was approximately 3 million people mostly from upper and middle class living in Gulshan and Mohammadpur area, respectively. Participants were selected purposefully from the study sites. In both the study areas, the data collector first selected a house nearest to a BTS and approached many adults living in the house meeting the inclusion criteria. The eligibility criteria included adult people of both sexes, living near a BTS for at least one year, and able to provide written informed consent. The use of mobile phone and migration was not considered as sample criteria. A total of 232 participants were approached with 12 refusals mentioning lack of time and not interested in the study with a response rate of 95.5%.

2.2. Data Collection. Data were collected from face-to-face interview using a structured questionnaire. The questionnaire was pretested in the fields and after necessary omission, addition, and language editing, used for data collection. Data were collected on demographic characteristics, duration of living in the current residence, use of mobile phone, knowledge and awareness about BTS and EMW, and self-reported health problems. Each participant was asked in local language if they noticed any recent changes of the following symptoms: sleeping pattern/habits, episodes of headaches/dizziness, changes in anxiety/depression, burning sensations, episodes of shaking/fits, and any other health changes over the past one year. Participants mentioning any other recent symptoms were collected and categorized into the following: mental health, cardiovascular diseases (CVD), gastrointestinal symptoms (GIT), and others/nonspecific symptoms. Participants were informed regarding the objective of the study and that participating in the study is voluntary and that they could stop at any time they wished. Also, confidentiality of the information provided was ensured that data collected will only be used for the study purpose and will not be shared with anyone else except the investigators. The study protocol was approved from the scientific and ethical review committee of School of Public Health and Life Sciences, University of South Asia, Dhaka, Bangladesh.

2.3. Data Analysis. The collected data were checked, edited, and verified to exclude any error or inconsistency. Data was coded and entered into an excel sheet. Data editing and analysis were done manually and using specific statistical software SPSS (Version 11, SPSS Corporation, Chicago, USA). Tables with frequency and percentage were prepared to demonstrate the findings.

3. Results

3.1. Sociodemographic Profile. Data was collected from adults aged 18 years and above from the households surrounding a BTS. The mean age of the respondents was 37.27 years. Out of 220 respondents, the majority 73 (33.2%) was in the age group 35–44 years, 54 respondents (24.5%) were in 25–34 years age group, and the rest were in other age groups. Most of the respondents (112) reported to be living in the current residence for 12–36-month duration (50.9%). The mean duration of living in current residence is 38.95 months. Most of respondents were married (64.5%) and had graduate or upper level of education (73.2%) and service holders (57.8%) (Table 1).

3.2. Awareness Regarding BTS and Electromagnetic Waves (EMW). Almost all the respondents (98.6%) reported using at least one mobile phone. The majority of respondents (92.7%) reported to have seen a BTS either from far, on a television, or in a picture. Half of the respondents have never seen the parts of a BTS (53.2%). About one-third of respondents (29.5%) claimed to know how the BTS works. Respondents were not asked to explain what they knew about the BTS in technical terms and whether their knowledge

TABLE 1: Sociodemographic characteristics of the respondents ($n = 220$).

Variables	Number	Percentage
Male	111	50.5
Female	109	49.5
Age group (years)		
18–24	36	16.4
25–34	54	24.5
35–44	73	33.2
45–59	47	21.4
60 and above	10	4.5
Duration of living in current residence (months)		
12–36	112	50.9
37–48	36	16.4
49–60	35	15.9
>60	37	16.8
Religion		
Muslim	197	89.5
Hindu	13	5.9
Christian	8	3.6
Others	2	0.9
Marital status		
Married	142	64.5
Unmarried	60	27.3
Divorcee/separated	18	8.2
Education		
None	6	2.7
Primary	12	5.5
Secondary	41	18.7
Graduate/masters	161	73.2
Occupation		
Unemployed	9	4.1
Student	31	14.1
Service	127	57.8
Business	18	8.2
House wife	35	15.9

was correct. The majority of the respondents (74.5%) had no knowledge about the EMW (74.5%). Anyone who self-reported that they knew about EMW was reported as Yes and thus this does not explain their exact knowledge about EMW (Table 2).

3.3. Self-Reported Health Problems. During the past one year almost half of the respondents experienced problems in sleeping patterns (49.1%), recent episodes of headache or dizziness (47.3%), and mood change, anxiety, or depression (41.4%). Only 11 respondents experienced some generalized burning sensation and 4 reported episodes of shaking or fits. However, these effects were not ruled out by taking

personal history of any existing previous medical conditions or diseases (Table 3).

Apart from the symptoms mentioned above, 48 respondents 21.8%) mentioned one or more other health effects, such as mood changes/problem, buzzing in the head, hopelessness, palpitation, tachycardia, heaviness of chest, anorexia, diarrhoea, and skin diseases. These symptoms mentioned as other health effects were classified and are shown in Table 4.

4. Discussion

The results of our study show that awareness of EMW and BTS is low among most of the respondents. Almost half of the respondents complained of sleep disturbances, episodes of headache or dizziness, and changes in mood or anxiety/depression while smaller number of respondents mentioned other heath complaints. Respondents were selected purposely from Gulshan, an elite area of Dhaka city and Mohammadpur where most of the people are highly educated and thus the awareness of the possible harmful effects of EMW from BTS can be assumed to be much lower at the national level. A survey report from European Union showed that about one-fourth of Europeans (23%) know that power lines, mobile communication masts, mobile phones, computers, radar equipment, household appliances, wireless computer networks, induction heaters, and antitheft devices are sources for EMW [12]. Two-thirds or more of those polled said that EMW is generated by mobile telephones (71%) and mobile communication masts (66%). In our study, lower rates of awareness of the harmful effects of BTS were reported.

The report published in May 2000 on "Mobile Phones and Health" by the "Independent Expert Group on Mobile Phones (IEGMP)" under the direction of Sir William Stewart describes under paragraph 3.5 various symptoms which were most commonly attributed to the base stations at the hearings: "headaches, sleep disturbance, depression, stress and tiredness" [4]. Paragraphs 3.22 and 3.23 of the report list the main concerns reported in the media about base stations: "The distance at which they were 'safe', and about the proximity to schools, homes, hospitals and residential accommodation for the elderly. Adverse aesthetic impacts were also noted. The health effects most often alleged were sleep disorders, fatigue, anxiety, stress, epileptic fits, burning sensations and shaking" [13]. In Austria there have also been various reports from the population attributing different disturbances of health and well-being to exposure to BTS [14]. The symptoms reported corresponded to a large extent to those listed in the IEGMP report. In addition, cardiac dysrhythmia, high blood pressure, forgetfulness, hearing difficulties, burning of the eyes, and susceptibility to infections were reported, which generally improved or disappeared when residents moved. Detailed clarification of these symptoms has not been performed [15]. Abdel-Rassoul and colleagues in 2007 concluded that inhabitants living nearby BTS are at risk for developing neuropsychiatric problems and some changes in the performance of neurobehavioral functions either by facilitation or inhibition [16].

TABLE 2: Awareness of BTS according to area of residence ($n = 220$).

	Gulshan	Mohammadpur	Total number	Percentage
Seen BTS	104	100	204	92.7
Seen parts BTS	50	53	103	46.8
Knowledge BTS	38	27	65	29.5
Knowledge EMW	32	24	56	25.5

TABLE 3: Self-reported health problems by area of living.

	Gulshan	Mohammadpur	Total number	Percentage
Sleeping disturbances				
Yes	54	54	108	49.1
No	40	46	86	39.1
Do not know	16	10	26	11.8
Headache/dizziness				
Yes	53	61	104	47.3
No	51	45	96	43.6
Do not know	6	4	20	9.1
Changes in anxiety/depression				
Yes	41	50	91	41.4
No	57	52	109	49.5
Do not know	12	8	20	9.1
Generalized burning sensation				
Yes	7	4	11	5.0
No	98	103	201	91.4
Do not know	5	3	8	3.6
Episodes of shaking/fits				
Yes	3	1	4	1.8
No	123	88	211	95.9
Do not know	4	1	5	2.3
Any other effects				
Yes	27	21	48	21.8
No	73	83	156	70.9
Do not know	10	6	16	7.3

TABLE 4: Classification of any other effects.

Any other effects	Number	Percentage
Mental health (mood disorders)	15	25.4
CVD (palpitation, tachycardia)	9	15.2
GIT (anorexia, diarrhoea)	6	10.2
Others/nonspecific (skin rash)	29	49.2
Total	59	100%

CVD = cardio vascular diseases, GIT = gastro intestinal systems.

Röösli et al. in 2004 concluded that "sleep disorders (58%), headaches (41%), nervousness or distress (19%), fatigue (18%), and concentration difficulties were most common complaints [17]. The results of the Röösli study comply with our study where sleep disorders were reported by 49% respondents and headache or dizziness by 47%. However, the presence of nervousness or distress, fatigue and concentration difficulties were also mentioned by the respondents of this study as other symptoms and the proportion is in line with Röösli study. A study by Santini in France showed increasing frequency of complaints among participants in relation with [sic] distance from base station who reported that they were living within 300 meters of BTS in rural areas, or within 100 meters of BTS in urban areas [18]. The most common complaints were irritability, depression, loss of memory, dizziness, libido decrease, and so forth. Women significantly more often than men ($P < 0.05$) complained of headache, nausea, loss of appetite, sleep disturbance, depression, discomfort and visual perturbations. Other studies reported people living in the vicinity of base stations report [sic] various complaints mostly of the circulatory system, but also of sleep disturbances, irritability, depression, blurred vision, concentration difficulties, nausea, lack of appetite, headache and vertigo" [19–21].

In our study the distance from BTS was not measured. Also comparison between the differences in terms of males and females was not performed. But the complaints were almost similar which shows the importance of conducting further research to determine the effects of EMW from BTS on human health. Also, studies need to be conducted to measure the safety distance of BTS from human living and recommend national authority for policy implications. Navarro and colleagues in 2003 showed that people more exposed to radiation from mobile phone antennas in La Nora (operating at 1800 MHz) had more symptoms than those who were less exposed. Exposure was associated with discomfort, irritability, appetite loss, fatigue, headache, difficulties concentrating, and sleep disturbance. Previous studies have reported that the most exposed people had a higher incidence of fatigue, irritability, headaches, nausea, loss of appetite, sleeping disorders, depression, discomfort, difficulties concentrating, memory loss, visual disorders, dizziness, and cardiovascular problems that are almost similar with our findings [22–26]. However, most of these population based studies did not show statistically significant association of the physical symptoms reported with exposure to BTS and the adverse effects might be due to nocebo effect.

Researchers in Austria found that volunteers exposed to radiation typical of that experienced at 80 meters from a BTS experienced changes in the electrical activity of their brains and feelings of unwellness [27]. Subjects reported buzzing in the head, palpitations of the heart, unwellness, and light-headedness. The Hutter report showed that, in homes with highest exposures, people reported more unpleasant symptoms including three times as many headaches, 2.3 times the incidence of tremor, 2.5 times the incidence of cold hands/feet and concentration problems, 2.4 times the incidence of appetite loss, twice as much exhaustion, and twice as much fatigue [22]. We could not make such comparisons in this study as we did not have a control group.

There are concerns, nevertheless, about whether the emissions from all BTS are uniformly low, about whether the emissions could cause unknown health effects, and whether, with the increased use of mobile telecommunications, their output will have to rise [28]. The International Agency for Research on Cancer showed that extremely low-frequency magnetic fields are possibly carcinogenic to humans (Group 2 B) [29]. EMF was demonstrated as a possible cause for the following health outcomes by the California EMF-Program 2002: leukaemia in children and adults, brain tumor in adults, miscarriage among pregnant mothers, and motor neuron disease (MND) [30–34]. Although several risk factors have been investigated, most studies on exposure from BTS could not find a direct association between RF-EMF and health complaints but several studies found health complaints associated with concern about (visible) RF-BTS. In addition, standardized blinded experimental studies were not able to confirm associations between EMF exposure and the physical complaints of the respondents.

Limitations of the Study. This study had several limitations. First, the study was conducted in two selected areas of Dhaka city with limited sample size and convenient sampling. So the results cannot be generalized and chances of sampling bias might occur. Second, health effects mentioned by the participants were self-reported and association of the symptoms with other conditions was not ruled out. Third, there was no exclusion criteria based on personal and medical histories including those having a history of epilepsy, psychiatric disorders, or specific causes of headache. Fourth, other sources of other RF such as microwave use, duration of mobile use, and wireless devices use were not included in the study and exposure contribution from BTS and other sources could not be measured due to lack of technical expertise. Also we were not able to measure the frequency, distance, and duration of exposure from BTS due to lack of technical skills. This lack of validated and reliable exposure assessment methods challenges the feasibility of such studies. Finally, we did not include any control group, so comparison of the responses could not be made.

5. Conclusions

From the results of our study we cannot conclude that the health effects are direct results of the BTS. However, various studies showed the association of health hazards with EMW radiation from BTS which cannot be ignored and should be considered as a public health concern. Further studies with appropriate sample size involving a control group and measuring the source and power of the radiation according to distance from source will validate the results of this study. Bangladesh Telecommunications Regulatory Authority should take measures to ensure that the BTS are set up following international standards and at a distant that is within the safety range. The exposure limits of the EMW should be restrictive to a safety limit with regular monitoring. The health authority should ensure that the BTS have no effect on human health.

Conflict of Interests

The author declares that there is no conflict of interests regarding the publication of this paper.

Author's Contribution

Sheikh Mohammed Shariful Islam initiated the study design, data collection, data management, and analysis. The author contributed to data interpretation, critically revised the drafts, and approved the final version.

Acknowledgments

The author gratefully acknowledges the support from the study participants to provide data for the study. This study was carried out as the partial fulfillment of the degree of Masters in Public Health, UniSA School of Public Health and Life Sciences, University of South Asia.

References

[1] International Telecommunication Union, *The World in 2013 ICT Facts and Figures*, International Telecommunication Union, Geneva, Switzerland, 2013.

[2] "Bangladesh Telecommunication Regulatory Commission," 2014, http://www.btrc.gov.bd/facts-and-stats.

[3] G. Neubauer, H. Haider, K. Lameds et al., "Measurement methods and legal requirements for exposure assessment next to GSM base stations," in *Proceedings of the 15th International Zurich Symposium on Electromagnetic Compatibility*, 2003.

[4] Independent Expert Group on Mobile Phones, "Mobile phones and health," in *Independent Expert Group on Mobile Phones*, S. W. Stewart, Ed., 2000.

[5] World Health Organization, *Electromagnetic Fields and Public Health*, 2014, http://www.who.int/peh-emf/publications/facts/fs296/en/.

[6] International Commission on Non-Ionizing Radiation Protection, "Guidelines on limits of exposure to static magnetic fields," in *Health Physics*, pp. 504–514, 2009.

[7] M. Otto and K. E. von Mühlendahl, "Electromagnetic fields (EMF): do they play a role in children's environmental health (CEH)?" *International Journal of Hygiene and Environmental Health*, vol. 210, no. 5, pp. 635–644, 2007.

[8] A. W. Preece, S. Goodfellow, M. G. Wright et al., "Effect of 902 MHz mobile phone transmission on cognitive function in children," *Bioelectromagnetics*, vol. 26, no. 7, pp. S138–S143, 2005.

[9] M. Blettner, B. Schlehofer, J. Breckenkamp et al., "Mobile phone base stations and adverse health effects: phase 1 of a population-based, cross-sectional study in Germany," *Occupational and Environmental Medicine*, vol. 66, no. 2, pp. 118–123, 2009.

[10] A. P. M. Zwamborn, S. H. J. Vossen, B. J. A. Leersum, M. A. Ouwens, and W. N. Makel, "Effects of global communication system radio-frequency fields on well being and cognitive functions of human subjects with and without subjective complaints," TNO-Report FEL-03-C148, 2003.

[11] P. Elliott, M. B. Toledano, J. Bennett et al., "Mobile phone base stations and early childhood cancers: case-control study," *British Medical Journal*, vol. 340, articla c3077, 2010.

[12] R. Santini, P. Santini, P. Le Ruz, J. M. Danze, and M. Seigne, "Survey study of people living in the vicinity of cellular phone base stations," *Electromagnetic Biology and Medicine*, vol. 22, no. 1, pp. 41–49, 2003.

[13] A. Huss, J. Küchenhoff, A. Bircher et al., "Symptoms attributed to the environment—a systematic, interdisciplinary assessment," *International Journal of Hygiene and Environmental Health*, vol. 207, no. 3, pp. 245–254, 2004.

[14] G. Oberfeld, *Precaution in Action—Global Public Health Advice Following BioInitative 2007*, BioInitative Working Group, 2012.

[15] S. J. Regel, S. Negovetic, M. Röösli et al., "UMTS base station-like exposure, well-being, and cognitive performance," *Environmental Health Perspectives*, vol. 114, no. 8, pp. 1270–1275, 2006.

[16] G. Abdel-Rassoul, S. Aalto, C. Haarala et al., *Mobile Phone Affects Cerebral Blood Flow*, 2012.

[17] M. Röösli, M. Moser, Y. Baldinini, M. Meier, and C. Braun-Fahrländer, "Symptoms of ill health ascribed to electromagnetic field exposure—a questionnaire survey," *International Journal of Hygiene and Environmental Health*, vol. 207, no. 2, pp. 141–150, 2004.

[18] R. Santini, P. Santini, J. M. Danze, P. Le Ruz, and M. Seigne, "Investigation on the health of people living near mobile telephone relay stations: I/Incidence according to distance and

sex," *Pathologie-Biologie*, vol. 50, no. 6, pp. 369–373, 2002 (French).

[19] A. Bortkiewicz, M. Zmyślony, A. Szyjkowska, and E. Gadzicka, "Subjective symptoms reported by people living in the vicinity of cellular phone base stations: review," *Medycyna Pracy*, vol. 55, no. 4, pp. 345–351, 2003.

[20] G. Hyland, How exposure to mobile phone base-station signals can adversely affect humans, 2005.

[21] A. W. Preece, A. G. Georgiou, E. J. Dunn, and S. C. Farrow, "Health response of two communities to military antennae in Cyprus," *Occupational and Environmental Medicine*, vol. 64, no. 6, pp. 402–408, 2007.

[22] H. Hutter, H. Moshammer, P. Wallner, and M. Kundi, "Subjective symptoms, sleeping problems, and cognitive performance in subjects living near mobile phone base stations," *Occupational and Environmental Medicine*, vol. 63, no. 5, pp. 307–313, 2006.

[23] E. Mohler, P. Frei, C. Braun-Fahrländer, J. Fröhlich, G. Neubauer, and M. Röösli, "Effects of everyday radiofrequency electromagnetic-field exposure on sleep quality: a cross-sectional study," *Radiation Research*, vol. 174, no. 3, pp. 347–356, 2010.

[24] G. Berg-Beckhoff, M. Blettner, B. Kowall et al., "Mobile phone base stations and adverse health effects: phase 2 of a cross-sectional study with measured radio frequency electromagnetic fields," *Occupational and Environmental Medicine*, vol. 66, no. 2, pp. 124–130, 2009.

[25] G. Oberfeld, N. A. Enrique, P. Manuel, M. Ceferino, and C. Gomez-Perrretta, "The microwave syndromefurther aspects of a Spanish study," in *Proceedings of the 3rd International Workshop on Biological Effects of Electromagnetic Fields (EMFs '04)*, Kos, Greece, 2004.

[26] A. Bortkiewicz, E. Gadzicka, A. Szyjkowska et al., "Subjective complaints of people living near mobile phone base stations in Poland," *International Journal of Occupational Medicine and Environmental Health*, vol. 25, no. 1, pp. 31–40, 2012.

[27] A. Fragopoulou, Y. Grigoriev, O. Johansson et al., "Scientific panel on electromagnetic field health risks: consensus points, recommendations, and rationales," *Reviews on Environmental Health*, vol. 25, no. 4, pp. 307–317, 2010.

[28] A. Ahlbom, A. Green, L. Kheifets, D. Savitz, and A. Swerdlow, "Epidemiology of health effects of radiofrequency exposure," *Environmental Health Perspectives*, vol. 112, no. 17, pp. 1741–1754, 2004.

[29] IARC Working Group on the Evaluation of Carcinogenic Risks to Humans, "Non-ionizing radiation, part 1: static and extremely low-frequency (ELF) electric and magnetic fields," *IARC Monographs on the Evaluation of Carcinogenic Risks to Humans/World Health Organization, International Agency for Research on Cancer*, vol. 80, pp. 1–395, 2002.

[30] R. Neutra, V. d. Pizzo, and G. M. Lee, "An evaluation of the possible risks from Electric and Magnetic Fields (EMF) from power lines, internal wiring, electrical occupations, and appliances," in *California EMF Program—Final Report 2002*, 2002.

[31] H. Mild, "Meta-analysis of long-term mobile phone use and the association with brain tumours," *International Journal of Oncology*, vol. 32, no. 5, pp. 1097–1103, 2008.

[32] P. D. Inskip, R. E. Tarone, E. E. Hatch et al., "Cellular-telephone use and brain tumors," *New England Journal of Medicine*, vol. 344, no. 2, pp. 79–86, 2001.

[33] I. Deltour, A. Auvinen, M. Feychting et al., "Mobile phone use and incidence of glioma in the nordic countries 1979–2008: consistency check," *Epidemiology*, vol. 23, no. 2, pp. 301–307, 2012.

[34] J. Schüz, E. Böhler, G. Berg et al., "Cellular phones, cordless phones, and the risks of glioma and meningioma (Interphone Study Group, Germany)," *The American Journal of Epidemiology*, vol. 163, no. 6, pp. 512–520, 2006.

13

The Challenges Confronting Public Hospitals in India, Their Origins, and Possible Solutions

Vikas Bajpai

Centre for Social Medicine and Community Health, Jawaharlal Nehru University, New Delhi, India

Correspondence should be addressed to Vikas Bajpai; drvikasbajpai@gmail.com

Academic Editor: Gudlavalleti Venkata Murthy

Despite the implementation of National Rural Health Mission over a period of nine years since 2005, the public health system in the country continues to face formidable challenges. In the context of plans for rolling out "Universal Health Care" in the country, this paper analyzes the social, economic, and political origins of the major challenges facing public hospitals in India. The view taken therein holds the class nature of the ruling classes in the country and the development paradigm pursued by them as being at the root of the present problems being faced by public hospitals. The suggested solutions are in tune with these realities.

1. Introduction

Some authors have described the big modern day hospitals as "monuments to disease." Indeed, this is what they will be so long as they function as institutions only for curative care, detached from the larger social, economic, cultural, and political context of the people's lives which largely determines their health. Unfortunately, even this curative care has become unaffordable to many common people due to the policy framework governing health sector in the country.

The fact is that public hospitals have become increasingly detached from the larger context in which medicine operates. If the public hospitals are to be made responsive to the health needs of the people, then problems facing these institutions ought to be located in the broader conditions (we may call these structural problems) that influence their functioning, rather than locating these in their inner working alone. This also implies that the solutions to these problems ought to be socially oriented rather than being guided by narrow managerial or technocentric approaches.

Public sector healthcare shall continue having its relevance for a long time in order to reach out healthcare to vast sections of underserved populations in developing countries like India. In the context that the 12th Five-Year Plan Document has rolled out an ambitious scheme to achieve "Universal Health Care" in the country, this review sets out the following objectives before itself:

(i) elucidate the more important challenges facing public hospitals in India and document their enormity;

(ii) understand the social, economic, and political sources/factors leading to the emergence of these challenges;

(iii) in accordance with the aforementioned analysis, propose solutions that are feasible within the present political and economic system.

For the purpose of this paper, a public hospital shall include the most peripheral PHC (primary health center) to a tertiary care hospital located in a big city. Even though there are differences in the specific functions of these institutions, they constitute a continuum of care, both preventive and curative. While the lower levels ought to provide more direct preventive and curative services for most of the common diseases, the higher level institutions are supposed to cater to a more selected set of patients who are in need for more specialized services not available at the lower public health facilities. Apart from this, the higher public health facilities have an obligation on providing supervision, training, and technical support to facilitate smoother functioning of the primary level facilities. It follows then that there is a synthesis across different levels of public hospitals and breakdown at any level has consequences for all levels.

2. Structure and Methodology

After setting out what the author believes to be the main challenges facing public hospitals in India, different secondary sources of information were relied upon to authenticate these challenges. Apart from this, reliance has also been placed on the observations made by the author during his monitoring visits to various health facilities, primarily in the states of Uttarakhand and Uttar Pradesh, while working as a consultant with the National Health Systems Resource Center, a technical advisory body of the Government of India under the Ministry of Health and Family Welfare.

Having thus delineated the major challenges, relying on evidence from relevant literature, different social, economic, and political sources of these challenges have been profiled. The suggested solutions for rectifying some of these social, economic, and political sources have been formulated as per the analysis made in the review and as per the author's understanding. However, it is admitted that the suggested solutions are in deference to the present system's ability to allow changes in the given social, economic, and political structure of the society.

Further, an attempt to comprehensively review the challenges facing a public hospital does not afford the advantage of ostensible clarity that comes with taking up a single focus for study. Alternatively, a compartmentalized approach tends to lose sight of the essentially interrelated nature of different challenges that confront a public hospital in India today. It is our considered opinion that there cannot be a solution that is strictly limited in its scope to a particular aspect of the problem under consideration, without impinging on other aspects. Hence, this is a comprehensive review.

3. Main Challenges Confronting a Public Hospital

In our opinion, the main challenges confronting the public hospitals today are as follows:

(1) deficient infrastructure,

(2) deficient manpower,

(3) unmanageable patient load,

(4) equivocal quality of services,

(5) high out of pocket expenditure.

3.1. Deficient Infrastructure. The format of the public health structure in the country draws directly from the recommendations of the Bhore Committee Report, 1946. However, the public health infrastructure has evolved lags far behind in matching the content and the spirit of the committee's report. The committee proposed the implementation of its recommendations in two distinct phases—"three-million plan" and the "ten-year plan."

The "three-million plan" laid down the required health infrastructure to provide for the health needs of an average

district in India having a population of three million. This was to be implemented over a period of three to four decades. Anticipating resource constraints, both in terms of manpower and money to make such an infrastructure available in a short time, the committee recommended a shorter "ten-year plan" to be implemented first. Table 1 gives a comparison between the "ten-year plan," the "three-million plan," and the public health infrastructure available at present in the country.

As against the 0.24 beds per 1000 population that were available in British India, the committee's overall plan for development of health services in India provided for achieving 1.03 beds per 1000 population within ten years of implementation of the plan and a ratio of 5.67 beds/1000 population in thirty to forty years. The committee further stated that:

> "We consider moreover, that our recommendations constitute an irreducible minimum, and were it not for the limitation imposed by the inadequacy of staff and funds; we should unhesitatingly have proposed a more comprehensive scheme than the one indicated." [1, Page 31].

However, even a cursory look at Table 1 shows that what was considered as "irreducible minimum" by the committee proved to be a formidable task to achieve for the health planners of the country.

The UPA (United Progressive Alliance) Government launched the ambitious "National Rural Health Mission" (NRHM) in 2005 to bolster the rural health infrastructure. After completion of the first phase in 2012 the mission is now in the second phase of its implementation. To begin with, the mission was meant to bring the EAG (Empowered Action Group) states which lagged far behind the rest of the country in health infrastructure, at par with the rest of the country. Table 2 provides the rural infrastructure status in the EAG states (Jammu and Kashmir and Himachal Pradesh excluded) as of March 2012.

It is clearly evident from the table that the average shortfall for different types of facilities is between two to three times more in EAG states as compared to the non-EAG states. Similarly, the average population served per facility continues to remain much higher for EAG states as compared to non-EAG states. With the notable exceptions of Chhattisgarh, Odisha, Uttarakhand, and Jharkhand for the number of CHCs in position, the shortfall for different levels of facilities in the other five states is much higher than the all India average.

The relative advantage of states like Chhattisgarh, Odisha, and Uttarakhand may well be illusionary because, as we will see shortly, mere availability of infrastructure does not mean it is delivering the required services, which, along with infrastructure, also depend on availability of amenities like water, electricity, beds, medical and paramedical manpower, and spatial distribution of available infrastructure. Table 3 illustrates some of the other deficiencies of the available infrastructure which undermines its functional status.

Nonavailability of facilities like water and electricity can only be expected to deeply undermine the functioning of

TABLE 1: Comparison between "ten-year plan," the "three-million plan" and the presently available health infrastructure.

	"Ten-year plan" (targets to be met at the end of ten years)			"Three-million plan"			Present available infrastructure		
	Population norm	Medical officers	Hospital	Population norm	Medical officers	Hospital	Population per facility	Medical officers	Hospital bed norms##
Primary unit	40,000	2	15 beds	20,000 population	6	75 beds	34 and 641.3**	1.2	4 beds
Secondary unit	5,00,000	17	200 beds	6,00,000 population	140	650 beds	1, 72, and 375**	3.3	30
District headquarters/bigger secondary units	7,50,000	—	500 beds* (1.03/1000)	30,00,000 population	268	2,500 beds (5.67/1000)	17, 45, and 152 approximately#	—	100 to 500 beds (0.9/1000)

Note: the "three-million plan" laid down the required health infrastructure to provide for the health needs of an average district in India having a population of three million. This was to be implemented over a period of three to four decades. Anticipating resource constraints, both in terms of manpower and money to make such an infrastructure available in a short time, the committee recommended a shorter "ten-year plan" to be implemented first.

Source: details of the "ten-year plan" and "three-million plan" have been obtained from chapters III and IV of the Government of India [1]: "Report of the Health Development and Survey Committee (Bhore Committee), Vol. II," Government of India Press. *In the "ten-year plan," the Bhore committee did not recommend setting up of a district level tertiary health set-up. Instead, 4 of the 200-bed secondary units in the districts were to be elevated to the level of 500-bed secondary units.

** Figures obtained from Table 11 of the "Rural Health Bulletin, 2012," Ministry of Health and Family Welfare, Government of India [2].

Figure has been obtained by dividing the total population of the country in 2011 by the number of district hospitals.

Obtained from Rural Health Bulletin, 2012, Ministry of Health and Family Welfare [2].

Figures in parenthesis are the beds per thousand population set to be achieved in the "ten-year plan" and "three-million plan" and the ratio at present in India.

TABLE 2: Shortfall in health infrastructure as of March 2012 in EAG states as per 2011 census population (provisional) norms.

State	Subcenters (SC)				PHCs				CHCs			
	Req.	In pos.	% short.	Pop/SC	Req.	In pos.	% short.	Pop/PHC	Req.	In pos.	% short.	Pop/CHC
Bihar	18533	9696	48%	9,496	3083	1863	40%	49,423	770	70	91%	13,15,357
Chhattisgarh	4904	5111	−4.2%	3,836	776	755	3%	25,965	194	149	23%	1,31,568
Jharkhand	6043	3958	35%	6,326	964	330	66%	75,870	241	188	22%	1,33,175
Madhya Pradesh	12314	8869	28%	5,924	1977	1156	42%	45,448	494	333	33%	1,57,771
Odisha	8136	6688	18%	5,226	1308	1226	6%	28,508	327	377	−15%	92,709
Rajasthan	15172	11487	24%	4,487	2326	1528	34%	33,731	581	382	34%	1,34,922
Uttar Pradesh	31037	20521	34%	7,559	5172	3692	29%	42,013	1293	515	60%	3,01,186
Uttarakhand	2341	1848	21%	3,802	351	257	26.8%	27,337	87	59	32%	1,19,078
EAG states combined	98480	68178	30.8%	6,423	15957	10807	32.3%	40,518	3987	2073	48%	2,11,231
All India-EAG	90614	80188	11.5%	4,928	14608	13242	9.4%	29,845	3644	2760	24.3%	1,43,191
All India	189094	148366	23%	5,615	30565	24049	26%	34,641	7631	4833	40%	1,72,375

Source: all figures are taken/calculated on the basis of figures in Table 11, RHS Bulletin, 2012, MOHFW, GOI [2].

TABLE 3: Some of the deficiencies in the available infrastructure.

Indicator	Shortfall
% of subcenters without ANM	3.2%
% of PHCs without doctor	3.8%
% subcenters without regular water supply	25.5%
% subcenters without electric supply	25.5%
% subcenters without all whether motor able roads	6.6%
% of PHCs without regular electric supply	8%
% PHCs without regular water supply	10.7%
% PHCs without all-weather motor able roads	5.8%

Source: RHS Bulletin, 2012, MOHFW [2].

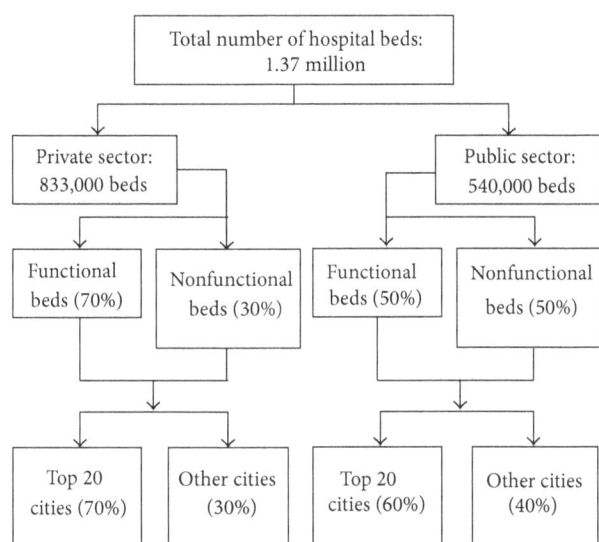

FIGURE 1: Distribution of available hospital beds in India. Source: [8].

existing facilities. It is very much possible that if the facility has one resource, it may not have other resources to optimally utilize the available resources; for example, if a health worker is available at the facility, it may not have water/electricity, thus undermining the ability of the health worker to perform his/her functions optimally.

Mismatch in the spatial distribution of infrastructure is another factor that magnifies the deficiency of infrastructure. Figure 1 illustrates this aspect very well. One can clearly see that there is a concentration of available beds in a tiny proportion of bigger cities. If the same beds were to be more equitably distributed between cities and between urban and rural areas, availability of the same infrastructure would have gone a longer way in ameliorating the curative needs of the people. However, this state of affairs is a logical outcome of the development paradigm pursued in the country rather than an inadvertent occurrence.

A comparison of availability of hospital beds per 1000 population between India and some of the much poorer countries (Table 4) offers a hitting comment on the sufficiency of country's health infrastructure. Many of the sub-Saharan countries and a country as impoverished as Timor-Leste seem to be doing much better.

3.2. Deficient Manpower. Deficiency of human resources in health adds further insult to injury caused by deficiency of health infrastructure. Deficiency of human resources in health occurs at several levels—between regions, between rural and urban areas, and between the public and private sectors. On the one hand, there is unwillingness of doctors and other health personnel to serve in rural areas; on the other hand, even in the urban areas, there is a preponderance of the health manpower in the dominant for profit private health sector in the country, thereby putting their services beyond the reach of the majority of poor in the country.

The deficiency of specialists in rural healthcare is as high as more than 90 percent in Chhattisgarh, Jharkhand, and Rajasthan, while being at nearly 86 percent in Uttarakhand, and Odisha. The interregional disparities are also explicit with there being a wide gap in the deficiency of both the specialist and graduate doctors between the EAG and the non-EAG states. Even though there seems to be an excess of GDMOs in Bihar and a relatively less shortfall in Jharkhand as against the required posts, this is highly misleading as the overall physicians per 10,000 population ratio remain dismal at .5 for both the states. The "required" here signifies required as against the sanctioned posts and not requirement as per some population norm. For example, the total rural population of Bihar was 92.07 million as per 2011 census, whereas the total number of required doctors (specialists and GDMOs) in rural health set-up as per Table 5 is only 2773. This would amount to only .3 doctors per 10,000 rural populations which by no standard is desirable. Even after seven years of implementation of NRHM (National Rural Health Mission), there remains a wide gap in the availability of allopathic doctors in the rural areas between the non-EAG states and EAG states. In the former, it is 2.25 times more.

Despite deficiencies in their training as managerial physicians, doctors have generally come to be perceived as responsible members of health care team comprising paramedical and other supportive staff. They are expected to lead the way in problem solving and supervising the work of other team members. As such, deficiency of doctors, besides impacting the delivery of curative services, may also reflect adversely in the overall functioning of the health team.

Deficiency of health personnel is by no chance limited to doctors alone. Figure 2 illustrates the shortfall in various categories of paramedical personnel in the public sector rural healthcare system. It may be pointed here that some of the countries such as Soviet Union in the immediate aftermath of Bolshevik revolution and China made up for the deficiency in strength of doctors by training and deploying a huge cadre of paramedical public health personnel in the poorly served areas.

Shortage of manpower is only made worse by the absence of a comprehensive and integrated health manpower policy dealing with health manpower requirement projection, manpower production, training, recruitment, career development, supportive supervision, skill enhancement, postings in underserved areas, retention and transfers, and so forth [16, 17]. This remains the state of affairs in spite of a number of official committees having stressed the need for such a policy

TABLE 4: A comparison of the availability of hospital beds for selected countries.

Country	Timor-Leste	Gabon	Equatorial Guinea	Djibouti	Kenya	Botswana	Zambia	India
Beds/1000 population	5.9	6.3	2.1	1.4	1.4	1.8	2	0.9

Source: World Development Indicators, World Bank DataBank [3].

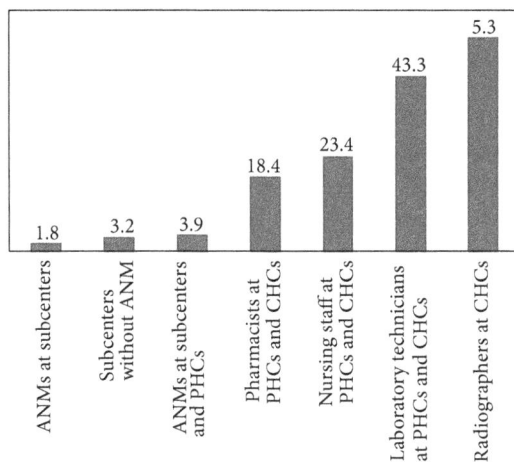

FIGURE 2: Shortfall in various categories of paramedical staff in rural healthcare set-up, all India. Source: based on figures in RHS Bulletin, 2012 [2].

beginning with the Bhore Committee Report of 1946 itself [18].

The skewed distribution of the available health cadre of different categories which has left the rural, tribal, and hilly areas grossly underserved is a direct consequence of deficiency of human resources and a lack of integrated health manpower resource development policy. The density of doctors is four times and that of nurses is three times higher in urban areas as compared to the rural areas [19]. According to WHO, of the 57 countries facing human resources in health crisis, India's ranking is 52nd [20].

Statistics by themselves may still not bring forth the acuteness of the challenges as perhaps the description of the ground realities can. While working as a consultant at the National Health Services Resource Center (NHSRC), the author had the opportunity to visit many health facilities in different districts of Uttar Pradesh and Uttarakhand. The following are observations from some of the visits.

(i) During a monitoring visit in June 2013 by the author to the district hospital in Pithoragarh district of Uttarakhand state, it was found that the doctors and the employees of the hospital were on strike in protest against roughing up of some hospital staff by the relatives of an 18- or 19-year-old boy who died the previous night of some complication following the operation for abdominal/inguinal hernia (a simple and routine surgery provided that there is no strangulation of the intestines at the hernia site).

At the time the boy died, there were only two nurses, one in the casualty of the hospital and the other to take care of admitted patients, in various wards, in a 120-bed hospital. After the regular working hours there is only one doctor available for all these patients, which is too in the emergency. So in the absence of doctors and nurses in the wards after routine hours, it is for the attendants to be able to locate them in the hospital in case their patient requires medical attention, provided of course that the attendants are able to judge the criticality of their patient's discomfort.

(ii) Likewise, in the 100-bed district women hospital at Jhansi, after four p.m., there is only one nurse (who was working on contract basis at the time of the author's visit) to take care of the labor room, the ward, and an occasional cesarean section that may take place. 100 beds do not mean only 100 patients, because one needs to count the babies of the delivered mothers as well, who require even greater medical attention.

(iii) The conditions at the 100 bed "Mahatma Gandhi Smarak District Hospital" at Naugarh, the district headquarter of Siddharthnagar district in UP, are even worse. The patients are pretty much on their own after 4 p.m. as the only available nurse is kept busy in the labor room, while the doctor mans the emergency. The hospital had just 5 nurses on its rolls at the time of writing to provide all the nursing care required at the hospital.

(iv) Almost similar conditions were to be found at district general and the district women hospital in Faizabad district of Uttar Pradesh. According to the information provided by the hospital authorities in February 2013, there had been 26 maternal deaths at the hospital in the last one year out of a total of 5860 deliveries that took place at the hospital. This works out to a maternal mortality rate of a whopping 443.7 per 100,000 live births.

(v) There was just one obstetrician and gynecologist in both Pithoragarh and Siddharthnagar districts to cater to cases requiring cesarean deliveries. The specialist in Pithoragarh was putting up around 580 km away from her family in Gwalior, situated in Madhya Pradesh state. She was forthright, "had I been posted in plain areas I could have at least visited my family easily; I am only biding my time and shall leave the moment I get a more suitable job."

Irrespective of the high tech nature of modern healthcare delivery, it is the personnel, who wield the technology to provide services, who matter the most. The impact of deficiency or absence of one category of health personnel is not restricted to "a particular service" delivery but impacts

TABLE 5: Number of specialists and MBBS doctors serving in public sector rural health care in the EAG states, non-EAG states, and all India.

State	CHCs Specialists		CHCs GDMOs*		PHCs GDMOs		Total GDMOs		Shortfall Specialists	Shortfall GDMOs	Physicians per 10,000 rural population
	Req.	In pos.	Req.	In pos.	Req.	In pos.	Req.	In pos.	%	%	
Bihar	420	151	490	451	1863	3532	2353	3983	64%	−69.3%	0.5
Chhattisgarh	894	71	1043	347	755	435	1798	782	92%	56.5%	0.4
Jharkhand	1128	86	1316	757	330	407	1646	1164	92.4%	29.3%	0.5
Madhya Pradesh	1998	267	2331	678	1156	814	3487	1492	86.6%	57.2%	0.3
Odisha	2262	317	2639	278	1226	1069	3865	1347	86%	65.15%	0.5
Rajasthan	2292	148	2674	265	1528	1755	4202	2020	93.5%	51.9%	0.4
Uttar Pradesh	3090	1740	3605	167	3692	2861	7297	3028	43.7%	58.5%	0.3
Uttarakhand	354	51	413	40	257	205	670	245	85.6%	63.4%	0.4
EAG states total	12438	2831	14511	2983	10807	11078	25318	14061	77.2%	44.5%	0.4
Non-EAG states	6894	3027	19320	6928	13242	17906	32562	24834	56.1%	23.7%	0.9
All India	19332	5858	33831	9911	24049	28984	57880	38895	69.7%	32.8%	0.6

Source: based on data taken from RHS Bulletin, 2012 [2]. Note: to calculate the required strength of specialists and GDMOs, we have multiplied the strength recommended as per the IPHS (Indian Public Health Standard) norms, given in Annexure 1 of the same source, with the number of CHCs and PHCs given in Statement 1 of the same source. The required strength of doctors at PHC and CHC as given in Statements 6 and 7, respectively, of the same source has not been considered here as the same is grossly below the recommended IPHS norms. GDMO* is the general duty medical officer and in the case of CHCs it includes one dental officer.

TABLE 6: Deficiencies in functioning of PHCs and CHCs in India.

Primary health centers	
PHCs without residential quarter for medical officer	45.5%
PHCs that did not provide 24-hour services	47.3%
PHCs conducting less than 10 normal deliveries in a month	50%
Community health centers	
CHCs not performing even normal delivery services	10%
CHC not designated as first referral units (FRUs)	48%
CHCs functioning without an obstetrician/gynecologist	74.8%
CHCs without a functional operation theatre	34.8%
FRUs having blood storage facilities	9.1%
FRUs without 24-hour new born care facilities	23.9%

Source: GOI, 2010 [4]. Note: these statistics are of a time of the beginning of NRHM; there may have been marginal improvement over the period of implementation of NRHM but comparable national level statistics for a later period are not available. Anyhow, it is nobody's claim that the implementation of NRHM has reduced the workload on public health facilities in bigger urban centers, especially, as almost the entire focus of NRHM has been on improving the maternal and child health services and in that also on improving the rates of institutional deliveries with the objective of reducing the maternal and infant mortality. Unfortunately, even the delivery of these services remains far from desirable and of equivocal quality.

the integrated nature of functioning of a modern hospital. Moreover, deficiency of personnel means overburdening of the personnel who are present and who have to work under intense pressure of various kinds. This cannot but have a negative impact on the morale of the health workers. The medical officer in charge of the CHC at Baijnath in district Bageshwar, Uttarakhand, lamented that: "given the patient load and strength of doctors at my facility I am hardly able to give a minute per patient in the OPD; this makes me wonder what the worth of my work is; what quality of services are we providing?"

3.3. Unmanageable Patient Load. Secondary or tertiary level public hospital in bigger cities is today bursting at seams due to a heavy rush of patients. The huge unplanned increase of Indian cities has resulted in urbanization of rural poverty causing expansion of slums and marginal populations starved of health and other basic amenities. Deficiency of urban health infrastructure, overcrowding in hospitals, lack of outreach, and functional referral system, standards, and norms for urban health care delivery system, social exclusion, unavailability or ignorance of information for accessing modern health care facilities, and lack of purchasing power are some of the issues that have been identified as challenges to urban healthcare in the country [21]. These factors are further complicated by poorly functioning subcenters, PHCs, and CHCs resulting in people from rural areas having to increasingly depend on hospitals in the bigger cities and towns for their curative needs thereby stretching the infrastructure at these hospitals to limits. Some idea of the level of functioning of peripheral health facilities in India can be had from Table 6.

Problems reflected in Table 6 are further accentuated by high rates of absenteeism among health workers. According to a nationally representative survey conducted in 2003, nearly 40 percent of the doctors and other health service providers were found to be absent from their posts on a typical working day. While absenteeism among doctors varied between 30 percent in Madhya Pradesh and 67 percent

in Bihar (the figure on availability of GDMOs, given in Table 5, in excess of requirement out to be viewed in this context); it was found to be 30% among pharmacists and laboratory technicians [22].

The pattern of organization of the health services into primary, secondary, and tertiary levels implies a referral system between these levels such that the patients who cannot be handled at the primary or secondary levels can be referred to the higher levels for appropriate management. Referral system, however, does not imply exclusivity between different levels of health care. Rather it entails an active cooperation between them which is necessary for the development of the health services system as a whole. In this respect, the Bhore Committee Report states the following.

"The heads of different sections in the district hospitals dealing with medicine, surgery and so on ... it will be of advantage if they can occasionally visit the secondary unit hospitals and a certain number of primary unit hospitals and inspect and guide the professional work of officers discharging corresponding duties in these hospitals. Such contacts should help to improve the standard of professional work carried out in the hospitals of the districts generally" [1, Page 21].

Apart from this, the committee also laid stress on the need for the tertiary level hospitals to play a role in the training and continuing skill enhancement for different categories of health personnel [23, Page 22].

Contrary to this there is hardly a "referral system" worth its name that operates in the public health set-up of the country. Rather the poor functioning or even the absence of the peripheral health services in large parts leaves no alternative before the people but to throng to the already overstretched facilities of bigger hospitals in towns and cities, bringing about a marked deterioration in their functioning.

A study conducted at three referral hospitals in Lucknow district showed that nearly 90 percent of the patients coming to these hospitals were new patients and, of these, two thirds had reached directly without any referral. Overall, only around a tenth of all patients attending these hospitals had been referred by someone, while the rest were all self-referred [24].

This trend is further worsened by some of the policy prescriptions of the government. For example, during a field visit to one of the "empowered group states" of north India by the author, the principal secretary health of the state in a meeting acknowledged the immense pressure on the largest public hospital in the capital of the state on account of the "Janani Suraksha Yojana," an institutional delivery scheme, under NRHM (National Rural Health Mission), sponsored by the central government to reduce the maternal mortality and the neonatal mortality rates. Because of the nonfunctioning or under performance of the peripheral health institutions as delivery points and the assistance of a government sponsored ambulance service, there had been such a rush of maternity cases to the hospital that the doctors pleaded: "for God's sake stop this madness." Another fall out of this scenario has been that the ambulance service sponsored by the state has established a world record in "deliveries conducted on way" to the hospital [25].

While decline in the maternal and infant mortality rates due to this scheme is circumspect, it has surely stretched the services of the state's tertiary healthcare services beyond capacity.

3.4. Equivocal Quality of Services. Patient load much in excess of what the infrastructure is capable of handling is bound to undermine the quality of care. "Chacha Nehru Bal Chikitsalaya," a Delhi government run child care hospital in east Delhi had much to celebrate when it became the first public hospital in the capital to be accredited by the National Accreditation Board for Hospitals (NABH). However, with the patient load bursting at its seams, the hospital soon found itself struggling to survive. Till date it has been difficult to arrange sufficient resources for the much required expansion of infrastructure to cope with the rush of patients [26].

Apart from general deficiencies in the development of public health infrastructure in the country, there has been a particularly marked deterioration in services of public hospitals in more than two decades of pursuit of neoliberal policies in general and in health sectors as well which have been oriented towards the strengthening of private health care. The growing dominance of private healthcare has resulted in the molding of public hospitals also in the image of the private hospitals. Some of the steps in this direction have been outsourcing of many services in public hospitals such as security, laundry, cleaning, kitchen services, and, in later stages, even the diagnostic and curative facilities on public-private partnership mode. Progressive imposition of user charges is another of such features [27].

While there is no evidence of these measures having resulted in improvement of the services of public hospitals, there is every reason to believe that these measures have made the services of public hospitals more inaccessible to the common man. Despite the persistent rush of patients. Figure 3 shows that the proportionate share of public hospitals in

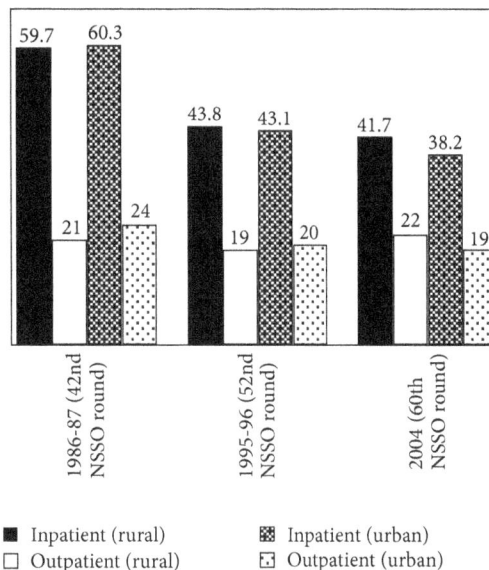

FIGURE 3: Inpatient and outpatient share of public hospitals in rural and urban areas. Source: [6].

hospitalized care has continued to decrease while it is about stagnant for outpatient care. Apart from this, the private sector has been poaching on the trained manpower of public hospitals to its expertise [28, 29] which cannot but be at a cost to the quality of services in public hospitals.

3.5. High Out of Pocket Expenditure. The last "National Health Accounts" for India published in 2004-05 unambiguously stated: "Among all the sources, households contributed a significant portion at 71.13% of total health expenditure for availing health care services from different health care institutions. This covers expenditure on inpatient, outpatient care, family planning, and immunization, and so forth" [30]. Table 7 gives some health spending patterns for selected group of countries, India and for India's neighboring countries. The only saving grace for India is that, among its neighbors, Pakistan and Myanmar spend lesser public resources on health than India. India's public health expenditure fails to match even that of the least developed countries and sub-Saharan Africa.

It is well acknowledged that catastrophic health expenditure is a significant cause for people being pushed below poverty line in India. Table 8 shows that 2.13 percent more people were pushed below poverty line on account of the out of pocket (OOP) expenditure on health between 1993-94 and 2004-05. The decade between 1993-94 and 2004-05 was the period when neoliberal economic reforms were on their zenith. The reading of the data in Tables 8, 9, 10, and 11, therefore, cannot but be with reference to the impact of these reforms on people's health condition.

During this period, there was increase in OOP expenditure as a proportion of the total household (HH) consumption expenditure across expenditure quintiles. Maximum increase was seen in the "richest" quintile.

Table 9 makes it evident that both inpatient and outpatient care is much costlier in private sector. If we see the

TABLE 7: Health spending indicators for selected group of countries, India and India's neighbors, 2010.

Country/Group of countries	Public health expenditure as % of GDP	Private expenditure on health as % of total expenditure on health	Out of pocket expenditure as % of private expenditure on health	Out of pocket expenditure as % of total expenditure on health
South Asia	1.08	70.9	80.7	61.5
India	1.06	71.8	86.0	61.8
Afghanistan	2.35	77.5	94.0	72.8
Bangladesh	1.35	63.5	96.6	61.3
Bhutan	3.60	15.4	94.7	14.5
China	2.70	45.7	77.2	35.3
Maldives	3.80	39.2	71.6	28.1
Myanmar	0.24	87.9	92.7	81.5
Nepal	1.89	62.6	90.4	56.6
Pakistan	0.79	71.8	88.0	63.2
Sri Lanka	1.57	54.4	81.9	44.6
Cuba	9.70	4.8	100	4.8
USA	8.49	51.8	22.7	11.8
OECD countries	7.94	37.4	—	—
Lower middle income countries	1.51	64.6	85.8	56.4
Low income countries	2.11	62.9	75.9	49.6
Least developed countries	2.18	60.9	80.7	50.5
Sub-Saharan Africa (developing countries)	2.8	56.8	62.8	30.9

Source: Health Nutrition and Population Statistics in World Bank DataBank. Available at http://databank.worldbank.org/data/views/variableselection/ selectvariables.aspx?source=health-nutrition-and-population-statistics on 15th August 2013.

findings of Tables 8 and 9 in light of Figure 3, it becomes clear that increasing share of private sector in provisioning of healthcare is, to a large extent, responsible for increasing OOP expenditure on health. With the position of public healthcare becoming even more dwarfed, the private sector has increasingly come to set the standards both for the care and its cost at terms congenial to its profits. Increasing commercialization of the services of public hospitals through measures like imposition of user charges at all levels under the impact of dominant private sector has heightened the challenges facing a public hospital in meeting the people's curative needs.

4. The Social and Political Origins of the Crisis of a Public Hospital

The present always originates from the womb of the past. In order to understand the origins of the challenges facing a public hospital, we need to put things in their historical perspective. It is instructive here to recall the famous minute of Thomas McCulay on education in India delivered on 2nd February 1835. Addressing the British Parliament, he said:

> "We must at present do our best to form a class who may be interpreters between us and the millions whom we govern; a class of persons, Indian in blood and color, but English in taste, in opinions, in morals, and in intellect" [31].

How well the designs of colonial masters have fructified is epitomized by the following words of our present Prime Minister which he said in Oxford on a visit during his first tenure as Prime Minister:

> "Today, with the balance and perspective offered by the passage of time and the benefit of hindsight, *it is possible for an Indian Prime Minister to assert* that India's experience with Britain had its beneficial consequences too. Our notions of the rule of law, of a constitutional government, of a free press, of a professional civil service, of modern universities and research laboratories have all been fashioned in the crucible where an age-old civilization met the dominant Empire of the day. These are all elements which we still value and cherish. Our judiciary, our legal system, our bureaucracy, and our police are all *great institutions*; derived from British-Indian administration and they have served the country well" [32].

Peoples' long experience of governance over 65 years since independence attests to the truthfulness of these words. There is much that can be said and demonstrated by way of highlighting the essentially reactionary character of India's ruling classes towards the overwhelming mass of impoverished Indians. Not all of that need be gone into here. Our intent is only to bring out this reactionary character since this

TABLE 8: Out of pocket (OOP) expenditure as a % of total household expenditure and impoverishment due to OOP.

Year	Mean OOP as % of total HH expenditure	Mean OOP as % of total HH expenditure by expenditure quintile					% HH having catastrophic expenditure at OOP expenditure >10% of total HH expenditure	People impoverished due to OOP
		Poorest	2nd poorest	Middle	2nd richest	Richest		
1993-94	4.39	3.25	4.19	4.68	5.23	5.45	15.12%	4.0%
2004-05	5.51	4.00	5.01	5.92	6.69	7.09	17.25%	4.4%

Source: Ghosh S., 2010 [5]. Note: the cross-sectional data taken by the author are taken from the fiftieth (1993-94) and sixty-first (2005) rounds of national and state representative surveys on "consumption expenditure," collected by the National Sample Survey Organization, India.

TABLE 9: Average medical expenditure (Rs) per hospitalization and nonhospitalization case.

Type of hospital	Expenditure per hospitalization case (Rs)				Expenditure per nonhospitalization case (Rs)	
	Rural		Urban		Rural	Urban
	2004	1995-96	2004	1995-96	2004	2004
Government hospital	3,238	2,080	3,877	2,195	11	7
Private hospital	7,408	4,300	11,553	5,344	246	299
Any hospital	5,695	3,202	8,851	3,921	—	—

Source: GOI, 2006 [6], Statements 28 and 32.

TABLE 10: Availability of allopathic doctors in the rural healthcare set up in India.

Year	2005[**]	2007	2008	2010	2011
Rural population	78,14,88,000[*]	79,99,05,000[*]	80,88,43,000[*]	82,61,73,000[*]	83,30,87,662
Total government doctors in rural health sector (a)	23,858	27,725	28,654	42,584	45.062
Doctors/1000 rural population	0.03	0.03	0.04	0.05	0.05
Total number of government allopathic doctors (b)	67576	76542	84852	85254	97648
Total number of allopathic doctors registered with IMC/SMCs in the country (c)	660801	731439	761429	846172	921877
Total number of allopathic doctors in urban areas (c−a)	636943	703714	732775	803588	876815
Ratio of the rural to urban allopathic doctors (c−a)/a	1 : 26.7	1 : 25.4	1 : 25.6	1 : 18.9	1 : 19.5

Source: [*] Figures for rural population for the respective year have been calculated from tables Projected Total Population by Sex in India (As on 1st March, 2001 to 2026) and Projected Urban Population by Sex in India (As on 1st March, 2001 to 2026) available from http://indiastat.com. [**] Figures for the year 2005 have been taken from the comparative tables available in Bulletin of Rural Health Services (RHS), 2011 [7]. Figures for the respective years have been taken from the RHS bulletin for the respective year. Note: It need be noted that the availability of doctors in rural health services is the availability as on records. However, there are large variations in the actual availability of doctors in the rural health institutions due to problems like absenteeism, unequal posting of doctors at different institutions. In some of the states, among the allopathic medical graduates posted at rural healthcare institutions, there are a good number of dental graduates who would find it difficult to handle many of the health problems of the people not covered by their discipline.
To calculate the total allopathic doctors (excluding dental surgeons) in urban areas we have presumed that the govt. doctors posted in rural areas are the only allopathic doctors in rural areas, which is largely true with some variations. As regards the availability of allopathic doctors in urban areas, the figures are only approximations because we have presumed that all the doctors registered with the medical councils and who are not serving in rural health services to be working in urban areas, whereas the fact is that a good number of them migrate out of the country.

has had implications for formulation of development policy in the country.

The very fact that Indian ruling classes have retained the colonial coercive machinery in letter and in spirit speaks volumes regarding their sincerity towards ensuring the welfare of India's impoverished masses. The following passage regarding the "Indian Police Act of 1861" brings forth the true meaning of "Our notions of the rule of law" that the Prime Minister spoke of at Oxford.

"The Indian Police Act of 1861 was primarily a mechanism to subjugate the people, and the traditional cooperation of the community was lost sight of in the concerns for law and order. The imperative need was to develop a sense of fear of authority in the entire population, and it was achieved through this system of ruler's police. The police were to be shaped as an instrument of the Raj, one where men were disciplined, armed and without hesitation would follow British officers' orders" [33].

The act per se continues to be in force ipso facto. The only difference is that the place of "British officer" has been taken by the "Brown Sahib." Little wonder then that between 2001 and 2010, 14,231 custodial deaths were recorded by National

TABLE 11: Top 5 countries for international medical graduates (IMG) physicians working in the United States.

Country	Total IMG physicians	% of total IMG population
India	51,447	20.7
Philippines	20,601	8.3
Mexico	13,834	5.6
Pakistan	12,111	4.9
Dominican Republic	7,979	3.2%

Source: Tables 1 and 2 in AMA, 2010 [9].
Total number of physicians in the USA: 985,375.
Total number of IMG physicians: 254,396 (from 127 countries).
% IMG physicians in USA: 26.0%.

Human Rights Commission (NHRC); that is, on an average, 4.33 person died in police and judicial custody in India every day [34]. We hope that this example would have carried through the point intended to be made. If not, we would further attempt to bring it home through examples specific to health policy paradigm that has been pursued in the country.

The recommendations of the Bhore Committee (its report was accepted by the government in 1946) constitute the most elaborate, liberal, and, by far, the most desirable of the schemes for the development of health sector in the country till date. And, yet, expressing its concerns regarding the population problem, the committee said:

"A reduction in the rate of growth of population may be brought about by permitting the death rate in the community to rise. Our social instincts militate against this … One of the objectives universally accepted in all civilized countries is the reduction of morbidity and mortality in the community. We have, therefore, to turn to other means of decreasing the rate of growth of population" [1, Pages 483-484].

It seems, but for the norms imposed by the civilized countries, that it might as well have recommended "letting the death rate to rise" as a means of controlling population growth. Their contempt for the people, nonetheless, is rather forthright. The committee states further:

"A birth control campaign has certain inherent dangers … Contraceptive practices are, therefore, more likely to be used by the more successful and intelligent sections of the community than by those who are improvident and mentally weak. It may also be mentioned that a certain number of defects, and diseases are known to be inheritable … The classes (emphasis ours) which processes many of these undesirable characteristics are known to be generally improvident and prolific (emphasis ours). A continued high birth rate among these classes, if accompanied by a marked fall in the rate of growth of the more energetic, intelligent and ambitious sections of the population, which make much the largest

contribution to the prosperity of the country, may be fraught with serious consequences to national welfare" [1, Page 487].

There need be no confusion as to which class is being despised—precisely, the one which depends most on the services of public sector healthcare. There is a continuum, between 1946 and today, in the contempt that the rulers reserve for the commonest of the common Indians. In 2009, our present *honorable* minister for health and family welfare at the centre had commented:

"If there is electricity in every village, then people will watch TV till late at night and then fall asleep. They won't get a chance to produce children … When there is no electricity there is nothing else to do but produce babies" [35].

4.1. Class Character of the Ruling Elite and the Development of Health Services in India. Unlike the bourgeoisie democracies of the West, the democratic form of government in India did not evolve as a result of a thorough going struggle encompassing commonest of the common Indians in struggle for their liberation. The bourgeoisie democratic "format" of polity in India was imposed by the colonial rulers from above and adopted as such by the native *"McCulaian"* elite. So while the better off among different sections of the society are coopted in the ruling structure, the vast base of the society remains undemocratic with there being little scope for the subaltern sections to assert themselves except within the limits defined by and the ways prescribed by the ruling classes.

True to their comprador class character, the rulers in India developed the healthcare system in the image of these systems as prevalent in the developed capitalist countries rather than develop a "healthcare system" that was sensitive to the local needs and relied on the resources available in the country.

India and China set out to meet their "tryst with destiny" as modern states almost at the same time, with China in fact being two years late in this regard, 1949 as against 1947 for India. Both were ancient civilizations and repositories of some of the most long standing indigenous systems of medicine that were rooted in popular culture and enjoyed widespread credibility among the people. The size of their populations, poverty, very low levels of development, widespread hunger, and disease were other features common to both. And yet the trajectories that health systems development took in either country were remarkably divergent.

China relied on a mix of modern medical knowledge and the indigenous knowledge systems to turn around the health of its predominantly rural masses, and the agents of this change were not the "medical doctors" imbued with the technical finesse and rigor of modern medicine but were the millions of "barefoot doctors" mobilized from among the impoverished, often illiterate peasant men and women, selected by their communities based on their willingness to serve the communities, educated and trained utilizing the resources the communities could afford with active support of the state. The indigenous medical knowledge systems were integrated on an equal footing with the modern medicine at all levels of health care, primary, secondary, and tertiary; and the science underlying these systems was developed and made explicit. Many of the barefoot doctors were supported by the state to go on and become full-fledged medical doctors only to come back to serve their communities [36, 37]. Most importantly this development was purely home grown, placing reliance almost exclusively on the indigenous resources.

India's trajectory provides a study in contrast. The Bhore Committee, which otherwise made some laudable recommendations, many of which flowed from the recommendations made by the Dawson Committee and the Beveridge Committee reports produced in England in the years 1920 and 1942, respectively, for the development of health services in the country, put its bet on "production of only one and that most highly trained type of doctor, which we have termed the "basic" doctor" (graduate of modern medicine) [1, Page 340]. As opposed to this the committee on "national health" of the "National Planning Committee" of the Indian National Congress proposed the following. "If medical advice and treatment to the mass of the people is [sic] to be provided on the necessary scale free of charge, the National Plan will have to bring the indigenous Vaidya, Hakim, or Dai into line with more elaborately or pretentiously trained physician or surgeon, gynecologist or obstetrician" [38].

That the rulers privileged the gold standard "basic doctor" over the latter could not have been without consequences; after all, which class of people could access and afford the opportunities to reach such a gold standard?

Mudaliar Committee opined "integration of Modern Medicine and Ayurveda is eminently desirable and all steps towards achieving that end should be promoted. Such integration should result in the development of a system of medical knowledge and practice based on all the best that is available in Modern Medicine and in Ayurveda" [39, Page 457]. But that such statements were meant for public consumption is evident from the assertion that "Participation in international health activities requires that the national health service in India should be based on modern medicine; ... the core of India's health service must continue to consist of persons adequately trained in Modern Medicine" [39, Page 458].

The policy proactively sought to make medical education the exclusive preserve of the well off. The Mudaliar Committee that followed the Bhore Committee endorsed the "opinion of the conference of principles of Medical Colleges that English should continue to be the medium of instruction in the medical colleges" [39, Page 327]. A further reflection of the mindset of the policy planners is evident from the following comment in the Mudaliar Committee report:

> "reservation for scheduled castes and backward communities, which is incumbent under the Constitution, have all tended to limit the number of well-qualified students being admitted to colleges" [39, Page 317].

Neither in 1960, when the Mudaliar Committee came out with its report, nor even today the vast multitudes of the working masses in India is endowed with proficiency in English language and indeed the worst of sections among them belong to the scheduled castes and the scheduled tribes. Hence, it is only the English speaking, urban based rich upper class, upper caste students who can aspire for the commanding positions in the health services/Health Policy System of the country or, for that matter, in any other field of governance or white collar professions.

This automatically divides the population into two sections: a miniscule minority of the well-endowed, urbane, civilized, intelligent, capable and meritorious herd of technocrats, bureaucrats, judiciary, industry captains, officers of the armed forces, doctors, engineers, academics, and so forth upon whom falls the task of caring for, tending, educating, civilizing, and developing the vast multitudes of the laboring poor who are deemed to be capable of doing little else than sell their labor. Much less than harness the energy and the potential of the poor to take their destiny in their own hands, such an institutionalized demarcation of the people places the downtrodden in perpetual positions of dependency. The "White Man's Burden" thus turned into the "Brown Sahib's Burden."

Elitism is not just a matter of social status or class one belongs to, but also how one conceptualizes the problems and their solutions. For the elite who came to occupy dominating positions in the health systems hierarchy of the country, setting up large tertiary care hospitals and medical colleges with sophisticated machinery/technology was a far greater priority than setting up primary healthcare centers and subcenters in rural areas; they had greater faith in technology driven vertical disease control programs, often imposed by international donor agencies, as an instrument of eliminating diseases rather than the general health systems strengthening down to the village level as the strategy of choice to overcome morbidity and mortality [40]. Banerji writes that the rulers quoted the recommendations of the Bhore Committee, often out of context, to draw legitimacy for their own plans to "establish a very large number of medical colleges with sophisticated teaching hospitals in urban areas. They also invoked the Bhore Committee to justify setting up an even more sophisticated All India Institute of Medical Sciences in New Delhi on the model of the Johns Hopkins Medical Centre of U.S.A (quoting Mudaliar committee report, Vol I, p 191 [39]). A number of other postgraduate centers for medical education were also set up in due course. It however, took them over seven years even to start opening primary health centers to provide integrated curative and preventive services to rural populations of the country. These primary health centers were a very far cry from what was suggested by the Bhore Committee" [41].

There is at times a tendency to get swayed by the "socialist" notions and phrase mongering regarding the leading role of the state in healthcare that were sought to be appendaged to these policies. With the benefit of hindsight, one can say that the great power rivalry of the bipolar world afforded our rulers the luxury of appropriating notions of welfarism unto themselves even as they persistently pursued policies to favor the big capital and the semifeudal forces in the country. The relative shifts between the left and the right in terms of policies were guided more by the desire to extract concessions from one or the other super power. However, the demise of Soviet Union has rendered the true nature of our ruling elite explicit, especially with the attendant ascendency of the neoliberalism as the dominant economic and social policy since early 1990s.

4.2. Elitist Medical Education. Banerji mentions two dia-metrically opposite social objectives of medical education: firstly, "to ensure that educational system prepares physicians who are specially molded to serve the requirements of the country" and, secondly, "to train professional physicians who are well versed with the knowledge of modern medicine in its most sophisticated forms and who are trained mostly to provide services to those who can afford to pay for such services" [42].

Tables 10 and 11 help us decipher which of the two social objectives has been met by the medical education system in this country. With concerted efforts to bring about "structural corrections" in the rural healthcare system in the country through NRHM, the doctors per 1000 population ratio in the country have barely gone up from .03 to .05. The total number of doctors available to serve more than 833 million rural population in the country in 2011 was a measly 45,062 while, in 2007, this figure was only 27,725. It is sobering to note that, in 2007, the number of Indian medical graduates working in the USA alone was more than 50,000 when the population of the USA was just above 300 million.

AIIMS, the medical institute modeled along the lines of John Hopkins Institute to train the model modern doctors for India, has indeed led from the front in bolstering the trend of migration of Indian doctors to greener pastures in the West. From 1989 to 2000, nearly 54% of the medical graduates from the institute migrated out of the country. From within these graduates, also, the ones from more well to do social backgrounds (the general category graduates were twice more likely to migrate than those coming from reserved categories) and the ones who performed better academically had a 35% greater chance of migrating compared to those who performed not so well [43].

Of the remaining graduate doctors in the country, nearly 74% live in urban areas serving a mere 28% of the population [44], assuming that the urban poor have the wherewithal to access their services. The elite capture of medical education has meant that doctors being produced in the country are largely from the privileged sections of the bigger cities. Present medical education inculcates in them an affiliation for technology driven costly curative care in the increasingly corporatized healthcare of the cities in India or the western shores. The rather drab illnesses of the rural folk that have their origins mainly in their poverty and malnutrition naturally fail to attract attention.

The careerist and commercial motivations inherent in such an education naturally undermine the more holistic concerns like the impact of poverty, caste, class, gender, and ethnic discrimination on health. This situation can only worsen further due to increasing commercialization of higher education that has already made it almost an exclusive preserve of the rich. There have been murmurs of

"reorienting" medical education and improving the clinical skills of medical graduates to address the health needs of the poor. However, these promises have proved illusionary till now.

4.3. Rural Urban Dichotomy in Health Services. It is in the nature of the systems based on exploitation that the backyards of exploitation be maintained to preserve the privileges of the privileged. Greater concern for the government is to first satisfy the needs of the urban elite. It is little wonder then that while the more affluent sections of the rural society have gained upward mobility and have managed to come closer to affording the amenities of the cities, including expensive curative facilities, but largely speaking, the colonial paradigm of rural urban dichotomy in provision of health services has continued till this day.

CEHAT (Center for Enquiry into Health and Allied Themes) undertook an exercise to disaggregate the health budget allocated to rural and urban areas from the finance accounts of five states from different parts of the country for the year 2002-03. The results are shown in Table 12.

In the rural urban distribution of health budget, it is noteworthy that, with the exception of Mizoram, in no other state is the rural health budget allocated in proportion to the size of the rural population which by far is much more than the urban population. Secondly, it may be noted that rural health budget is predominantly constituted of family welfare budgets, while, for the curative care, the budget is heavily loaded in favor of urban areas. It is our villages that are the forte of poverty, caste, illiteracy, malnutrition, and disease. Apparently, our planners are concerned about the proliferation of this population, hence, the need for increased allocation for family planning, whatever may become of the slogan, "development as the biggest contraceptive." Even if we were to disregard the concerns for functionality of rural beds, Table 13 further shows the preponderance of curative facilities in the urban areas, meaning thereby that rural urban dichotomy is intertwined with what may be called the curative-preventive dichotomy.

4.4. Curative-Preventive Dichotomy in Health Services. Beginning with Chadwick's sanitary reforms in England, the history of modern medicine is replete with evidence of how preventive measures have played a defining role in man's continuing struggle against disease, resulting in elimination of many diseases as public health problem in the industrialized West. Much later, countries like China and Cuba showed the way to improve the health of entire populations by prioritizing disease prevention through comprehensive public health measures and at a cost that is a fraction of spending otherwise incurred on cost intensive technological interventions.

In India, we seem to have learnt the lessons the other way around where medical technologies have become a substitute for taking action on more basic issues like water, sanitation, and nutrition. For example, the massive "Pulse Polio Program" has been pushing unprecedented doses of polio vaccine, disregardful of its impact on the disease epi-demiology, while it has nothing to offer as regards intervening

Table 12: Rural urban inequities in public health expenditure of selected states for the year 2002-03.

State/Type of expenditure		Medical care*	Public health	Family welfare#	MCH	Capital**	Total	Rural/Urban population
Maharashtra	Rural	5.71%	60%	49.97%	60%	0.78%	32.51%	66.57%
	Urban	94.29%	40%	50.03%	40%	99.2%	67.49%	42.43%
Mizoram	Rural	51.9%	51%	63.87%	51%	100%	55.68%	50.47%
	Urban	48.1%	49%	36.13%	49%	0.00%	44.32%	49.53%
Orissa	Rural	46.89%	80%	90.20%	80%	53.4%	58.89%	85.01%
	Urban	53.11%	20%	09.80%	20%	46.5%	41.11%	14.99%
Punjab	Rural	42.47%	66%	65.46%	0	0.00	45.00%	66.08%
	Urban	57.53%	34%	34.54%	0	100%	54.60%	33.92%
Tamil Nadu	Rural	18.96%	54%	73.07%	54%	75.0%	35.01%	55.96%
	Urban	81.04%	44%	26.49%	44%	24.7%	64.66%	44.04%
Madhya Pradesh	Rural	39.47%	73%	72.80%	73%	90.6%	50.03%	73.54%
	Urban	60.53%	27%	27.17%	27%	9.34%	49.96%	26.46%

Source: CEHAT, 2006 [10]. *Including health services both allopathy and other system of medicines, minor head includes ESIS, medical education department drug manufacture; #excluding MCH Program; **including capital expenditure of medical, public health, and family welfare. Proportions of rural and urban population are taken from CBHI, 2005 [11]. Note: demarcation for the rural and urban health budget was done from finance accounts 2002-03 for respective states. For about two-thirds of the expenditure, there is a clear rural-urban indication in the budget; for the rest, CEHAT used their functional knowledge of program implementation to allocate proportions to rural and urban areas.

Table 13: Number of government hospital beds in rural and urban areas.

State	Rural hospital beds (government)	Urban hospital beds (government)	Total beds (government)	Proportion of rural and urban beds
Bihar	1830	16686	18516	10 : 90
Chhattisgarh	3270	6158	9428	35 : 65
Jharkhand	N.A.	N.A.	N.A.	N.A.
Madhya Pradesh	10040	18493	28533	35 : 65
Odisha	7099	8715	15814	45 : 55
Rajasthan	13754	12236	25990	53 : 47
Uttar Pradesh	15450	40934	56384	27 : 73
Uttarakhand	3746	4219	7965	47 : 53
EAG states	55189	107477	162630	34 : 66
Non-EAG states	114673	511187	622310	18 : 82
All India	169862	618664	784940	20.5 : 79.5

Source: GOI, 2011 [12].

in the principle mode of transmission of polio that is fecooral transmission through contaminated water supply [45, 46]. Tackling the later would have benefits for host of other public health problems like diarrheal diseases, typhoid, and malnutrition. Likewise, the Revised National Tuberculosis Control Program (RNTCP) has placed its bet only on providing DOTS (directly observed therapy short course) while leaving untouched the conditions that give rise to tuberculosis. The result has naturally been a rising mortality due to TB [47] and an increasing morbidity due to multidrug resistant tuberculosis [48]. Undermining disease prevention only leaves us to tackle greater burden of morbidity and mortality at later stages and thereby bringing the curative facilities under severe strain.

Table 14, based on figures given in Table 3.7, National Health Accounts of India, 2004-05, gives the health expenditure by different ICHA (International Classification of Health Accounts) functions. Of the total health budget, the preventive functions command barely 20.78 percent of the budget while curative services corner close to 50 percent of the budget. The relatively higher proportion of preventive health care spending of the central government is on account of the fact that all the "National Disease Control Programs" are funded by the center.

Nutrition program is included in "Health and Related Functions" but has been mentioned separately over here on purpose. It would hardly be an exaggeration to say that that "food is the basic medicine of public health" and yet, at conceptual and programmatic level, the health planners seem to have completely divorced themselves from this fact. It is true that there are supplementary nutrition programs run by other departments of the government, but should that be the reason why health policy establishment should almost give up on such a fundamental aspect, the impacts on the health of the people as nothing else does, only to focus on narrow technocentric approaches to alleviate the health problems of the people? It is anybody's guess as to the efficacy of complete immunization in a malnourished child.

TABLE 14: Health expenditure by ICHA functions, National Health Accounts, 2004-05.

Health care function		Proportion of budget spent		
		Center*	State	Total
HC.1	Curative care	22.16%	46.92%	42.67%
HC.2 and 3	Rehabilitative and long term nursing care	1.02%	0.13%	0.28%
HC.4	Ancillary services related to medical care	1.46%	2.50%	2.33%
HC.5	Medical goods dispensed to outpatients	2.01%	0.69%	0.92%
Subtotal	Curative health care services	**26.65%**	**50.24%**	**46.2%**
	Prevention and public health services			
HC.6	RCH and family welfare	24.23%	9.55%	12.07%
	Control of communicable diseases	14.64%	5.20%	6.82%
	Control of noncommunicable diseases	01.63%	0.76%	0.91%
	Other public health activities	1.24%	0.93%	20.78%
Subtotal	Preventive health care services	**41.74%**	**16.44%**	**20.78%**
HC.7	Health administration and insurance; health and related functions (medical education and training of health personnel, research and development, capital formation, and food adulteration control); functions from other sources; and functions not specified.	31.61%	33.21%	31.86%
	Nutrition program	—	0.10%	0.08%
Subtotal	Health functions other than curative and preventive	**31.61%**	**33.31%**	**31.94%**
Total		100	100	100

Source: GOI, 2004-05 [13].
Note: *is related to Ministry of Health and Family Welfare only.
(1) Services of curative care include expenditure on teaching hospitals, specialty hospitals, ESI dispensaries, homeopathic hospitals and dispensaries, ayurvedic hospitals and dispensaries, and primary health centers, community health centers, and expenditure on dental care.
(2) Rehabilitative care includes expenditure on rehabilitative centers for TB and leprosy patients, institute for rehabilitation of physically handicapped, and drug deaddiction programs.
(3) Ancillary services related medical care includes expenditure on blood banks, blood transfusion council, regional diagnostic centers, ambulance related expenditure, and medical store depot.
(4) RCH and family welfare covers expenditure on RCH and family welfare programs.

4.5. Market Led Growth of Health Care in India. There is a large body of literature internationally and from India [27, 49–55] that attests to the devastating effects of market led growth of healthcare. The biggest blow that globalization has delivered to healthcare systems is that it uprooted healthcare from its moorings in "social justice" and "service" to humanity and legitimized it as a source of extracting profits. As already mentioned above, this paradigm shift governs not only the private sector but has extended to the public sector healthcare in form of commercialization of its components/ services. Paradoxically the public sector has proved to be a supporting pillar for private health care in the country. Public sector medical colleges contributed hugely to the growth of the private sector with 80 percent of the doctors passing out of these colleges either joining the private sector or migrating abroad [53, Page 24].

Even though the private healthcare always constituted larger part of the healthcare system in India, with the advent of globalization, big corporate houses entered into healthcare provisioning and have increasingly came to influence health policies and set standards of care that are far removed from the real life conditions of common Indians. Private sector constitutes eighty percent of the health sector in India [56]. Corporate healthcare is pushing high end technologies in both diagnostics and treatment irrespective of their desirability for the profile of public health problems in India. Additionally, pushing of unjustifiable high end technologies is a drag on precious public resources for health in the form of either direct or indirect tax concessions on their import and operation and through public-private partnerships doled out to the private sector.

Now, there is talk of the government turning itself into net purchaser of curative healthcare from the private sector while restricting itself to providing a small package of preventive services. This has been euphemistically termed as "managed care" [57]. Imposition and successive escalation of "user charges" levied for the services of publically financed health institutions is another feature of neoliberal economic policies that is the bane of the poor [58]. User charges have been beaten back to the extent people have forced the governments, through their struggles, to do so. The latest 7th Common Review Mission Report, which went into the implementation of National Rural Health Mission (NRHM) in different states, says that the governments in the states of Kerala and

Jharkhand have withdrawn user charges from public facilities [2].

With corporate healthcare becoming the "prima donna" of healthcare industry in the country, this has consequences for the motivation of public sector health workers in dedicating themselves to the more holistic motives of public healthcare. Motivation of workers critically impacts the performance of health sector since efficiency, equity, and service quality, all, are directly transacted by the willingness of the workers to dedicate themselves to their tasks [59]. Apart from individual level determinants, worker motivation is determined by "organizational (work context) level, and determinants stemming from interactions with the broader societal culture" [59].

The "broader societal culture" of healthcare today is being tempered by the commercialized ethos of private healthcare. For example, while the healthcare system allows (implicitly or explicitly) a number of extraneous incentives, varying from systems of commissions from private diagnostic labs to outright bribes by drug and medical equipment manufacturers for the doctors, not because of the work that they may do towards furthering patient care but because of the position they occupy in the medical system, similar opportunities, however, are not available to the other categories of hospital staff, who may then feel tempted to resort to more crude and direct extraction of money from the patients.

In either case, personal aggrandizement becomes the desired social objective and any improvement in the societal wellbeing becomes contingent upon the fulfillment of the former. These are not inadvertent outcomes but are the result of the policies that have been pursued over the years. Developing markets in healthcare have become the conscious objective of the economic and health policy of the state. Today, the price for which the private sector plucks top notch consultants from the public hospitals is considered a measure of the doctor's professional capabilities. The government, on its part, feigns helplessness in spite of the fact that it spent a considerable sum of people's money in, first, training these consultants and, then, providing them with the facilities of public hospitals to hone their clinical skills. The private sector gobbles up the talent for virtually no cost to it.

Another insult to injury that has been added during the implementation of the neoliberal economic policies since the beginning of the 1990s has been the large scale hiring of the contractual staff at all levels for work profiles that are perennial in nature. The contract paramedical and medical staff feels exploited even as they do more work compared to the regular health workers for lesser remuneration and facilities. Such medical and paramedical health workers hardly visualize their future with the growth of the public hospital or public health system. For them, such an engagement is a stop gap measure which they must utilize for maximizing personal welfare rather than the welfare of their patients.

In all these years, there has not been a single study to show that hiring staff on contractual basis has helped in increasing the patient care or efficiency of the hospitals. Yet the myth keeps getting reinforced that contractual staff can be made to work better than the regular staff, because it suits the convenience of the government and the administrators.

The "private medical sector" has proved to be the proverbial "camel" that has pushed the Arab (the "public medical sector") out of the tent.

4.6. Deficiency of Political Will. As goes the adage—"where there is a will, there is a way"; equally true is our contention— *"where there is no will, there are alibis and subterfuge, albeit in the form of elaborate schemes."* No government in India since 1947 transfer of power has failed in expressing its solidarity with the Indian masses in terms of alleviating their suffering. On the face of it, they still remain committed to increase welfare spending cutting across political spectrum. However, failure to achieve, till date, even the goals and targets laid out for the first ten-year period after independence in the Bhore Committee Report is equally eminent.

In 1977, the India's ruling classes committed themselves to the Alma Ata Declaration on achieving "Healthcare for All by the year 2000" through the strategy of "primary health care." No sooner than this commitment was made that our ruling elites jumped on to the bandwagon of "selective primary health care" that was sponsored by the American foundations and multinational vaccine corporations. The year 2000 came and went, but the goals of neither the "primary health care" nor its "selective" variant were achieved.

In 2002, the then Bhartiya Janata Party led National Democratic Alliance government at the Centre came up with the "National Health Policy." This was followed soon by the "National Common Minimum Program" of the first "United Progressive Alliance" government at the Centre that was eminently supported by the Parliamentary Left in 2004. The "National Health Policy, 2002" and the "Common Minimum Program" of the first "United Progressive Alliance" government at the Centre promised to increase the health spending to a level of 2 to 3 percent of the GDP by 2010 [60]. A huge program for the renewal of rural health care in the country was launched in the form of National Rural Health Mission (NRHM) in 2005. Having finished its first phase of seven years in 2012 without having been able to achieve even one of the goals set before it, NRHM is now into its second phase. Yet the pious objective of taking the public health expenditure in the country to 2 to 3 percent of the GDP continues to evade the country.

At the time of rolling out the process of preparing their "Program Implementation Plans" (PIP) for the implementation of NRHM during the financial year 2013-14, the states were instructed that they could increase their expenditure under NRHM up to 30 percent over the baseline of 2012-13. However, the economic slowdown hit back in the meanwhile and, by the time of actual allocation of central assistance to different states, the officials of the Ministry of Health and Family Welfare bluntly told the states that no increase in allocation would be possible (the author was privy to these developments while working as a consultant with National Health Systems Resource Center, Government of India).

Apart from indicating the financial resources committed for health, the health budget is also the single most important measure of the political commitment of the rulers to improve the health of the people. Government's backing off from offering even a very modest increase in the budget for rural

TABLE 15: Cuba's total government expenditure and expenditure on social services (including health) and defense during the special period (in millions of current Cuban Pesos).

Year	Total government expenditure	Expenditure on defense/internal order	Expenditure on social services (education and health)
1989	14041	1269 (9.04%)	2576 (18.35%)
1990	13852	1120 (8.1%)	2492 (18.00%)
1991	15436	925 (6.0%)	2548 (16.50%)
1992	14312	746 (5.2%)	2395 (16.70%)
1993	12564	615 (4.9%)	2123 (16.90%)
1994	10035	461 (4.6%)	1696 (16.90%)
1995	8866	392 (4.42%)	1584 (17.90%)
1996	8326	323 (3.9%)	1697 (20.4%)
1997	8368	421 (5.03%)	1797 (21.50%)
1998	8344	343 (4.1%)	1823 (21.80%)

Source: based on data given in Table V, Dunning, 2001 [14].

TABLE 16: India's total government expenditure and expenditure on social services (including health) and defense during the economic crisis of early 1990s (in billion current Rupees).

Year	Total government expenditure	Defense expenditure	Social services expenditure
1989-90	929.08	144.16 (15.5%)	30.61 (3.3%)
1990-91	1052.98	154.26 (14.6%)	32.74 (3.1%)
1991-92	1114.14	163.47 (14.7%)	35.69 (3.2%)
1992-93	1226.18	175.82 (14.3%)	40.09 (3.3%)
1993-94	1418.53	218.45 (15.4%)	48.30 (3.4%)
1994-95	1607.39	232.45 (14.5%)	58.73 (3.7%)
1995-96	1782.75	268.56 (15.1%)	76.55 (4.3%)
1996-97	2010.07	295.05 (14.7%)	96.72 (4.8%)
1997-98	2320.53	352.78 (15.2%)	118.45 (5.1%)
1998-99	2793.4	398.97 (14.3%)	146.56 (5.2%)

Source: based on figures taken from Tables 103 and 104, RBI, 2012-13 [15].

healthcare in the country at the first whiff of an economic slowdown, even as it continues to offer tax exemptions to the most wealthy in the country to the tune of lakhs of crores of rupees, shows the shakiness of their political commitment to the welfare of the people.

As to the possibility of doing things differently, we present the comparison between Cuba and India to underscore what political commitment to health care means. It is well known that Cuba went through a sudden and catastrophic economic crisis in the early 1990s due to the collapse of the Soviet Union and, along with it, the collapse of preferential trade and economic aid Cuba received from the Soviets. The Cuban economy contracted suddenly and rapidly. These are the kind of trying circumstances that test the commitment of governments to ensure human well-being as reflected by the resources committed for the same. Generally speaking, the experience is that, in times of economic crisis, expenditure on welfare (health, education, and food) is the first to come under knife, precisely, at a time when the people, especially the poor, need greater protection.

Beginning 1990s, India also faced an onerous economic crisis which queered the pitch for neoliberal economic reforms in the country. Tables 15 and 16 present the response of the governments of Cuba and India towards ensuring human welfare under such trying circumstances. After the economic crisis, during the special period, the total government expenditure declined continuously till 1998 in comparison to the base year of 1989, except for a marginal increase in 1991 and 1992. There was also an absolute decline in expenditure on social services, almost continuously till 1994, after which the absolute budgetary allocation for social services started increasing once again even though the total budget of the government was still contracting in comparison to that of the base year. As a proportion of total government expenditure, however, expenditure on social services started recovering from 1992 itself. The budget on social services varied between 16.5 and nearly 20 percent. Cuba severely compromised on its defense budget which reduced from 9.04 percent of the total government expenditure in 1989 to 4.1 percent in 1998. This is exceptional given the geopolitical situation of Cuba, especially at a time when it was most vulnerable to US hostility.

With respect to India, the situation is almost the reverse. Our defense expenditure has consistently varied between 14 and 15.5 percent during the 1990s, whereas expenditure on social services hovered between 3 and 5 percent.

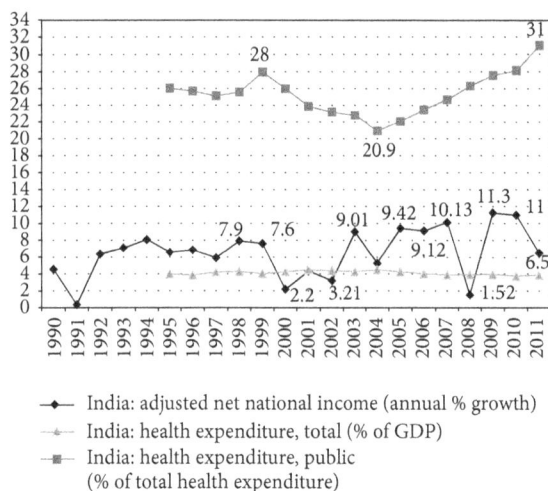

FIGURE 4: Variation in India's health expenditure with GDP growth rate. Source: all the figures have been obtained from Health Nutrition and Population Statistics in World Bank DataBank. Available at http://databank.worldbank.org/data/views/variableselection/selectvariables.aspx?source=health-nutrition-and-population-statistics since 15th August 2013.

Figure 4 shows that India's public expenditure on health reached its nadir in 2004 when it accounted for barely 21 percent of the total health expenditure. Between 2004 and 2011, this proportion increased from 21 percent to 31 percent, which can easily be attributed to NRHM. However, the overall impact of this increase can be judged from the fact that it has made little difference to the overall expenditure on health in India. In fact, there is a slight negative slope between 2004 and 2011 in the graph as regards this. What is particularly noteworthy is that the phenomenally high economic growth rates observed in the country during 1990s and 2000s seem to have made little difference to the overall resources being committed for health. An increase of 10 percent in public expenditure as a proportion of total expenditure on health is too little too late and even this could well be set to suffer rollback in face of economic uncertainties that currently face the country.

5. What Are the Solutions to Alleviating These Challenges?

Before we go on to discuss the possible solutions to the crisis under discussion, one has to be a bit discerning regarding what is remediable and what is remediable and what is not under the given social, political, and economic system in the country. Tackling factors like class character of the ruling elite and their orientation towards development issues is a far more complex issue that can hardly be remedied by some policy initiatives. The policy orientation of the ruling classes also depends on larger global geopolitics. Bringing about a longer lasting change in their character, however, entails a political process which is beyond the pale of our discussion here, except that an understanding of these issues enables us to make realistic assessments and policy choices that are

feasible, besides aligning ourselves with the larger processes of political change. As a corollary, it also follows that even the most liberal of the policy regime that can be pursued in the given system shall constitute only a partial solution of the crisis. However, even these partial solutions are worth pursuing in so far as they hold the promise of bringing some relief to the people from the present neoliberal policy regime.

Having placed this caveat we can say that the policy instruments to improve the functioning of the public hospitals cannot but flow from an understanding of the consequences of the factors that constitute the crisis and their social and political origins. The solutions would essentially lie in instituting policies that would reverse these consequences.

The most fundamental premise underling these solutions is that the provision of food, health care, water, sanitation, and education, the most important factors impacting on health outcomes, ought to be ensured as a matter of right, free from profit motives. Further, only such measures can be acknowledged as solutions that are primarily responsive to epidemiological needs of the patients, rather than those that suit the exigencies of the health administrators.

It would be worthwhile to point out here the experience of India's biggest and most reputed public health institution—the All India Institute of Medical Sciences (AIIMS).

The doctors at AIIMS have been complaining since long that the huge daily rush of patients in the institute's outpatient department not only has worsened the standard of clinical care at the hospital but also leaves hardly the faculty with time to concentrate on medical research and teaching. This is defeating the most important role that the institute is supposed to perform—that of setting up model of patient care and medical teaching in the country.

While one can be at variance with the models they may have in mind, this is a perfectly legitimate concern of the faculty and administration at AIIMS. However, in response to this, various departments have arbitrarily decided to limit the number of patients registered daily in their outpatient departments. While this may have been expedient for institute administration to get over its problem, the remedy has turned out to be the quintessential double whammy for the patients who come from far corners of the country to seek treatment at AIIMS. Meanwhile, it seems unlikely that this solution will change things in any meaningful way. To the contrary, some senior doctors discovered (as personally told to the author) that this "solution" resulted in outpatient cards being sold at high premium by some unscrupulous employees.

Worse still, developing models for excellence inpatient care or for medical research in the country do not seem to be the important motivation behind such decisions. Most of the doctors have been passive in opposing the commercialization of services of such institutions or in opposing attempts at privileging industry interest in their research. Doctors have been raising their economic demands but invariably fail to demand alternative strategies that are expedient in tackling the high patient load or raise the issue of reinvigorating the peripheral healthcare institutions such that institutions like AIIMS do not end up performing the functions of general hospitals. In fact, the height of cynicism on these issues can be judged from a comment made by a senior ex-faculty-member of the institute in a conversation with the author. While lamenting over falling standards of patient care due to huge patient load, he went as far as to suggest the following: "let the patients die (due to limited registration of the patients), but the Institute must not let its standards be diluted." It is not our assertion that this is a view generalizable to all doctors at AIIMS; but this does certainly show how retrogressive the sentiment can get.

5.1. Suggestions for Reinvigorating Peripheral Services and Improving the Services of Public Hospitals. The challenges that confront functioning of public hospitals are vexed and, as such, cannot be addressed in their entirety within the development paradigm of the present ruling classes which has its roots in the class character of the Indian state. A comprehensive redress of the issues raised above shall entail nothing short of the remaking of the Indian state itself, which is a political process and, as such, is out of the scope of this paper. Accordingly, the possible solutions suggested here concern with policies that can provide some relief under the present conditions. This too goes with the caveat that the arraignment of political forces internationally and nationally, as it obtains today, does not forebode well even for these policy changes, which should, otherwise, have been possible in a liberal bourgeoisie framework of a welfare state. This only highlights the primacy of the political task mentioned above; howsoever much, we may disagree with it.

5.1.1. For Rejuvenating Peripheral Health Services

(i) The task of making the primary and secondary level health institutions functional ought to be the utmost priority, such that people can access effective healthcare for common and easily treatable conditions nearest to their homes.

(ii) Urgent steps need be taken to provide working and living conditions in the peripheral areas that will encourage doctors and other health personnel to be willing for rural service. Family hostels should be built in the nearby urban centers to house the families of doctors and other medical personnel, while they are posted in remote areas. State should ensure admission of their children in best schools in the area and other such facilities. It may be noted that such steps are routinely taken in the case of defense personnel.

(iii) All the vacancies for medical and paramedical posts should be filled promptly and the administrative procedures should facilitate speedier permanent appointments. There is little evidence to show that provision of ad hoc/contract appointments has led to a sustained availability of health personnel in rural areas.

(iv) Consequent to fulfillment of the aforementioned conditions, rural service should be made compulsory for health personnel of varying categories immediately after their graduation. There should not be waivers of any kind to allow the personnel to avoid doing such service.

(v) A much greater reliance should be placed on the training of a large number of paramedical personnel or on reviving licentiate courses to fill in the gap in the availability of primary level healthcare.

(vi) The capacity of peripheral health services should be expanded to absorb the large number of health workers as full time workers in the health services system. Private practice for any category of workers should not be allowed.

(vii) There should be regular programs organized wherein the senior doctors from the secondary or tertiary level health facilities and medical colleges should mandatorily go to the rural areas to help the peripheral health workers improve their knowledge and skills.

(viii) Once these conditions are realized, certain administrative steps can be undertaken to ensure a proper referral system for the patients from the most peripheral to the tertiary level institutions.

(ix) The local communities, peoples organizations, and representative bodies should be involved in "the planning, organization, operation and control of primary healthcare, making fullest use of local, national and other available resources" in the true spirit of the "primary health care" as enunciated in the Alma Ata Declaration of 1977 [61]. However, it need be stressed here that unless a fundamental reordering is brought about in the power relations of caste, class, gender, and community in the rural society, such kind of control and participation shall only be exercised by the presently dominant sections of the rural society.

(x) Public hospitals associated with large institutes or medical colleges should be encouraged to further strengthen their outreach services.

(xi) In order to ensure that things work as they ought to, a system of accountability should be in place with the guiding principle, firstly, that responsibility has to be fixed for the most empowered functionary rather than the one which is least empowered and, secondly, that no system of accountability can be enforced through policing oversight as the principle mechanism. In order that people are willing to stand accountable, it is of utmost importance to provide working environment that harnesses people's enthusiasm to work as per their respective capabilities.

It need be emphasized here that it is the engrained logic of the systems based on exploitative relations of production to believe that people work either in response to fear of authority or for individual material incentives. The fact, that to work and to indulge in a socially productive work is a fundamental human want which is least recognized in such systems.

5.1.2. For Improving Services at Public Hospitals

(i) To reinvigorate the positive spirit of Bhore Committee, it need be stressed that national health organization ought to be a "whole time salaried service devoting itself to the development of the health of the people." Hence, the provision of allowing private practice by the government doctors should be banned forthwith.

(ii) For maximal utilization of the infrastructure of public hospitals, provision should be made for both morning and evening OPDs. The necessary staff, equipment, and space should be provisioned for running such clinics and diagnostic set-up. Evening OPDs shall have the added advantage of obviating "opportunity costs" for the poor who have to miss their daily wage to attend to the hospital in the morning. It may be noted that if the private hospitals or diagnostic centers can operate such facilities, why should it be difficult for a public hospital to do so?

(iii) A number of modern technologies have become available over the years to improve the functioning of public hospitals. The guiding principle for their use should be that these technologies should be used to maximize the patient welfare, rather than for curtailing patient services.

Diagnostic equipment, like autoanalyzers that are now available, have replaced the manual diagnostic processes and can be deployed to do laboratory investigations round the clock without necessarily having to deploy larger manpower as was necessary with manual processes. This can be most expedient in arriving at an early diagnosis of ailment and facilitate setting up of evening OPDs. Likewise, use of information technology for improving the hospital records; for example, the laboratory or radiological investigations can be uploaded on central portal such that they are readily available to those who have to use the results of the investigations. Such a measure can be very helpful in preventing harassment to the patients that they face in tracing their reports, often ending up wasting days on this without actual movement in the treatment that they seek.

(vi) Last but not the least, all measures directed at commercializing the use of hospital services through imposition of user fees on patients should be rolled back. These are highly inefficient in providing cross subsidies to the poor patients and have grave implications for equity and access to healthcare [58].

The World Bank was the chief proponent of the imposition of user fees in public health services throughout the world. However, addressing the 66th World Health Assembly at Geneva on 21st May 2013, the World Bank President Jim Yong Kim said:

"Anyone who has provided health care to poor people knows that even tiny out-of-pocket charges can drastically reduce their use of needed services. This is both unjust and unnecessary" [62].

5.2. Reversing the Market Led Growth of Healthcare. Market led growth of healthcare is part of the economic agenda of the ruling classes and is motivated by their "class interests" which are in antagonistic relationship with the "class interests" of the working masses. Besides harnessing healthcare as a source of profit, the interest of the ruling classes is to provide exclusive services for the affluent sections while relegating public health services to a secondary status. The interest of the overwhelming masses on the other hand lies in provisioning of universal healthcare as a "societal good" irrespective of the individual's ability to pay.

If there is willingness to search for policy options based on the empirical examination of different policies that have been implemented in different parts of the world in different contexts, as also in our own country over the last two decades, maybe there can be some scope of reasoning our way through to secure the interests of the common people. Unfortunately, as things stand today, such a possibility does not seem to exist.

The lack of political will on part of the government to act in the interest of the vast majority of poor people is linked to class interests of the people it actually represents. In other words, the question is of class struggle which is part of larger political process. Here, we can only reiterate the need to choose sooner than later the side on whose behalf we would like to pitch in, in this struggle.

As regards the government, it has made its intensions very clear by the fact that the Planning Commission rejected the "High Level Expert Group (HLEG) Report on Universal Health Coverage for India" that was instituted by the commission itself.

The report, while being agreeable to private sector involvement in health sector, had recommended "expansion and augmentation of primary healthcare, strengthening of district hospitals, expansion and upgrading the skills of the health workforce, free provision of essential medicines, abolition of "user fees", establishment of effective regulatory structures and support for active community participation as high priorities requiring early action" [63]. Apart from the recommendation of contracting out services to the private sector wherever necessary, HLEG made a recommendation in stating that "every citizen should be entitled to assured free access to a package of essential health services, which will be periodically defined by an expert body, through a national health entitlement card (India Health Card). Public facilities for healthcare will have to be the main delivery system of UHC" [63].

However, no sooner were these recommendations made by HLEG than the system struck back. World Bank is reported to have said, "There is a growing number of high-quality, low-cost providers that may be willing to engage with the government in providing defined packages of care to the poor. Policies need to be in place to foster more effective engagement with the private sector" [64].

The Planning Commission was quick to put its emergency brakes on. In a meeting on 3rd February 2012, it briefed the PMO (Prime Minister's Office): "The HLEG excludes the possibility of contracting out of services to qualified providers . . . With 80% of doctors, 26% of nurses, 49% of beds, 78% of ambulatory services, and 60% of inpatient care, the private sector has to be partnered with healthcare delivery" [65]. The representatives of private healthcare industry had this to say, "Specialty and super-specialty areas should be left to private sector since the government can afford neither the infrastructure nor the salaries to retain the talent required for tertiary care" [65].

These developments regarding HLEG recommendations, which in no way sought to establish "socialism" in the realm of healthcare delivery in the country, only point to the tenacity with which we need to pursue the propeople health agenda in the country.

5.3. Resolving the Question of Elitist Medical Education. As a measure of what is missing in our medical education today, we would like to offer the following quote from the Bhore Committee's report:

> "... a social outlook should be developed in every health worker and that a spirit of emulation be cultivated throughout the rank and file of service ... Understanding and sympathy, tact and patience are equally important for the proper handling of these persons and, in their absence, mere professional skill will fail to achieve satisfactory results. On the other hand the possession of these qualities will lift the efforts of the health worker to the plane of social service" [1, Page 27].

There is an important task at hand, that of "demystifying" medical education. In order to make medical education an exclusive preserve of the elite, there is a cultivated notion that medicine, as a field of study, is so complex that only those with exceptional intelligence and "merit" can become worthy doctors. Above all, becoming a worthy doctor is a matter of having the aptitude to serve and that the real merit of a doctor does not lie as much in his/her being able to acquire medical knowledge, as much it does in his/her ability to translate this knowledge into practice in highly challenging circumstances of our people and in the generation of new knowledge. These two latter aspects have been totally sidelined in the manner of selection of medical students and their training.

Like other biological sciences, medical knowledge is more of factual than logical or conceptual, which means that, as far as acquiring medical knowledge is concerned, one can do so by putting in reasonable hard work, provided of course other impediments to accessing medical knowledge can be overcome. In our opinion there are four major impediments in this direction that need to be tackled forthwith.

(i) Dual system of education.

The roots of the elite capture of medical profession and indeed other professional courses lie in the dual system of school education in the country, costly English medium education for the elite, and poor quality of government schools teaching in vernacular medium. Education is not just about the medium of instruction, it is about inculcation of social, moral, and ethical values; it is about how one relates to and aspires to improve the society one lives in.

The top notch English medium schools in the big urban centers have become a preserve of the rich who seek an exclusivist education for their children.

So long as this class with exclusivist nurturing exists, they shall seek and also manage almost exclusive access to top positions in all walks of life including the polity, the bureaucracy, the judiciary, and higher education. This is a class that is least desirous of sharing its privileges with common citizenry of the country and is by far the most potent force in the reproduction of the system as it stands today. Hence, the dual system of education must go.

(ii) The present system of selection of medical graduates is as follows.

The present system of medical entrance examination with its emphasis on memorizing more and more obscure facts and correctly recalling them while answering the multiple choice questions should be done away with. Over the years, this system has spawned a whole industry of coaching institutes which provide this specialized training to crack the exams at prices that are invariably beyond the capability of even many of the middle class families.

A system of selection needs to be developed that will test basic intelligence of the aspirants; their aptitude for serving the people, especially the underprivileged; their understanding regarding social issues impacting on the health of the people; and other such factors. Such kind of a process could entail multilevel selection process with each step being designed to sieve in the most deserving candidates.

Towards this end, we learn from the historical examples that are available from post-1917 Soviet Union and preneoliberal reform China, but even the more contemporary examples like the "National Training Program for Comprehensive Community Physicians" (NTPCCP) in Venezuela [66].

(iii) Decommercialization of medical education is as follows.

In order that men and women and boys and girls from the subaltern sections can easily afford to get educated in medicine, medical education should be entirely free for all students with strict conditions built into the program that the student shall have to serve the underserved populations once their training is completed. Such conditions should not be bartered for monetary or any other kind of fines.

The upper age limit should be liberally relaxed to enable even older persons to undertake medical education. For candidates from working class or poor rural backgrounds, the government should provide maintenance allowance for the family such that these students can complete their education without having to worry for the needs of their families. Such measures have currently been undertaken in Venezuela as part of the NTPCCP.

Such reforms in medical education would automatically disincentivize it for those candidates who look upon medicine as a lucrative career option and help in changing the class base of medical profession.

(iv) Changing the medium of instruction from English to the locally spoken languages is as follows.

In the Indian context, as perhaps might be true for many other developing countries, English is not just another language spoken by a certain section of people. It has come to represent a social class, is associated with certain social status and a cultural mindset, and above all is the language of governance in the country. All of this alienates overwhelming majority of Indians who do not have either the knowledge of the language or enough of a command over it, from vast areas of governance, higher education, and elite professions where English is the medium of transaction.

An impression is created that our education, especially technical education, shall lag behind the international standards if the medium of instruction were not to be English. One need only point out here that barring the Anglo-Saxon world, English is not the currency of academic exchange in large parts of the world like China, Japan, Russia, France, Germany, and the like; but can they be said to be lagging behind international standards?

We can devise some practical steps to make the transition as follows.

A national project should be instituted to translate/write medical books into local languages while retaining the English technical terms with or without the corresponding term in the local language. For example, gall bladder can remain gall bladder for instruction in all languages or the word enzyme can be retained as such.

Till such time that an Indian language can be developed to act as a truly pan Indian language, there will still be the need for imparting working knowledge of English or communication skills in it to all students such that medical professionals across the country can engage in a professional interaction.

While being discussed in the context of medical education, such measures need be initiated in almost all the disciplines of education. In fact, one such beginning has been made in the state of Madhya Pradesh that too by a right wing political force such as the BJP. The President Mr. Pranab Mukerjee laid the foundation stone of the Atal Bihari Vajpayee Hindi University at Mugalia Kot in the state on the 7th of June 2013. The university has been established with the promise of offering courses in medicine and engineering among others in Hindi [67]. It is to be seen, however, how far this move goes, but it is commendable to begin with.

Apart from the aforementioned measures another important policy thrust has to be—to bridge the gap between the medical and the paramedical branches of healthcare personnel. Policy measures should be devised to encourage the lower rungs of healthcare professionals like the nursing staff, ANMs, and community health workers to graduate to the higher levels. Necessary changes should be made in the medical curricula/courses to facilitate this.

A word need be said here regarding the "Rural Doctors" course that had been in discussion till sometime back. While being open to the desirability of such a course, we would caution that such a course should not end up being a "poor doctor" course for poor people and add another tier to the medical hierarchy. Instead, a possibility need be considered for devising a single uniform course at the undergraduate level that is much abridged and more focused on community level healthcare. The present M.B.B.S course incorporates too much of detailed information on many subjects that are of the best use to a specialist in those subjects rather than a public health physician. Subjects like forensic medicine can best be avoided at undergraduate level.

Our suggestions here are only suggestive. We are sure that if a systematic approach is taken in this direction, far more constructive opinions can come forth.

5.4. Resolving the Curative-Preventive Dichotomy. Curative-preventive dichotomy in health is intertwined with two aspects—the rural-urban dichotomy (preventive care for rural areas and costly curative care for urban areas) and the hierarchy between curative and preventive branches of medicine. While value of preventive medicine is little appreciated by people in the absence of disease, seeking care becomes incumbent upon falling ill and therein lies the higher market value of clinical disciplines. To this extent, clinical care serves as the convenient mode of profit generation. Hence, market driven growth of healthcare has widened the chasm between the clinical and preventive branches, thereby increasing the overall cost of improving people's health. Following policy measures can be helpful in bringing about a correction in this dichotomy.

(i) Overall development of public healthcare systems shall minimize the profit motive in medicine and can be expected to privilege application of preventive medical knowledge to reduce the overall cost of improving people's health.

To strengthen the curative care in rural areas by creating facilities that will encourage doctors and other paramedical personnel to accept postings in rural areas, government cannot shy away from providing decent boarding and lodging facilities for them besides taking care of the family needs like schooling of the children.

More and more training institutes for at least lower categories of paramedical staff should be located in the rural areas by upgradation of existing facilities.

(ii) A necessary change need be brought in the orientation of medical education as distinct from the efforts made hither to at reorienting medical curriculum. There is a need to include strong social science components in medical education such that the medical professionals can comprehend the complex social, economic, and political context in which medicine operates. Secondly, the clinicians should, as a matter of routine, be pulled out from their ivory towers to engage in preventive care/get involved in strengthening preventive and promotive services.

6. Conclusion

With respect to the challenges facing public hospitals in India, it need be remembered that the sorry state of affairs of public healthcare in the country is not for want of policies or managerial skills or for want of latest technologies. The situation is what it is because it suits the interests of the dominant classes in the society. To undo this conundrum ought to be much more than a bureaucratic or technocratic putsch. This is a situation which demands popular based mobilization of the widest possible sections of the society, especially the working masses to support policy initiatives directed at demolishing the elite capture of healthcare and medical profession in the country.

From a hospital administrator's point of view, our account would indeed be very disappointing as there are no ready-made shortcuts on the offer to improve the outcomes. Nonetheless, it is important to realize that health is a social phenomenon and a public hospital is a social institution which cannot be studied in isolation from the societal conditions in which it operates. The analysis presented here is in conformity with this reality. However, we are sure that there still are public hospitals that offer much to learn in terms of internal workings of these hospitals for improving the services of a public hospital.

Taken overall, the public healthcare system in the country stands at crossroads where there is little in the present system that is worth *emulating*. However, even as the adversities seem insurmountable, the solution lies in propagating and creating space for an alternative paradigm both in the realm of theory and practice. In order that theory gains in virility, it must develop the language to articulate people's struggles for an alternative development paradigm.

Conflict of Interests

The authors declare that there is no conflict of interests regarding the publication of this paper.

References

[1] Government of India (GOI), *Health Survey and Development Committee*, vol. 2, Government of India Press, 1946.

[2] Government of India (GIO), *Rural Health Statistics 2012*, Ministry of Health and Family Welfare, New Delhi, India, 2013.

[3] "Health Nutrition and Population Statistics," World Development Indicators, World Bank Data Bank, http://databank.worldbank.org/data/views/variableselection/selectvariables.aspx?source=health-nutrition-and-population-statistics.

[4] Government of India (GOI), *District Level Household and Facility Survey 2007-08*, Ministry of Health and Family Welfare, 2010.

[5] S. Ghosh, "Catastrophic Payments and Impoverishment Due to Out-of-Pocket Health Spending: The Effects of Recent Health Sector Reforms in India," Asia Health Policy Program Working Paper 15, 2010, Working paper series on health and demographic change in the Asia-Pacific, Stanford University Walter H. Shorenstein Asia-Pacific Research Center Asia Health Policy Program.

[6] Government of India (GOI), *Morbidity, Healthcare and the Condition of the Aged*, NSSO, Ministry of Statistics and Programme Implementation, 2006.

[7] (RHS), *Rural Health Statistics in India 2011*, Statistics Division, Ministry of Health and Family Welfare, New Delhi, India, 2011.

[8] R. Mehta, B. Gulshan, A. P. Singh, and M. Khejriwal, "A Peek into the Future of Healthcare: Trends for 2010, Technopak perspective: A quarterly report," Quoted in 'High Level Expert Group Report on Universal Health Coverage for India, Instituted by Planning Commission of India, 2010.

[9] American Medical Association (AMA), "International Medical Graduates in American Medicine: Contemporary challenges and opportunities," A position paper by the AMA-IMG Section Governing Council, 2010, http://www.ama-assn.org/resources/doc/img/international-medical-graduates-in-american-medicine.pdf.

[10] Center for Enquiry into Health and Allied Topics (CEHAT), "Changing Health Budgets," Centre for Enquiry into Health and Allied Themes, Research Centre of Anusandhan Trust, 2006.

[11] CBHI, "Table 1. 1. 3, National Health Profile, 2005," Ministry of Health and Family Welfare, Government of India, New Delhi, India, CBHI (Central Bureau of Health Intelligence), 2005, http://cbhidghs.nic.in/CBHI%20Book/chapter1.pdf.

[12] GOI, *Table 6. 2. 2 State/UT Wise Number of Govt. Hospitals and Beds in Rural and Urban Areas (including CHCs) in India (Provisional)*, in "Health infrastructure" in 'National Health Profile, 2011', Central Bureau of Health Intelligence, Ministry of Health and Family Welfare, 2011.

[13] "National Health Accounts 2004-05 (With Provisional Estimates from 2005-06 to 2008-09)," GOI 2004-05, National Health Accounts Cell, Ministry of Health and Family Welfare, New Delhi, India.

[14] T. Dunning, "Structural Reform and Medical Commerce: The Political Economy of Cuban Health Care in the Special Period," Department of Political Science, University of California, Berkeley, Paper was prepared for delivery at the 2001 meeting of the Latin American Studies Association, Washington, DC, USA, 2001, http://lasa.international.pitt.edu/Lasa2001/DunningThad.pdf.

[15] RBI: Reserve Bank of India, *Handbook of Statistics on Indian Economy*, 2013, http://rbidocs.rbi.org.in/rdocs/Publications/PDFs/FHB160913FLS.pdf.

[16] D. Nandan, K. S. Nair, and U. Datta, "Human resources for public health in India: issues and challenges," *Health and Population: Perspectives and Issues*, vol. 30, no. 4, pp. 230–242, 2007.

[17] M. Rao, K. D. Rao, A. S. Kumar, M. Chatterjee, and T. Sundara-raman, "Human resources for health in India," *The Lancet*, vol. 377, no. 9765, pp. 587–598, 2011.

[18] High Level Expert Group (HLEG), "Human resources for health," in *High Level Expert Group Report on Universal Health Coverage for India*, Planning Commission, Government of India, 2011.

[19] K. Rao, A. Bhatnagar, and P. Berman, "India's health work-force: size, composition and distribution," in *World Bank/Public Health Foundation of India*, J. La Forgia and K. Rao, Eds., India Health Beat, New Delhi, India, 2009.

[20] World Health Organization (WHO), *Global Atlas of the Health*, Workforce, Geneva, Switzerland, 2010.

[21] M. D. John, S. J. Chander, and N. Devadasan, "National Urban Health Mission: An analysis of strategies and mechanisms for improving services for urban poor," Background paper for National Workshop on Urban Health and Poverty, 2-3 July 2008, New Delhi, organized by Ministry of Housing and Urban Poverty Alleviation, Government of India, 2008, http://www.academia.edu/855928/National_Urban_Health_Mission_An_analysis_of_strategies_and_mechanisms_for_improving_services_for_urban_poor.

[22] K. Muralidharan, N. Chaudhury, and J. Hammer, "Is There a Doctor in the House? Medical Worker Absence in India," Working paper, Department of Economics, Faculty of Arts and Sciences, Harvard University, 2011, http://scholar.harvard.edu/files/kremer/files/is_there_a_doctor_in_the_house_-_12_april_2011.pdf.

[23] American Medical Association, "International medical graduates in American medicine: Contemporary challenges and opportunities," A position paper by the AMA-IMG Section Governing Council, AMA Press, Chicago, Ill, USA, 2012, http://nycsprep.com/pdf/international-medical-graduates.pdf.

[24] N. Bhola, R. Kumari, and T. Nidha, "Utilization of the health care delivery system in a district of North India," *East African Journal of Public Health*, vol. 5, no. 3, pp. 147–153, 2008.

[25] Government of Uttrakhand, "Department of Information and Public Relations," Press Note, 2011, http://www.cm.uk.gov.in/upload/pressrelease/Pressrelease-280.pdf.

[26] N. Chandra, "Delhi hospital pays high price for excellence," India today, 2012, http://indiatoday.intoday.in/story/delhi-hospital-pays-high-price-for-excellence/1/200025.html.

[27] Jan Swasthya Abhiyan, *Globalization and Health*, 2006.

[28] D. N. Jha, "All India Institute of Medical Sciences faces exodus of top doctors," Times of India, 2012, http://articles.timesofindia.indiatimes.com/2012-05-03/delhi/31555155_1_faculty-association-voluntary-retirement-faculty-members.

[29] B. S. Perappadan, "Private hospitals advertise at AIIMS to recruit doctors," The Hindu, 2012, http://www.thehindu.com/todays-paper/tp-national/private-hospitals-advertise-at-aiims-to-recruit-doctors/article3389387.ece.

[30] India, *National Health Accounts 2004-05 (with Provisional Estimates from 2005-06 to 2008-09)*, Ministry of Health and Family Welfare, New Delhi, India, 2004-05.

[31] T. B. MacCulay, "Minute on Indian Education," The British Parliament, 1835, http://www.columbia.edu/itc/mealac/pritchett/00generallinks/macaulay/txt_minute_education_1835.html.

[32] S. Manmohan, "Of Oxford, economics, empire, and freedom," The Hindu, 2005, http://www.hindu.com/2005/07/10/stories/2005071002301000.htm.

[33] D. K. Das and A. Verma, "The armed police in the British colonial tradition: the Indian perspective," *Policing*, vol. 21, no. 2, pp. 354–367, 1998.

[34] Asian Centre for Human Rights, *Torture in India, 2011*, Asian Centre for Human Rights, 2011.

[35] R. Blackely, "Ghulam Nabi Azad says late night TV will help slow India's birth rate," The Sunday Times, 2009.

[36] V. W. Sidel and R. Sidel, *Serve the People: Observations on Medicine in the People's Republic of China*, Becon Press, Boston, Mass, USA, 1973.

[37] R. Sidel and V. W. Sidel, *The Health of China*, Zed Press, London, UK, 1982.

[38] Sokhey Committee, *Sub-Committee on National Health, National Planning Committee*, Vora and Co Publishers, Bombay, India, 1948.

[39] Mudaliar Committee, *Health Survey and Development Committee*, Government of India, New Delhi, India, 1959.

[40] D. Banerji, *Health and Family Planning Services in India: An Epidemiological, Sociocultural and Political Analysis and a Perspective*, Lok Paksh, New Delhi, India, 1985.

[41] D. Banerji, "Evolution of health services in India," in *In Search of Diagnosis: Analysis of Present System of Health Care*, A. J. Patel, Ed., 1977, Published by Voluntary Health Association of India for Medico Friend Circle.

[42] D. Banerji, "Objectives of medical education," in *In Search of Diagnosis: Analysis of Present System of Health Care*, A. J. Patel, Ed., Medico Friend Circle, New Delhi, India, 1977.

[43] M. Kaushik, A. Jaiswal, N. Shah, and A. Mahal, "High-end physician migration from India," *Bulletin of the World Health Organization*, vol. 86, no. 1, pp. 40–45, 2008.

[44] K. Yadav, P. Jarhyan, V. Gupta, and C. Pandav, "Revitalizing rural health care delivery: can rural health practitioners be the answer?" *Indian Journal of Community Medicine*, vol. 34, no. 1, pp. 3–5, 2009.

[45] C. Sathyamala, O. Mittal, R. Dasgupta, and R. Priya, "Polio eradication initiative in India: deconstructing the GPEI," *International Journal of Health Services*, vol. 35, no. 2, pp. 361–383, 2005.

[46] Jan Swasthya Abhiyan, *New Technologies in Public Health: Who Pays and Who Benefits?* 1st edition, 2007.

[47] R. Dasgupta and I. Ghanashyam, "Connecting the DOTS: spectre of a public health iatrogenesis?" *Indian Journal of Community Medicine*, vol. 37, no. 1, pp. 13–15, 2012.

[48] A. K. Maurya, A. K. Singh, M. Kumar et al., "Changing patterns and trends of multidrug-resistant tuberculosis at referral centre in Northern India: a 4-year experience," *Indian Journal of Medical Microbiology*, vol. 31, no. 1, pp. 40–46, 2013.

[49] E. Hong, *Globalisation and the Impact on Health: A Third World View*, The Peoples' Health Assembly, Savar, Bangladesh, 2000.

[50] M. Gandy, "Deadly alliances: death, disease, and the global politics of public health," *PLoS Medicine*, vol. 2, no. 1, pp. e4.9–e4.11, 2005.

[51] R. Baru, A. Acharya, S. Acharya, A. K. Shiva Kumar, and K. Nagaraj, "Inequities in access to health services in India: caste,

class and region," *Economic and Political Weekly*, vol. 45, no. 38, pp. 49–58, 2010.

[52] R. Duggal, "Health Care and New Economic Policies, the Further Consolidation of the Private Sector in India," Paper Presented at the National Seminar on the Rights to Development, University of Mumbai, Mumbai, India, 1998.

[53] Jan Swasthya Abhiyan, "Health System in India: Crisis and Alternatives," Towards the National Health Assembly II, Booklet 2, 2006.

[54] S. Bhide and R. Shand, "Inequalities in income growth in india before and after reforms," *South Asia Economic Journal*, vol. 1, no. 1, pp. 19–51, 2000.

[55] A. Marriot, "Blind Optimism Challenging the myths about private health care in poor countries," Oxfam Briefing Paper 125, 2009.

[56] L. V. Gangolli, R. Duggal, and A. Shukla, *Review of Healthcare in india*, Centre for Enquiry into Health and Allied Themes, Research Centre of Anusandhan Trust, 2005.

[57] Arti Dhar, "Activists up in arms against new proposal on health care," The Hindu, 2012.

[58] V. Bajpai and A. Saraya, "User charges as a feature of health policy in India: a perspective," *National Medical Journal of India*, vol. 23, no. 3, pp. 163–170, 2010.

[59] L. M. Franco, S. Bennett, and R. Kanfer, "Health sector reform and public sector health worker motivation: a conceptual framework," *Social Science and Medicine*, vol. 54, no. 8, pp. 1255–1266, 2002.

[60] M. Chaudhary, "Public spending on health in low-income states and central transfers," Financing Human Development, Policy Brief 1, National Institute of Public Finance and Policy, 2006.

[61] WHO, *Primary Health Care: Report of the International Conference on Primary Health Care, Alma-Ata*, USSR, Geneva, Switzerland, 1978.

[62] J. Y. Kim, "World Bank Group President Jim Yong Kim's Speech at World Health Assembly: Poverty, Health and the Human Future," The World Bank, 2013, http://www.worldbank.org/en/news/speech/2013/05/21/world-bank-group-president-jim-yong-kim-speech-at-world-health-assembly.

[63] K. Srinath Reddy, "Universal Health Coverage in India: the time has come," *National Medical Journal of India*, vol. 25, no. 2, pp. 65–67, 2012.

[64] Arti Dhar, "Panel on health coverage addresses World Bank concerns," The Hindu, 2011.

[65] S. Makkar, "Universal healthcare plan may be nixed," The Wall Street Journal, 2012, http://www.livemint.com/.

[66] E. R. B. Cruz and R. S. S. Perea, "National training program for comprehensive community physicians, Venezuela," *MEDICC Review*, vol. 10, no. 4, pp. 35–42, 2008.

[67] Express News Service, "New MP varsity to teach medicine, engg in Hindi," The Indian Express, 2013, http://www.indianexpress.com/news/new-mp-varsity-to-teach-medicine-engg-in-hindi/1126170/.

14

Control of an Outbreak of *Acinetobacter baumannii* in Burn Unit in a Tertiary Care Hospital of North India

Shweta Sharma, Nirmaljit Kaur, Shalini Malhotra, Preeti Madan, and Charoo Hans

Department of Microbiology, Dr. Ram Manohar Lohia Hospital & PGIMER, Baba Kharak Singh Marg, New Delhi 110001, India

Correspondence should be addressed to Shweta Sharma; drshwetamicro@gmail.com

Academic Editor: Julio Diaz

Acinetobacter infection is increasing in hospitals and now it is considered as a global threat, as it can be easily transmitted and remain viable in the hospital environment for a long time due to its multidrug-resistant status, resistance to desiccation, and tendency to adhere to inanimate surfaces. Outbreaks caused by multidrug-resistant *Acinetobacter baumannii* (MDRAB) are difficult to control and have substantial morbidity and mortality, especially in vulnerable host. Here we are describing an outbreak of multidrug-resistant *Acinetobacter baumannii* in burn unit of a tertiary care hospital in India followed by its investigation and infection control measures taken to curtail the outbreak. Outbreak investigation and environmental sampling are the key factors which help in deciding the infection control strategies for control of outbreak. Implementation of contact precautions, hand hygiene, personnel protective equipment, environmental disinfection, isolation of patients, and training of health care workers are effective measures to control the outbreak of MDRAB in burn unit.

1. Introduction

Burn wound surface provides a favourable niche for microbial colonization and proliferation. Burn wound infections may originate from the patient's endogenous skin and gastrointestinal and respiratory flora (endogenous) or may also be transferred via contact with contaminated external surfaces and soiled hands of healthcare workers (exogenous). Burn patients are more susceptible to colonization from organisms in the environment as well as disperse organisms into the surrounding environment [1]. *Acinetobacter* spp. remain as normal skin flora, can be easily transmitted, and remain viable in the hospital environment for a long time due to its multidrug-resistant status, resistance to desiccation, and tendency to adhere to inanimate surfaces; hence *Acinetobacter* infection is increasing in hospitals and now it is considered as a global threat. Risk factors associated with *Acinetobacter* infection include invasive procedures which are commonly required in patients with burn injuries, like mechanical ventilation, central venous or urinary catheters, and broad-spectrum antimicrobials [2]. Outbreaks caused by multidrug-resistant *Acinetobacter baumannii* (MDRAB) are difficult to control and have substantial morbidity and mortality,

especially in vulnerable host. Here, we are describing an outbreak of multidrug-resistant *Acinetobacter baumannii* in burn unit of a tertiary care hospital in India, followed by its investigation and infection control measures taken to curtail the outbreak.

2. Materials and Methods

Burn unit in our hospital has both burn patients and plastic surgery patients or old burn cases. These are separated and are placed in different cubicles and also the dressing rooms for both the types of patients are different with different nursing staff. A total of 12 beds are allotted for new burn patients, which are distributed in various cubicles according to the severity of burn and condition of the patient. There are 2 beds in one cubicle, 4 beds in the second cubicle, and 6 beds in the third cubicle, with a distance of approximately 10 feet between two beds, with approximate total admissions of 20–25 burn patients in the month. The second cubicle with 4 beds is the intensive care unit with ventilator and cardiac monitor dedicated to all the beds, for critical patients with large burn surface area and infected with multidrug resistant organisms. Burn wound swabs which were received in microbiology department were processed according to standard microbiological techniques. MDRAB was defined as *A. baumannii* resistant to three or more antimicrobials of the following: aminoglycoside, β-lactam-β-lactamase inhibitor, antipseudomonal carbapenem, antipseudomonal cephalosporin, and fluoroquinolone [3]. For environmental sampling, sterile swabs moistened with sterile distilled water were used to swab items in the burn ward, like dressing room trolley, transport trolley, patient's beds, silver sulfadiazine ointment, water taps, and so forth. The hands of health care workers (HCWs), including burn dressers, doctors, nurses, were also sampled to assess the potential of hand carriage. They were immediately inoculated onto 5% sheep blood agar plates and in BHI broth and incubated overnight in air at 37°C. Microorganisms were identified by conventional methods and were tested for susceptibility to amikacin, aztreonam, ceftriaxone, cefotaxime, ciprofloxacin, cotrimoxazole, cefotaxime-clavulanic acid, colistin, gentamicin, imipenem, piperacillin-tazobactam, and tigecycline using Kirby Bauer disc diffusion method according to CLSI guidelines [4]. All the isolates were confirmed and also breakpoint MICs were done with automated system, Microscan WalkAway 40 plus system, as per manufacturer's guidelines.

3. Outbreak Investigation

Acinetobacter baumannii was common in causing burn wound infections, but its incidence was 1 to 2 isolates in one to two weeks till March 2014. However the isolation of the organism increased to 1 to 2 cases in two to three days, in April 2014, and *Acinetobacter* spp. was isolated in total of 12 cases. *Acinetobacter baumannii* was identified on the basis of various biochemicals like motility, oxidase, OF media, sugars, indole, methyl red, Voges Proskauer, citrate, urease, triple sugar iron agar, 10% lactose, hemolysis, growth at 44°C, and so forth. And also the isolates were confirmed as *Acinetobacter baumannii* in Microscan WalkAway 40 plus system. All the isolates were MDRAB with the same antibiogram, that is, resistant to amikacin (>32 μg/mL), aztreonam (>16 μg/mL), ceftriaxone (>32 μg/mL), cefotaxime (>32 μg/mL), ciprofloxacin (>2 μg/mL), cotrimoxazole (>2/38 μg/mL), cefotaxime-clavulanic acid (>4 μg/ mL), gentamicin (>8 μg/mL), and piperacillin-tazobactam (>64 μg/mL), and were sensitive to imipenem (≤4 μg/mL), colistin, and tigecycline by Kirby Bauer disc diffusion method and MICs by Microscan WalkAway 40 plus system. Hence, infection control team was informed about increase in number of cases and environmental samples were taken by infection control nurse especially from the dressing room of burn unit. Overall 18 swabs were collected, from various areas in the burn ward especially from the dressing room like dressing room trolley, transport trolley, patient's beds, silver sulfadiazine ointment, water taps, and so forth. Out of them, two swabs were positive for *Acinetobacter baumannii*, one collected from the burn dressing trolley and the other from the transport trolley, which was especially used for transport of patient from the bed to the dressing room. Both the isolates from swabs were showing the same sensitivity pattern as the MDRAB isolated from patient's wound swab. All the isolates were confirmed by Microscan automated system. Samples were also collected from the hands of eight health care workers including two burn dressers, and none of them were positive for *Acinetobacter baumannii*.

3.1. Outbreak Control Measures. The infection control team established the outbreak control strategies which were implemented in May 2014. All health care staff including dressers and nursing staff were taught probable routes of transmission, with emphasis on patient to patient cross-contamination and infection control measures such as hand hygiene, standard precautions, aseptic techniques, personnel protective equipment, environmental cleaning and disinfection, and also biomedical waste management. Proper steps of hand hygiene were demonstrated to health care workers and also the posters of hand washing were placed in various areas of the burn ward. Also the use of alcohol based hand rubs with automatic dispensers was reinforced in the ward so that hand hygiene could be improved before and after contact with the patient. The use of gloves wherever necessary was emphasised. Staff allocated for affected patients was not allowed to care for any unaffected patients, till three negative cultures were obtained from affected patient at weekly intervals. Burn dressers used sterile gloves, mask, and gowns for dressing of burn patients and gown and gloves were changed after every patient to be disinfected later, and hands were washed before and after removing gloves and wearing another glove in between each patient. Burn wounds were occlusively wrapped and never kept open to prevent cross-contamination of environment. All the bandages and dressing material used for dressing were preautoclaved; local agent like silver sulfadiazine was applied aseptically and separate nursing staff was provided to guide the dressers and for support during dressing. Dressing frequency was increased to be daily if total burn surface area was > 35–40% or if the dressings were soaked; otherwise with lesser burn surface area dressing was done on alternate days. Dressing rooms were disinfected with high level disinfectants like hydrogen peroxide with silver nitrate, which is dispersed with the help of a fogger-like device inside the dressing room for a contact time of 1 hour, before starting the dressings. Patients were shifted to dressing room in transport trolley and then shifted to dressing trolley which was thoroughly disinfected between each patient. The bed of the patient and the trolley of patient were disinfected regularly and the bed sheets for each patient were changed daily. In case of discharge or death of the patient, the area was cleaned and disinfected thoroughly before taking any new patient. The frequency of environmental cleaning and disinfection was increased to 3-4 times in a day, and hydrogen peroxide with silver nitrate was used for disinfection. Entry of visitors was limited in the ward, and only one person was allowed with each patient and shoe covers were made compulsory for entry in the ward. Patient relatives were also trained by nursing staff regarding infection control measures to be taken to control the spread of infection. Proper disposal of soiled linen and other biomedical waste was undertaken in the ward. Antibiotic usage was limited to short periods, and ceftazidime and amikacin were used empirically, and other antibiotic usage is according to the results of cultures and antibiotic susceptibility report. MDRAB patients were switched to carbapenems, as they were susceptible to imipenem.

3.2. Results of Outbreak Control Measures. After the introduction of infection control measures, the number of newly diagnosed cases began to decline by the end of May, and June 2014, to 1-2 *Acinetobacter baumannii* in two weeks. Also the environmental samples collected from the dressing room, dressing trolley, transport trolley, and so forth stopped growing *Acinetobacter baumannii*.

4. Discussion

An outbreak of MDR organism occurs in a particular unit due to lapses in infection control measures, resulting in an increased cross-transmission between patients [5]. The outbreak reported here appeared to be initiated from the dressing trolley or transport trolley, because the sensitivity pattern was exactly the same in the isolates cultured from these areas and from patient's burn wound swabs. Also the enhancement and appropriate implementation of barrier precautions, hand hygiene, and disinfection at the time of dressing of patients were found very effective in preventing the spread of MDRAB. Environmental sampling was found effective to find the source of spread of MDRAB in the ward and thus helped to make the outbreak control strategies in our study and to guide the cleaning and disinfection of environmental sites and to check the quality of environmental cleaning after thorough disinfection of environment. Many previous studies have reported isolation of *Acinetobacter* species from environmental sites and hence environmental cleaning is a major part of infection control strategy [6–8]. However, it is difficult to curtail the outbreak of multidrug resistant organisms by merely environmental disinfection especially in the burn unit as these patients are more susceptible to infections due to loss of normal skin barrier and large colonised burn area can easily spread the MDR strains in the environment and also to other patients due to cross-contamination. Hence isolation of patients and contact precautions along with proper disposal of soiled linen and education of patient's relatives and dressers are equally important for the control of outbreak as seen in our study [9].

The outbreak in our burn unit was controlled after implementation of various measures, and it is not possible to describe which measure ultimately controlled the outbreak; however, control of environmental reservoir by disinfection and barrier precautions at the time of dressing of patients with education of dressers were considered as the major factors in controlling the outbreak. In some previous studies, complete closure of units was necessary to control outbreaks [10]. However, it was not done in our hospital as it is a very renowned tertiary care centre for burn patients with a load of referrals, and still the outbreak was controlled. Hence strict precautions and environmental disinfection may control the outbreak without closure of the unit. The limitation of this study was that the molecular typing of strains by pulsed field gel electrophoresis (PFGE) was not done in our study; hence it is difficult to say that the outbreak was caused by a single clone. However, the sensitivity pattern was the same in the isolates from environment and from patients, suggesting the possibility of transmission of a single clone responsible for this outbreak.

To conclude, this study shows that outbreak investigation and environmental sampling are the key factors which help in deciding the infection control strategies for control of outbreak. Implementation of contact precautions, hand hygiene, personnel protective equipment, environmental disinfection, isolation of patients, and training of health care workers as well as patient's attendants are effective measures to control the outbreak of MDRAB in burn unit.

Conflict of Interests

The authors declare that there is no conflict of interests regarding the publication of this paper.

References

[1] S. Erol, U. Altoparlak, M. N. Akcay, F. Celebi, and M. Parlak, "Changes of microbial flora and wound colonization in burned patients," *Burns*, vol. 30, no. 4, pp. 357–361, 2004.

[2] K. J. Towner, "Acinetobacter: an old friend, but a new enemy," *Journal of Hospital Infection*, vol. 73, no. 4, pp. 355–363, 2009.

[3] WHO, "Multidrug-resistant *Acinetobacter baumannii* (MDRAB)," Fact Sheet 1, World Health Organisation, Metro Manila, Philippines, 2010.

[4] Clinical and Laboratory Standards Institute, "Performance standards for antimicrobial susceptibility testing," Twenty-Third Informational Supplement M100-S23, 2013.

[5] E. M. C. D'Agata, V. Thayer, and W. Schaffner, "An outbreak of Acinetobacter baumannii: the importance of cross-transmission," *Infection Control and Hospital Epidemiology*, vol. 21, no. 9, pp. 588–591, 2000.

[6] M. Denton, M. H. Wilcox, P. Parnell et al., "Role of environmental cleaning in controlling an outbreak of *Acinetobacter baumannii* on a neurosurgical intensive care unit," *Journal of Hospital Infection*, vol. 56, no. 2, pp. 106–110, 2004.

[7] M. E. Falagas and P. Kopterides, "Risk factors for the isolation of multi-drug-resistant *Acinetobacter baumannii* and *Pseudomonas aeruginosa*: a systematic review of the literature," *Journal of Hospital Infection*, vol. 64, no. 1, pp. 7–15, 2006.

[8] C. Landelle, P. Legrand, P. Lesprit et al., "Protracted outbreak of multidrug-resistant *Acinetobacter baumannii* after intercontinental transfer of colonized patients," *Infection Control and Hospital Epidemiology*, vol. 34, no. 2, pp. 119–124, 2013.

[9] J. D. Naranjo, J. I. V. Navarro, M. S. Busselo et al., "Control of a clonal outbreak of multidrug-resistant *Acinetobacter baumannii* in a hospital of the Basque country after the introduction of environmental cleaning led by the systematic sampling from environmental objects," *Interdisciplinary Perspectives on Infectious Diseases*, vol. 2013, Article ID 582831, 9 pages, 2013.

[10] A. Markogiannakis, G. Fildisis, S. Tsiplakou et al., "Cross-transmission of multidrug-resistant Acinetobacter baumannii clonal strains causing episodes of sepsis in a trauma intensive care unit," *Infection Control and Hospital Epidemiology*, vol. 29, no. 5, pp. 410–417, 2008.

15

Patients' Compliance with Tuberculosis Medication in Ghana: Evidence from a Periurban Community

Evans Danso, Isaac Yeboah Addo, and Irene Gyamfuah Ampomah

Department of Population and Health, Faculty of Social Sciences, University of Cape Coast, Cape Coast, Ghana

Correspondence should be addressed to Isaac Yeboah Addo; yebaddo9@yahoo.com

Academic Editor: Gudlavalleti Venkata Murthy

Globally, an estimated 2 million deaths occur every year as a result of tuberculosis. Ghana records over 46,000 new cases annually despite numerous efforts to curb the disease. One major challenge associated with the control of the disease is patients' noncompliance with medication. Despite the noncompliance setback, not much information is available on the issue. This paper, therefore, examines patients' compliance with medication at the Suhum Kraboa Coaltar District in Ghana. A cross-sectional descriptive study was carried out using interview schedules. Data were primarily retrieved from 40 treatment supporters, in addition to 110 previously treated persons registered in 2010 and 2011 with cases of pulmonary tuberculosis. Evidence from the study indicates that 63 percent of the previously treated persons complied with medication which is below the expected national target of at least 85 percent. However, those with treatment supporters significantly complied with medication. Depression, substance abuse, financial problems, and long duration of treatment were other issues that discouraged patients' adherence to medication. Some patients also attributed supernatural explanations to the source of the disease which negatively affected compliance. Conclusively, future approaches aimed at controlling/eradicating tuberculosis in the district should consider counselling, economic empowerment packages, and detailed education for patients.

1. Introduction

One-third of the world's population is infected with tuberculosis (TB) with nearly 2 million deaths occurring each year. Among those infected annually, more than 1.5 million occur in Sub-Saharan Africa [1]. In Ghana, about 46,000 cases are reported in health facilities yearly, but the treatment of the disease had been erratic since 1900 until the introduction of TB services in 1959 [2]. Many infected people apply both homeopathic and allopathic medicines as treatment since 1900, but the World Health Organization has recommended medicines for treatment [3, 4]. After diagnosing someone with the disease, chemotherapy is administered to interrupt transmission to others [5]. Ghana adopts the directly observed treatment strategy (DOTS) when a case is identified. Initially, multiple doses were given for treatment between eight and eighteen months until the introduction of fixed dose combination (FDC) in which two or more drugs are combined to form a single tablet. FDC involves the amalgamation of first-line drugs: ethambutol, isoniazid,

rifampicin, and pyrazinamide into one dosage [3]. Initial treatment duration is six months for all new cases with intensive phase of two months and continuation phase of four months. Patients are usually assigned a treatment supporter who supervises the in-take of medication to prevent cases of default [6, 7]. From 1960 to 1990, programmes designed to combat TB in the country decreased. However, in 1994, a National TB Control Programme began with the aim of eradicating the disease from the country through set of related activities and services such as free supply of drugs to patients [1, 3, 8].

Despite all efforts to eradicate the disease, TB persists in the country largely because of patients' noncompliance with medication [9–12]. Studies in New Juabeng Municipality, Tamale Metropolitan Assembly, and Agogo in Ghana identified patients' noncompliance with medication as a challenge [9–12]. With the inception of the community TB care in the Eastern Region of Ghana in the year 2007, Suhum Kraboa Coaltar District has achieved a compliance rate of 70 percent in 2009 and 71 percent in 2010 which is below the national

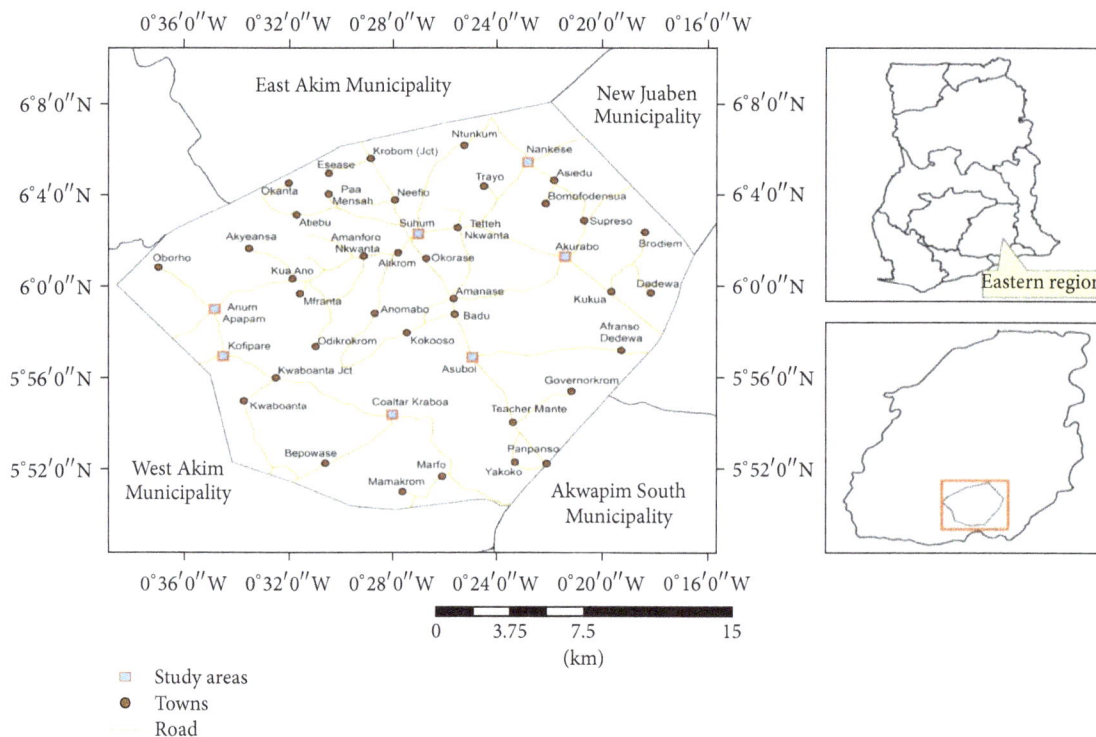

FIGURE 1: Map of Suhum Kraboa Coaltar District. Source: Cartographic Unit, Department of Geography and Regional Planning, UCC (2013).

target of at least 85 percent [11, 13, 14]. Patients' noncompliance with TB medication is gradually becoming a health burden in the country, but most studies focus on the medical aspects of the disease rather than looking at it from a social viewpoint [10, 13]. Patients' noncompliance with medication is a behavioural issue which requires research to generate knowledge that would help District Health Management Teams (DHMT) to design effective approaches to solving the problem. This paper, therefore, examines indices influencing patients' compliance with medication, using Suhum Kraboa Coaltar District in Ghana as the study setting.

2. Theoretical Guide

Patients' compliance with medication is well understood in the context of self-determination theory, because it considers individual and societal matrixes in explaining behaviour. Self-determination theory postulated by [15] measures a person's inherent resources for personality development and regulation of behaviour. According to the theory, society has persistent effects on the motivation and psychological well-being of an individual to perform behaviour. However, this is mostly reliant on the innate psychological needs of the person, namely, self-perceived competence, autonomy, and relatedness. An individual first perceives himself/herself as competent and gets intrinsic motivation to perform a particular behaviour. For behaviours that are not intrinsically motivated, the individual adapts to his/her existing values and needs. In the social context, an individual's feeling of relatedness to "significant others" influence behaviour. Thus people

who are important to the person in question provide motivation which becomes a function of his/her innate capability to perform behaviour. For instance, a patient's family member (treatment supporter) may influence the patient to either take or neglect his/her medication depending on whether the family member is revered by the patient. Therefore, greater internalisation is associated with the ability to comply with medication given the importance of motivation in producing lasting behavioural change. Autonomy refers to the extent to which behaviour is performed under volition. The theory considers that performing behaviour is not a matter of using force, but rather a person "marries" views from revered people with his/her own values and needs before performing behaviour. It may signify a situation where patients take independent decisions to comply with medication after they have received motivation from treatment supporters [16].

3. Data and Methods

The study was conducted in the Suhum Kraboa Coaltar District in the Eastern Region of Ghana (Figure 1). The district has a population of about 167,551 people comprising 82,402 males and 85,149 females [17]. A cross-sectional descriptive study was conducted after reviewing patients' records for 2010 and 2011 in the district [13]. The total number of registered patients was 127; but 17 had died and hence were exempted from the study. The remaining 110 previously treated persons together with 40 available treatment supporters were contacted for interview schedules. The data collection instruments (interview schedules) were reviewed by the University of Cape Coast Ethical Review Board before they were administered. Factors affecting patients' compliance with medication, roles played by treatment supporters and background characteristics of respondents were the main issues discussed in the interview schedules. Eight research assistants from the Social Science Faculty in the University of Cape Coast were recruited and trained for the collection of data. The training lasted for two days and centred on issues relating to the objectives of the study, contents of the survey instruments, recording of data, and observing community entry protocols.

Ethical considerations and translation of instruments into Twi language which was widely spoken by most respondents were discussed during the training. Pretesting of the interview schedules was conducted in the West Akim District in the Eastern Region from 16 to 18 October 2013. West Akim District was chosen because it is a Twi-speaking community and has a number of tuberculosis patients with similar characteristics as the study area. Ten tuberculosis patients were randomly selected for the pretest using the West Akim district tuberculosis register and the results showed that the content of the interview schedule was comprehensive. The actual fieldwork took place from 16 November 2013 to 7 January 2014. Right of entry into the community was gained after sending an advanced letter to the Suhum Kraboa Coaltar District Director of Health Administration. The District Tuberculosis Coordinator introduced the researchers to the subdistrict heads to assist in locating the houses of the previously treated patients for the collection of data. After establishing a rapport with the patients, informed consents were sought before the administration of the interview schedules. Patients were assured of confidentiality and the services of a counsellor were employed in case of any unexpected psychological discomfort. Data were made anonymous by using codes on the interview guides instead of names and phone numbers. Epi Info software version 3.4.2 was used to analyse the data. Frequency distribution tables for all variables were run to identify and correct missing values. Write and merge commands were used to merge patients and treatment supporters' interview schedules. Frequency tables, cross tabulations, chi-square, and independent sample t-test were the main statistical applications used in the study. One major challenge during the data collection was that most of the respondents had changed their locations. This challenge was overcome after telephone numbers were collected from neighbours and various calls were made to meet the study participants.

4. Results and Discussion

4.1. Background Characteristics of Previously Treated TB Patients and Treatment Supporters. Wide disparity in background characteristics between patients and their treatment supporters can affect acceptance of health directives provided by the treatment supporter [8, 9]. Specific background characteristics of respondents captured in the study were sex, age, educational attainment, marital status, and main occupation (Table 1). The results show that males who were previously treated (71%) were more than females (29%). This confirms

TABLE 1: Background characteristics of respondents.

Background characteristics	Previously treated patients (%) ($N = 110$)	Treatment supporters (%) ($N = 40$)
Total	73.3	26.7
Sex		
Males	71.0	42.5
Females	29.0	57.5
Age (years)		
<20	4.5	0.0
20–29	14.6	7.5
30–39	24.4	20.0
40–49	29.0	42.5
50–59	15.6	22.5
60+	11.9	7.5
Highest level of education attained		
No formal education	8.2	10.0
Primary	20	10.0
Middle/JHS/JSS	62.7	42.5
Senior secondary/SHS	9.1	15.0
Tertiary	0.0	22.5
Marital status		
Never married	28.2	12.5
Married	58.2	75.0
Divorced	9.1	0.0
Widowed	4.5	12.5
Main occupation		
Farmer	50.9	47.5
Trader	16.9	12.5
Artisan	15.5	0.0
Unemployed	16.7	15.0
Public servant	0.0	25.0

Source: fieldwork, 2013.

the findings of [5, 11] that male TB patients are more than females in many districts in Ghana. In contrast, more than half (58%) of the treatment supporters were females (Table 1).

Their ages ranged from 18 years to 79 years and their mean age was 44 years. Similar to our findings, [11] reported a mean age of 35 years in their study in the Eastern Region of Ghana. The most populous age group among the respondents was 40–49 years. Twenty-nine percent of the previously treated TB patients were aged between 40–49 years while 43 percent of the treatment supporters were aged within the same age cohort (Table 1). This is an indication that treatment supporters were relatively older than the previously treated TB patients and hence positively influenced compliance with medication as supported by the findings of [9]. The highest percentage of the previously treated TB patients (63%) and their treatment supporters (43%) had attained at least middle/junior high/junior secondary school (Table 1). Table 1 shows that majority of the respondents were married, but more treatment supporters (75%) were married compared with previously treated TB patients (58%). Reference [9] also found that more patients and treatment supporters are married in Ketu Municipality.

Farming was the dominant occupation among the respondents, but more previously treated TB patients (51%) were engaged in farming compared with the treatment supporters (48%). This is consistent with the 2010 Population and Housing Census of Ghana which indicate that more than half of the people in the Suhum Kraboa Coaltar District engage in agriculture [17].

5. Patients' Compliance with Tuberculosis Medication

It is often held that compliance with tuberculosis treatment is influenced by background characteristics of patients [10, 18]; but the chi-square tests show that there were no significant relationships between patients' background characteristics (sex, age, educational level, marital status, and occupation) and compliance with medication. Nonadherence to TB medication was found among a substantial proportion of the previously treated patients. In general, 63 percent complied with their medication and had been consequently declared cured while the remaining 37 percent defaulted and were being treated after failure. In a study of New Juabeng Municipality in Ghana, 62 percent of the respondents similarly complied with medication [11]. Our findings show 22 percent failure in compliance using Ghana's expected compliance rate for 2008 as the baseline. Found explanations to this are that more than three-quarters of the patients were burdened with financial problems (77%) as many had to still engage in active work (particularly farming) for survival. Sometimes, their working activities made them either miss the correct times to take their medicines or visit a health centre for injections. Claims of financial burden on households infected with TB were correspondingly reported by [19] in a study of the Western Region of Ghana. Other ramifications such as depression (46%), alcoholism (24%), smoking of cigarettes (11%), and long duration of treatment (26%) were identified as other factors affecting patients' adherence to medication. Some patients resorted to drinking of alcohol and smoking as means of managing depressions resulting from the disease. As they become intoxicated, they usually miss the indications of their medicines because treatment supporters did not have the required expertise in managing such behaviour which consequently affected adherence to medication. Others (17%) complained that the duration for treatment is too long and hence they are tempted to ignore their medicines when they begin to feel better. This emphasizes the findings of [3] that treatment period was initially too long for patients until the introduction of a fixed dose combination therapy.

Despite the point that people accept the "germ theory" of disease causation, people had spiritual explanations to why the disease occurred at that particular point in time. Slightly less than a quarter (24%) proclaimed that their infection was caused by "witchcraft" and hence 19 percent visited spiritual/fate healers for spiritual healing. Spiritual centres such as churches and shrines were consulted with

the hope of finding spiritual remedies to the disease. This led to noncompliance with medication depending on their surety of cure from these spiritual sources. This confirms the works of [12, 20] in Ghana. They found that some diseases have been given supernatural explanations. In line with the self-determination theory, this group of defaulters made decisions based on their needs and beliefs.

There were variations in compliance with regard to age differences. Patients' compliance with medication increased from 56 percent among those aged 20–29 years to 71 percent among those aged 60 years and above. Our findings suggest that aged patients adhere to their medications more than young patients which echo the submissions of [11, 21] that older people comply with medication more than younger people. Education promotes good health not only by generating economic resources through better employment but also by providing knowledge and skills by which people are able to manage illnesses and diseases themselves [22, 23]. Conversely, 89 percent of patients who had no formal education complied with medication compared with those who had attained some form of formal education. Similar findings were revealed by [12] in their study of Agogo in Ghana. Possible explanation to this is that those uneducated benefited more from the services of treatment supporters.

More patients who had never married (68%) complied with medication compared with those who were married (59%). From this finding, marriage does not relatively serve as a form of social support for compliance with medication. This corresponds with findings of [24] that marital status is not a sole predictor of health behaviour. However, the findings contradict a study conducted by [9] in Ghana where marriage was found as a stimulus for compliance with medication. Reference [22] argues that females are naturally more likely to utilise health care services than males. Likewise, more females (69%) than males (63%) complied with medication, although the margin of difference was small. This conforms to findings of [25] that women make a greater use of health care resources than men. In addition, more than three-quarters of respondents who were unemployed (83%) complied with medication compared with farmers (61%), traders (55%), and artisans (65%); purporting that work negatively affects compliance with medication. The findings provide useful knowledge about socioeconomic and psychological factors affecting patients' compliance with medication. A limitation was that the previously treated patients were cases of only pulmonary tuberculosis (PTB). Subsequent studies can consider people who have experienced relapses, new episodes of TB strains, and HIV to ascertain whether there would be differences in compliance.

6. Effects of Roles Played by Treatment Supporters on Patients' Compliance with Medication

In many developing countries, tuberculosis treatment services reach a small proportion of the population because of inadequate health service infrastructure [26]. This prompted interest in assessing the contribution of Community Tuberculosis Care (CTC) to curtailing the disease. CTC which is

TABLE 2: Roles of treatment supporters by patients' compliance with medication.

Roles of treatment supporters and their effects on patients' compliance with medication (N = 110)	Mean	Standard deviation	T value	Significant level ≤0.05	Degree of freedom
Directly observed therapy by health professional***			2.619	0.010	108
Compliant	1.59	0.495			
Noncompliant	1.34	0.480			
Treatment supporter accompany patient to fetch medicine			1.977	0.065	35
Compliant	1.26	0.447			
Noncompliant	1.60	0.516			
Regular visit of patient by treatment supporter***			4.733	0.000	108
Compliant	1.13	0.339			
Noncompliant	1.51	0.506			
Treatment supporter serve patient with medication***			5.534	0.000	108
Compliant	1.32	0.469			
Noncompliant	1.80	0.401			
Treatment supporter reminds patient of clinic days***			3.258	0.001	108
Compliant	1.45	0.501			
Noncompliant	1.76	0.435			
Treatment supporter advise patient on the in-take of medication***			3.357	0.001	108
Compliant	1.32	0.469			
Noncompliant	1.63	0.488			

Source: fieldwork, 2013; ***significant.

quite an extension of DOTS envisages that when community members are trained they could provide DOT at the community level. This strategy makes TB services accessible beyond a health facility which is very crucial [14]. Therefore, we used independent sample t-test to compare significant differences between roles played by treatment supporters and patient's compliance with medication. Results in Table 2 point out that patients who were offered DOT by a health professional in a health centre significantly [$t(108)$ = 2.619; P = 0.010] complied with their medication (M = 1.59, SD = 0.495) which substantiates findings of [8]. However, treatment supporters' escort of patients to a health care centre is not largely associated with compliance with medication [$t(35)$ = 1.977; P = 0.065].

For patients who were served with medication by their treatment supporters, there is significant difference [$t(108)$ = 5.534, P = 0.000] between those who complied with medication (M = 1.32, SD = 0.469) and the noncompliant group (M = 1.80, SD = 0.401). Similarly, [9] found that treatment supporters administering drugs to patients promote compliance. The implication is that "social support" in the form of offering medicines directly to patients promotes patients' compliance with medication as highlighted in the self-determination theory. Those who were regularly visited by treatment supporters significantly [$t(108)$ = 4.733, P = 0.000] complied with their medication. Correspondingly, [3] found that community involvement has helped to reduce rates of default because treatment supporters within patients' immediate environment help to supervise treatment.

Reminding patients about the days for visiting a health centre significantly influenced [$t(108)$ = 3.258; P = 0.001]

compliance with medication (M = 1.45; SD = 0.501), suggesting that patients who are not prompted to visit health centres regularly are likely to be defaulters. Significant difference in scores [$t(108)$ = 3.357; P = 0.001] was also identified among those who were advised and motivated by treatment supporters about the in-take of their medications. The inference is that when treatment supporters advise patients, they are likely to comply with medication and vice versa as noted by [3]. Generally, the findings show that the services of treatment supporters contributed to adherence to treatment.

7. Conclusions

Patients' compliance with tuberculosis medication is of great importance so far as the problem of tuberculosis remains a global health concern. Ghana and for that matter Suhum Kraboa Coaltar District has participated in DOTS to control the menace of tuberculosis. Yet, the target of Ghana to achieve a compliance rate of 85 percent by the year 2008 and beyond has not been accomplished within Suhum Kraboa Coaltar District which records a 22 percent failure. However, the administration of DOT by health professionals alone shows positive influence on patients' compliance with medication. Depression, patients' engagement in work for survival, substance abuse, and the long duration for treatment negatively affect adherence to TB medication. Spiritual inclinations to the disease also discourage compliance with medication. Contrary to what was expected, patients' compliance with medication is not largely influenced by their background characteristics (sex, age, formal education, marital status, and occupation). Rather, assistance given by treatment supporters had emphatic positive effects on compliance with medication. For instance, patients who were monitored and reminded of their clinical days significantly complied with their medication and those who were offered counselling and advice on their medication also notably complied. In conclusion, treatment supporters should be galvanised more in order to ensure a better control of the disease. Patients' noncompliance with medication in the district is an issue and requires new approaches to solve the problem. Future approaches to ensuring patients' adherence to medication could consider skills training, counselling for substance abuse, and pharmacotherapy which were recommended by some respondents.

Conflict of Interests

The authors declare that there is no conflict of interests regarding the publication of this paper.

References

[1] World Health Organization, *Global Report on Tuberculosis*, WHO, Geneva, Switzerland, 2005.

[2] World Health Organization, *Global Tuberculosis Control Report*, World Health Organization, Geneva, Switzerland, 2006.

[3] J. Amo-Adjei and K. Awusabo-Asare, "Reflections on tuberculosis diagnosis and treatment outcomes in Ghana," *Archives of Public Health*, vol. 71, no. 1, article 22, 2013.

[4] K. K. Addo, D. Yeboah-Manu, M. Dan-Dzide et al., "Diagnosis of tuberculosis in Ghana: the role of laboratory training," *Ghana Medical Journal*, vol. 44, no. 1, pp. 31–36, 2010.

[5] E. A. Dodor, "Evaluation of nutritional status of new tuberculosis patients at the Effia-Nkwanta regional hospital," *Ghana Medical Journal*, vol. 42, no. 1, pp. 22–28, 2008.

[6] World Health Organisation, *Management of Tuberculosis Training for Health Facility Staff*, World Health Organisation, Geneva, Switzerland, 2nd edition, 2010.

[7] E. Johansson, N. H. Long, V. K. Diwan, and A. Winkvist, "Attitudes to compliance with tuberculosis treatment among women and men in Vietnam," *International Journal of Tuberculosis & Lung Disease*, vol. 3, no. 10, pp. 862–868, 1999.

[8] A. Salisu and V. Prinz, *Health Care in Ghana*, 2009, http://www.roteskreuz.at/accord.

[9] C. K. Azagba, *Tuberculosis Treatment Outcomes Using Treatment Supporters in Ketu South Municipality of Volta Region in Ghana*, 2013, http://hdl.handle.net/123456789/5535.

[10] A. Yahaya and S. Acquah, "Impact of DOTS plus on treatment outcome among TB patients undergoing DOTS at the Tamale Teaching Hospital (TTH)," *European Journal of Biology and Medical Science Research*, vol. 3, no. 3, pp. 1–9, 2013.

[11] A. S. Boateng, T. Kodama, T. Tachibana, and N. Hyoi, "Factors contributing to tuberculosis defaulter rate in New Juabeng Municipality in the Eastern Region of Ghana," *Journal of the National Institute of Public Health*, vol. 59, pp. 291–297, 2010.

[12] T. S. van der Werf, G. K. Dade, and T. W. van der Mark, "Patient compliance with tuberculosis treatment in Ghana: factors influencing adherence to therapy in a rural service programme," *Tubercle*, vol. 71, no. 4, pp. 247–252, 1990.

[13] Suhum-Kraboa-Coaltar District Health Administration (2013), *Health Facilities at Suhum-Kraboa-Coaltar District*, District Health Directorate, Suhum, Ghana, 2013.

[14] World Health Organization, *Community Involvement in Tuberculosis and Prevention*, World Health Organization, Geneva, Switzerland, 2008.

[15] R. M. Ryan and E. L. Deci, "Self-determination theory and the facilitation of intrinsic motivation, social development, and well-being," *The American Psychologist*, vol. 55, no. 1, pp. 68–78, 2000.

[16] E. L. Deci, H. Eghrari, B. C. Patrick, and D. R. Leone, "Facilitating internalization: the self-determination theory perspective," *Journal of personality*, vol. 62, no. 1, pp. 119–142, 1994.

[17] Ghana Statistical Service, *2010 Population and Housing Census of Ghana: Demographic and Economic Characteristics*, Ghana Statistical Service, Accra, Ghana, 2010.

[18] I. Ajzen, "The theory of planned behavior," *Organizational Behavior and Human Decision Processes*, vol. 50, no. 2, pp. 179–211, 1991.

[19] H. K. Blankson, *Economic burden of tuberculosis (TB) in Ghana, case of western region [M.S. thesis]*, Kwame Nkrumah University of Science and Technology, Kumasi, Ghana, 2012.

[20] K. Awusabo-Asare and J. K. Anarfi, "Health-seeking behaviour of persons with HIV/AIDS in Ghana," *Health Transition Review*, vol. 7, pp. 243–256, 1997.

[21] I. Aboderin, "Understanding and advancing the health of older populations in sub-Saharan Africa: policy perspectives and evidence needs," *Public Health Reviews*, vol. 32, no. 2, pp. 357–376, 2010.

[22] M. K. Murithi, "The determinants of health-seeking behaviour in a Nairobi slum, Kenya," *European Scientific Journal*, vol. 9, no. 8, pp. 156–157, 2013.

[23] D. P. Goldman and J. P. Smith, "Can patient self-management help explain the SES health gradient?" *Proceedings of the National Academy of Sciences of the United States of America*, vol. 99, no. 16, pp. 10929–10934, 2002.

[24] A. McNamara, C. Normard, and B. Whelan, *Patterns and Determinants of Health Care Utilisation in Ireland*, Trinity College, Dublin, Ireland, 2013.

[25] E. Fernandez, A. Schiaffino, L. Rajmil, X. Badia, and A. Segura, "Gender inequalities in health and health care services use in Catalonia (Spain)," *Journal of Epidemiology and Community Health*, vol. 53, no. 4, pp. 218–222, 1999.

[26] J. Ogden, "Improving tuberculosis control—social science inputs," *Transactions of the Royal Society of Tropical Medicine and Hygiene*, vol. 94, no. 2, pp. 135–140, 2000.

16

Prevalence of Stunting among Children Aged 6–23 Months in Kemba Woreda, Southern Ethiopia: A Community Based Cross-Sectional Study

Eskezyiaw Agedew[1] and Tefera Chane[2]

[1]*Department of Public Health, Arba Minch University, Southern Ethiopia, Ethiopia*
[2]*Department of Public Health, Wolaita Sodo University, 251138 Southern Ethiopia, Ethiopia*

Correspondence should be addressed to Eskezyiaw Agedew; esk1agid@gmail.com

Academic Editor: Ronald J. Prineas

Background. Stunting is a public health problem in developing countries. Stunting (HAZ < −2 Z-score) is a major cause of disability preventing children who survive from reaching their full developmental potential. *Objective*. To assess stunting and associated factors among children aged 6–23 months in Southern Ethiopia. *Methods*. Community based cross-sectional study was carried out among 562 mothers who have children from 6 to 23 months in 2014/15 in Kemba district. Multivariate analyses were applied to identify predictor variables and control effect of confounding. *Results*. The study revealed that out of 562 children, 18.7% (95% CI (15.6–22.1)) of children were stunted. In multiple logistic regressions, boys [AOR: 2.50; 95% CI (1.60–4.01)], older mothers [AOR: 2.60; 95% CI (1.07–6.35)], mothers who have no formal education [AOR: 2.76; 95% CI (1.63–4.69)], mothers who work as daily workers [AOR: 3.06; 95% CI (1.03–9.12)] and have private work activity [AOR: 2.39; 95% CI (1.61–3.53)], mothers who have no postnatal follow-up [AOR: 1.64; 95% CI (1.05–2.55)], and maternal illness encountered after delivery [AOR: 1.56; 95% CI (1.05–2.32)] were identified as significant independent predictors of childhood stunting. *Conclusion and Recommendation*. A significant number of children had chronic undernutrition in critical periods. An organized effort should be made at all levels to solve the problems of chronic undernutrition (stunting) in children.

1. Introduction

Poor linear growth, or stunting (low length- or height-for-age), in young children is the result of multiple circumstances and determinants, including antenatal, intrauterine, and postnatal malnutrition, more commonly due to inadequate or inappropriate nutrition and the impact of infectious disease. Childhood stunting continues to be a public health issue in many African countries [1, 2].

Stunting in early life is associated with adverse functional consequences and growth failure during infancy and early childhood is often irreversible, leading to short stature during adolescence and adulthood. Stunting is associated with an elevated risk of child mortality, increased susceptibility to infection, and poor cognitive and psychomotor development. The long-term consequences of stunting include deficits in school achievement, reduced work capacity, and adverse pregnancy outcomes. Worldwide, stunting affects nearly one-third of children under 5 years of age, with the prevalence being higher in low-resource countries in sub-Saharan Africa and South Asia [3–5]. Stunting is a multifactorial phenomenon with a high prevalence in developing countries [6]. Globally, it is estimated that undernutrition is responsible, directly or indirectly, for at least 35% of deaths in children less than five years of age. Stunting (deficit in height/length-for-age of at least −2 Z-score) affects close to 195 million children under five years of age in the developing world [7].

Appropriate weaning and complementary feeding behaviors, nutritional interventions, and disease control and treatment programs are strategies to prevent stunting. However, their effectiveness also depends on counteracting the environmental and socioeconomic circumstances that allow infection and suboptimal nutrition to persist [1, 6].

The period from birth to two years of age is particularly important because of the rapid growth and brain development that occurs during this time. The period is often marked by growth faltering, micronutrient deficiencies, and common childhood illnesses [8].

Infant-feeding practices constitute a major component of child caring practices apart from sociocultural, economic, and demographic factors. Somehow, these practices constitute one of the most neglected determinants of young child malnutrition in spite of their important role in growth pattern of children [9].

Data exists in Ethiopia showing the problem of malnutrition beginning early in life, primarily during the first 12 months, when growth faltering takes hold due to suboptimal infant feeding practices. Stunted infants grow to be stunted children and stunted adults [10]. At national level, 44% of children under age of five are stunted and 21% of children are severely stunted [11]. In order to effectively accomplish the goals of Accelerated Stunting Reduction, identifying the potential determinants of chronic undernutrition is a vital step to reduce the burden of stunting. Therefore, the aim of this study was to have detailed and concrete data that fill these gaps and would add a value that directs policy makers to draw appropriate intervention measures to improve and flourish the health of future generation.

2. Methods and Materials

2.1. Study Setting and Source Population. This community based cross-sectional study was carried out in December 7–27/2014 on 562 mothers who have young child from 6 months to 2 years of age in Kemba Woreda located in Southern parts of Ethiopia. The Southern Nations Nationalities and People's Regional State (SNNPRS) consists of 13 zones and 104 woreda. The region has an estimated 15,042,531 (20.4% of the national estimate) people. Close to 90% of the population are estimated to be rural inhabitants, while 1,545,710 or 10.3% are urban. Kemba Woreda is one of the administrative woreda in Gamo Gofa Zone, South Ethiopia, 100 km away from zonal town Arba Minch. From the total population around 44,000 are women in reproductive age group. The health institution distribution in the woreda is 39 health posts and 9 health centers providing health services including maternal and child health care.

2.2. Inclusion and Exclusion Criteria. Mothers/care givers who have young children from 6 months to 23 months old who live in the selected Keble for at least 6 months were included in the study and those who had mental illnesses interfering with the interview were not considered in study.

2.3. Sample Size Determination and Sampling Methods. The sample size was determined by using single population proportion formula by the following assumption for prevalence of stunting (chronic malnutrition) as 44% in SNNPR,

Southern Ethiopia [12], desired precision (*d*) as 5% and 95% as confidence interval:

$$N = \frac{((z/2)\,\alpha)^2\,p\,(1-p)}{d^2}. \tag{1}$$

The final sample size was calculated by taking 1.5 as design effect which is 567.

2.4. Sampling Methods. Interviewed mothers were selected from eight kebeles which were selected by using lottery method from all kebeles. Then the number of study participants was allocated for each kebele based on proportional to population size allocation methods by using community based demographic and health related information registration prepared by Health Extension workers as the sampling frame. Rapid censuses were conducted first to identify the target household. Finally infant-mother pairs were selected from each kebele by using simple random sampling methods after giving code for each household which has young child from six months to 24 months (Figure 1).

2.5. Data Collection Methods, Measurement, and Quality Control. Data was collected from mothers/care givers who have one child in age 6 months to 23 months from each household by direct interviewing. Pretested structured questionnaire adapted from different literature was used to collect sociodemographic and other variables. The questionnaire were arranged and grouped according to the issue addressed.

First the questionnaire was prepared in English and translated to Amharic and pretested on 5% of mothers before actual data collection outside the selected kebeles; correction and modification was done based on the gap identified during interview. Six Grade 12 completed students were recruited as data collectors and supervised by 3 nurses. Three-day training was given on the aim of the research, content of the questionnaire, and how to conduct interview for data collectors and supervisor to increase their performance in field activities. The collected data were checked every day by supervisors and principal investigator for its completeness and consistency.

Anthropometric measurements such as weight and height were measured using standard technique and calibrated equipment. The weight of each child was taken by using digital scale wearing light cloth, checking the calibration using 2 kg rod during each instant of weight measuring, and the measurement was approximated to the nearest 10 g. Children were not in fasting condition and each subject was weighted twice and the average weight was taken. Length was measured in recumbent position using sliding board by two data collectors and taken to the nearest 1 mm [2, 13, 14]. The data collectors were trained efficiently on how to take the anthropometric measurements.

2.6. Data Analysis and Management. Data was coded and entered into Epi-Info version 3.5.1 and exported to SPSS version 20 for analysis. Exploratory data analysis was done to check missing values, potential outliers, and the normality distribution for those continuous variables. The presence of

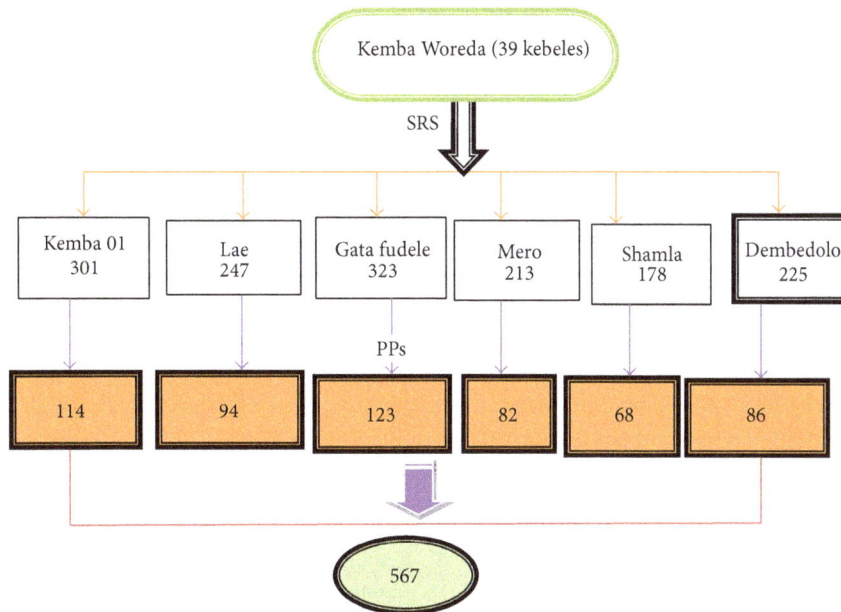

FIGURE 1: Schematic presentation of sampling procedure in Kemba Woreda, Southern Ethiopia, 2014/15.

multicollinearity also was checked and effort was made to incorporate different models to cross check. Anthropometric index (HAZ) was analyzed by using WHO Anthro software version 3.2.2 and categorized as stunted if HAZ < −2 Z-score and as normal if HAZ > −2 Z-score; stunting is defined as HAZ < −2 SD [13]. Extreme outlier of <−6 Z-score of HFA was omitted from the analysis. Descriptive frequencies were calculated to describe the study population in relation to relevant variables. Bivariate logistic regression analysis was calculated to assess the crude association between dependent and independent variables. Finally variables which show association in bivariate logistic regression analysis and have P value less than 0.25 (not to miss some of important variables that are not significant in the bivariate analysis) were entered into multivariate logistic regression model, to identify significant independent predictors of stunting and to control the possible effect of confounding. Variables with P value less than 0.05 were identified as significant predictors of stunting.

2.7. Ethical Consideration.

2.7. Ethical Consideration. Ethical clearance was obtained from Research Ethics Committee (REC) of Addis Continental Institute of Public Health. Permission letter was obtained from Kemba Woreda Health Office. Verbal informed consent from each study participant was obtained after clear explanation about the purpose of the study. All the study participants were reassured that only anonymous data were taken. They were given the chance to ask anything about the study and made free to refuse or stop the interview at any moment they want if that was their choice.

3. Result

3.1. Sociodemographic Characteristics of the Mothers and Young Child. A total of 562 women having young child aged 6

months to 23 months were interviewed in the study from 567 sampled mothers with 99.11% response rate. The mean age of children were 13.82 months with ±5.85 standard deviation and 53% of them were found in age range from 6 months to 1 years and 273 (48.6%) were boys and 289 (51.4%) were girls with sex ratio of 0.94. Almost half of the mothers, 271 (48.2%), were in age range 25–29 years. About one-third of respondents (30.8%) had no formal education and 46% of them were farmers and daily workers in their occupational status. About two-thirds of the respondent mothers 348 (61.9%) were Protestant followers and the rest were Orthodox and Muslims (Table 1).

3.2. Prevalence of Chronic Undernutrition (Stunting). From 562 interviewed mothers-child pair 18.7%, 95% CI (15.6–22.1), out of all children, 25.8%; 95% CI (20.8–31.4) boys and 12.5%; 95% CI (8.5–16.0) girls had chronic undernutrition. The level of moderate stunting was 10.4%; 95% CI (7.9–12.9). Among all boys, 14.4%; 95% CI (10.2–18.6) and among all girls, 6.8%; 95% CI (3.9–9.7) boys and girls had moderate chronic undernutrition respectively. The prevalence of severe stunting (HAZ < −3 Z-score) was 8.4%, 95% CI (6.1–10.7). In the overall scenario, boys were more affected than girls. There were higher numbers of stunted boys than stunted girls (Figure 2).

3.3. Factors Associated with Chronic Undernutrition (Stunting). Variables like sex of child [AOR: 2.50; 95% CI (1.60–4.01)], age of mothers those in age group ≥30 years [AOR: 2.60; 95% CI (1.07–6.35)], education level those who have no formal education [AOR: 2.76; 95% CI (1.63–4.69)], occupational of mothers those who work as daily workers [AOR: 3.06; 95% CI (1.03–9.12)] and Private work activity (merchant, farmers) [AOR: 2.39; 95% CI (1.61–3.53)], mothers who have

TABLE 1: Sociodemographic characteristics of mothers, who had infant aged from 6–23 months, who live in Kemba Woreda, 2014/15.

Variables	Frequency ($n = 562$)	Percent (%)
Age of child		
6–8 months	125	22.2
9–12 months	172	30.6
13–17 months	119	21.2
18–23 months	146	26.0
Sex of child		
Male	273	48.6
Female	289	51.4
Residence of mother		
Rural	205	36.5
Urban	357	63.5
Age of mother		
15–19	97	17.3
20–24	165	29.4
25–29	256	45.6
≥30	44	7.7
Religion status		
Orthodox	197	35.1
Protestant	348	61.9
Muslim	17	3.0
Education		
No education	173	30.8
Primary education	202	35.9
Secondary and above	187	33.3
Occupational status		
Daily laborer	20	3.6
Private (merchant, farmers)	259	46.1
Government worker	27	4.8
Housewife	256	45.6
Ethnicity		
Gamo and Gofa	491	87.4
Wolaita	58	10.3
Amhara	11	2.0
Others	2	0.4

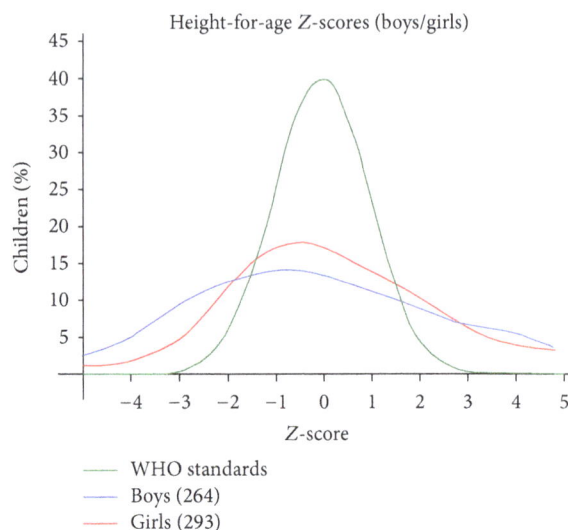

FIGURE 2: Distribution of chronic undernutrition/stunting by sex among children 6–23 months of age residing in Kemba Woreda, Southern Ethiopia, 2014/15.

no postnatal follow up for their child in Health service [AOR: 1.64; 95% CI (1.05–2.55)], and maternal illness encountered after delivery [AOR: 1.56; 95% CI (1.05–2.32)] were significantly associated with chronic undernutrition. However, variables such as place of residence, place of delivery, and ANC followup did not show statistical association with chronic undernutrition (Table 2).

4. Discussion

The result of this study showed that the prevalence of stunting (HAZ < −2 SD) was 18.7% 95% CI (15.6–22.1). Boys were more likely to be stunted than girls (25.8% versus 12.5%). The prevalence of stunting in this setting was much lower than findings from different parts of Ethiopia (Bule Hora (47.6%), Jimma arjo (41.4%)) [14] and even lower than the

regional stunting levels of Ethiopian demographic and health surveillance report [11], Eastern Kenya (33.3%) [15], and this finding was consistent with finding from Johannesburg (18%) [16]. In contrast to the above findings, the magnitude of stunting in the our study area was higher than report from Latin America and Caribbean countries (11%) [17]. The reason why the finding in our setting is lower than the others may be due to the narrowing of age of children in the study making the magnitude of stunting declined as compared to studies having wide target children <5 years of age. The reason goes in line with findings from Eastern Kenya showing that stunting is more prevalent in children >2 years [15].

In this study, child sex, maternal age, maternal educational level and occupational status, and postnatal followup were statistically significant with chronic undernutrition. Having no formal education of mothers and older mothers (>31 years) were negatively associated with the nutritional status of children. Similarly the findings are supported with findings from Johannesburg, Tanzania, and Kenya [15, 16, 18]. Having maternal illness and not attending postnatal care were also independent predictors of stunting.

5. Strength and Weakness of the Study

This study is community based showing real nutritional condition of children 6–23 months of age. Thus it has strong generalization power because other studies were conducted with relatively small sample size and were institutional based. Recall bias may be introduced even if it was minimized by probing mothers to report by association with different life events may not remember events occurred in the past, and possibility of interviewer bias and misreporting of events were the potential limitation. Another limitation of the study was failing to incorporate wealth index, dietary diversity, and household food security.

TABLE 2: Factors associated with stunting among mothers who have 6–23 months of young child in Kemba Woreda in 2014/15.

Explanatory variable	Chronic nutritional status		Crude OR (95% CI)	Adjusted OR (95% CI)	P value
	Normal (%)	Stunted (%)			
Residence					
Rural	159 (77.6)	46 (22.4)	1.50 (1.04–3.33)	1.34 (0.82–2.19)	0.24
Urban	298 (83.5)	59 (16.5)	1	1	
Sex of child					
Male	204 (74.2)	69 (25.8)	2.43 (1.56–3.80)	2.50 (1.60–4.01)	0.001
Female	253 (87.5)	36 (12.5)	1		
Age of mother					
≤19	74 (76.3)	23 (23.7)	1	1	
20–24	144 (87.3)	21 (12.7)	1.03 (0.60–1.74)	1.15 (0.647–2.08)	0.620
25–30	203 (79.3)	53 (20.7)	1.20 (0.74–1.95)	0.97 (0.54–1.75)	0.924
≥31	36 (81.8)	8 (18.2)	1.96 (0.94–4.09)	*2.60 (1.07–6.35)	0.035
Maternal education level					
No formal education	102 (75.6)	33 (24.4)	3.08 (1.98–4.79)	*2.76 (1.63–4.69)	0.001
Primary education	199 (80.9)	47 (19.1)	1.72 (1.15–2.57)	1.42 (0.89–2.25)	
Secondary and above	156 (86.2)	25 (13.8)	1	1	
Occupational status					
Daily laborer	16 (72.7)	6 (17.3)	3.55 (1.40–9.09)	*3.06 (1.03–9.12)	0.045
Private (merchant, farmers)	216 (80.9)	51 (19.1)	0.41 (0.28–0.59)	*2.39 (1.61–3.53)	0.001
Government worker	30 (88.2)	4 (11.8)	0.34 (0.12–0.96)	0.44 (0.16–1.18)	0.103
Housewife	195 (81.6)	44 (18.4)	1	1	
Media exposure					
Yes	251 (83.7)	49 (16.3)	1		
No	206 (78.6)	56 (21.4)	1.91 (1.35–2.69)	0.86 (0.53–1.39)	0.54
Place of delivery					
Home	153 (78.9)	41 (21.1)	1.25 (0.87–1.78)	1.41 (0.89–2.24)	0.14
Health facility	304 (82.6)	64 (17.4)	1	1	
ANC followup					
Yes	404 (81.3)	93 (18.7)	1	1	
No	53 (81.5)	12 (18.5)	1.66 (0.95–2.89)	0.82 (0.44–1.57)	0.55
PNC followup					
Yes	132 (84.1)	25 (15.9)	1	1	
No	325 (80.2)	80 (19.8)	1.80 (1.48–3.2)	*1.64 (1.05–2.55)	0.029
Maternal illness					
Yes	19 (79.2)	5 (20.8)	1.40 (0.99–1.96)	*1.56 (1.05–2.32)	0.027
No	437 (81.4)	100 (18.6)	1	1	

*Significant factors.

6. Conclusion and Recommendation

A significant number of young children were affected by chronic malnutrition. Stunting was significantly associated with child sex, maternal illiteracy, mothers who work as daily workers and have private work, and those having no postnatal followup and maternal illness encountered after delivery. An organized effort should be made at all levels to improve maternal education, postnatal care practice, and maternal health status to solve the problems of chronic undernutrition (stunting) in children, especially in such critical periods, to avoid its effect on future development of young children. Appropriate and early intervention should be designed at health facility and community level for mothers to have postnatal followup since it is an opportunity for health professional to give nutrition education for mothers. Further research should be conducted to investigate specific nutrient deficiency status in body serum by using laboratory methods.

Abbreviations

AOR: Adjusted odds ratio
SAM: Severe acute malnutrition
MUAC: Mid-upper-arm circumference
CI: Confidence interval
SD: Standard deviation
TFU: Therapeutic feeding unit.

Conflict of Interests

The authors declare that they have no conflict of interests.

Authors' Contribution

Eskezyiaw Agedew initiated the research, wrote the research proposal, conducted the research, did data entry and analysis, and wrote the paper. Tefera Chane contributed in the designing of methodology and writing of proposal.

Acknowledgments

The authors would like to thank Arba Minch University for funding their research work. Their deepest gratitude goes to data collectors, kebeles leaders, and Kemba Woreda Health Center Manager for his cooperation starting from the beginning till the end of data collection time.

References

[1] B. A. Willey, N. Cameron, S. A. Norris, J. M. Pettifor, and P. L. Griffiths, "Socio-economic predictors of stunting in preschool children—a population-based study from Johannesburg and Soweto," *South African Medical Journal*, vol. 99, no. 6, pp. 450–456, 2009.

[2] M. de Onis, M. Blössner, and E. Borghi, "Prevalence and trends of stunting among pre-school children, 1990–2020," *Public Health Nutrition*, vol. 15, no. 1, pp. 142–148, 2012.

[3] J. H. Rah, N. Akhter, R. D. Semba et al., "Low dietary diversity is a predictor of child stunting in rural Bangladesh," *European Journal of Clinical Nutrition*, vol. 64, no. 12, pp. 1393–1398, 2010.

[4] UNC's Fund, *The State of the World's Children 2009*, UNICEF, 2008.

[5] C. G. Victora, L. Adair, C. Fall et al., "Maternal and child undernutrition: consequences for adult health and human capital," *The Lancet*, vol. 371, no. 9609, pp. 340–357, 2008.

[6] M. T. Ruel and P. Menon, "Child feeding practices are associated with child nutritional status in Latin America: innovative uses of the Demographic and Health Surveys," *Journal of Nutrition*, vol. 132, no. 6, pp. 1180–1187, 2002.

[7] World Health Organization, *Global Data Bank on Infant and Young Child Feeding, World Health Statistics*, World Health Organization, Geneva, Switzerland, 2010.

[8] T. Wolde, E. Adeba, and A. Sufa, "Prevalence of chronic malnutrition (stunting) and determinant factors among children aged 0–23 months in Western Ethiopia: a cross-sectional study," *Journal of Nutritional Disorders & Therapy*, vol. 4, article 148, 2014.

[9] D. Kumar, N. K. Goel, P. C. Mittal, and P. Misra, "Influence of infant-feeding practices on nutritional status of under-five children," *Indian Journal of Pediatrics*, vol. 73, no. 5, pp. 417–421, 2006.

[10] E. W. Kimani-Murage, N. J. Madise, J.-C. Fotso et al., "Patterns and determinants of breastfeeding and complementary feeding practices in urban informal settlements, Nairobi Kenya," *BMC Public Health*, vol. 11, article 396, 2011.

[11] Central Statistical Agency and ICF Macro, *Ethiopia Demographic and Health Survey 2011*, Central Statistical Agency, Addis Ababa, Ethiopia; ICF Macro, Calverton, Md, USA, 2012.

[12] Central Statistical Agency and ORC Macro, *Ethiopia Demographic and Health Survey*, Central Statistical Agency, Addis Ababa, Ethiopia; ORC Macro, Calverton, Md, USA, 2011.

[13] WHO, *WHO Multicenter Growth Reference Study Group. WHO Child Growth Standards: Length/Height-for-Age, Weight-for-Age, Weight-for-Length, Weight-for-Height and Body Mass Index-for-Age: Methods and Development*, World Health Organization, Geneva, Switzerland, 2006.

[14] M. Asfaw, M. Wondaferash, M. Taha, and L. Dube, "Prevalence of undernutrition and associated factors among children aged between six to fifty nine months in Bule Hora district, South Ethiopia," *BMC Public Health*, vol. 15, no. 1, p. 41, 2015.

[15] Z. N. Bukania, M. Mwangi, R. M. Karanja et al., "Food insecurity and not dietary diversity is a predictor of nutrition status in children within semiarid Agro-Ecological zones in Eastern Kenya," *Journal of Nutrition and Metabolism*, vol. 2014, Article ID 907153, 9 pages, 2014.

[16] B. A. Willey, N. Cameron, S. A. Norris, J. M. Pettifor, and P. L. Griffiths, "Socio-economic predictors of stunting in preschool children—a population-based study from Johannesburg and Soweto," *South African Medical Journal*, vol. 99, no. 6, pp. 450–456, 2009.

[17] UNICEF, *Improving Child Nutrition: The Achievable Imperative for Global Progress*, UNICEF, 2013.

[18] C. M. Mcdonald, R. Kupka, K. P. Manji et al., "Predictors of stunting, wasting and underweight among Tanzanian children born to HIV-infected women," *European Journal of Clinical Nutrition*, vol. 66, no. 11, pp. 1265–1276, 2012.

Eating Behaviours and Body Weight Concerns among Adolescent Girls

Nadira Mallick,[1] **Subha Ray,**[1] **and Susmita Mukhopadhyay**[2]

[1] *Department of Anthropology, University of Calcutta, 35 Ballygunge Circular Road, Kolkata 700 019, India*
[2] *Biological Anthropology Unit, Indian Statistical Institute, 203 B.T. Road, Kolkata 108, India*

Correspondence should be addressed to Nadira Mallick; r09mullick@gmail.com

Academic Editor: Julio Diaz

This paper presents a global review of research done on adolescent eating behaviours and food choices and the probable factors underlying it. Worldwide adolescent girls tend to develop moderate to high level of disordered eating behaviour as a result of their excessive concern with body weight or obsession with thinness. The objective of the review is to understand the concerns over body weight and the current eating patterns of adolescent girls in the developed and developing countries.

1. Introduction

Adolescent eating behaviour is a function of individual and environmental influences [1]. Individual influences are psychological as well as biological, whereas, environmental influences include immediate social environments such as family, friend, and peer networks and other factors such as school meals and fast food outlets. In addition, another important factor is social system or macrosystem which includes mass media, marketing and advertising, social and cultural norms of the society [1]. Adolescent girls in particular, because of their excessive concern with body weight or obsession with thinness, are reported with moderate level of disordered eating behaviours [2]. Disordered eating behaviours refer to many disturbed eating patterns [3] which affect the nutritional status of adolescent girls [4]. The literature shows that adolescent girls are more prone to adopt various forms of eating behaviours than boys [5, 6], because they become preoccupied with and sensitive to their changing body size, shape, and physical appearance. This growing concern has led many of them to adopt dietary modifications that potentially throw serious threat on psychosocial development, nutritional status, and development of eating disorder. A number of factors like family environment [7–9], peer pressure [10–12], media habits [13, 14], concern over body image [15–17], sociocultural and economic context [7, 16, 18], gender [6], and

age [19] make them feel dissatisfied with their body shape and weight.

Many studies have found that adolescent girls are interested in losing weight and more than 40% have even tried to lose weight due to concern over their body weight [20, 21]. A report of Youth Risk Behavioural Surveillance System (YRBSS) showed that more than 11% of high school girls in the United States reported taking diet pills, powders, or liquids to lose weight [22]. The data of this study also revealed that about 8% of the girls reported vomit their food after having it in the past month.

Study reports from USA and Europe suggested that the prevalence of disordered eating behaviours is increasing in western countries [23]. Disordered eating behaviours are associated with a number of harmful behaviours such as smoking, alcohol consumption, drug use, and suicide [24, 25] as well as physical and psychosocial consequences like poorer dietary quality [26, 27], depressive symptoms [28], weight gain and onset of obesity [29, 30], and finally the onset of eating disorders [31].

Obesity and eating disorder among adolescents are of serious public health concern owing to their high prevalence and adverse influence on psychological [32, 33] and physical health [34, 35]. The prevalence of overweight [body mass index (BMI) > 95th percentile for age and sex] based on Centre for Disease Control and Prevention Growth charts

[36] among children and adolescents has increased steadily over the past three decades. Currently, 15% of youth aged 6–19 years are found to be overweight [37]. On the other hand, eating disorders like anorexia nervosa, bulimia nervosa, and binge eating affect a much small percentage of adolescent population (1–3%) but are of great concern given their serious health consequences [3]. Another form of eating disorder called eating disorder not otherwise specified (EDNOS) affects much larger segment of adolescent population, with prevalence estimates as high as 15% [38]. Eating habits of adolescents, in general, are in process of changing from more traditional to more westernized one. Yannakoulia et al. [39] observed that eating behaviours like skipping meals, snacking, eating away from home, consumption of fast food, and following alternative dietary patterns (in terms of dieting) are the common eating behaviours of Greek adolescents. This type of eating habits may lead to nutritional deficiency during adolescence [40, 41] which may have long term consequences such as delayed sexual maturation and lower final adult height [42].

The aim of this review is to understand the current eating patterns and body weight concerns among adolescent girls in global and Indian context. Secondly, an attempt has been made to explore those factors influencing eating behaviours and body weight concerns.

2. Western Scenario

In western countries thin body is the most preferred body shape [43]. However, exceptions observed in certain ethnic groups [44]. Thinness is a symbol of beauty, success, control, and sexual attractiveness, while obesity represents laziness, self-indulgence, and lack of willpower [45]. To achieve thin body image, adolescent girls of western countries often remain engaged with their body weight and shape [46]. They may even deny the requirement of important nutritional components in their body when they need it most [47]. For example, in the United States, Killen et al. [48] found that 11% of female adolescents regularly vomit their food after having it and 13% of them reported some form of purging behaviours like use of laxatives or diuretics for body weight control due to excessive concern over body weight. A Minnesota school-based survey suggested an association between dieting and later onset of obesity and eating disorders [30]. Another study carried out in Minnesota revealed that 56% of 9th grade females and 28% of 9th grade males reported disordered eating behaviours such as fasting, vomiting, or binge eating. These behaviours were found to be high among both 12th grade females and males [49]. In Europe, study reported that adolescent who practiced disordered eating such as dieting had less self-esteem compared to those who practiced normal eating [50]. Many studies carried out in Australia also showed the existence of disordered eating behaviours and unhealthy weight reduction practices among adolescent girls [46, 47, 51, 52]. Both young and older adolescent girls reported significantly more disordered eating behaviours than their male counterparts of these two age groups [19, 53]. Study carried out in America found that rates of disordered

eating were highest among overweight and obese youth school students [19, 54, 55]. Wichstrom [56] found that perceived obesity is associated with depression and unstable self-perceptions among general adolescent population of Norway.

3. Situation in Nonwestern Countries

The western concept of thinness as a symbol of beauty and attractiveness is not confined to western countries anymore. The western concept of beauty and attractiveness in thinness is diffusing among the youth of some nonwestern countries like Philippines [57] and Thailand [58]. Lorenzo et al. [59] found in his study that disordered eating attitude and behaviour among adolescents are becoming a significant problem in Philippines. Studies on Chinese population show that adolescents who were concerned about their body weight suffered from depression [60] and high level of psychological distress [61]. A study from Singapore reported that about 7.4% of women are at risk of developing eating disorder [62]. Study concluded that western media might have a negative impact upon body image and eating pattern among women in Singapore.

Taiwan and Japanese females show higher incidence of dieting [63]. Chang et al. [64] found that about 17.11% of Taiwanese adolescent girls reported disordered eating behaviours. Results of the same study showed that intake of energy, protein, carbohydrate, zinc, and vitamins B6 and B12 was significantly lower in those adolescent girls who followed disordered eating behaviours compared to those who showed normal eating behaviours. The adolescent girls who followed disordered eating consumed higher amount of fiber rich foods than those who did not. The study concluded by saying that disordered eating behaviours markedly affect nutritional status of these adolescent girls.

Internalization of thin body weight and mass media play an important role in the development of disordered eating behaviours among Arabian adolescents living in the United Arab Emirates [65]. Study reported that about 66% of adolescents perceived themselves as overweight and desired to be thin. Study also revealed that about 78% of adolescents expressed dissatisfaction with their current body weight and attempted to reduce it through restricting food intake, avoidance of certain food groups, excessive exercise, and self-induced vomiting. Such types of eating behaviours among adolescents were found in past studies, carried out in Saudi Arab and Oman [66, 67]. Another west Asian country, Israel, showed higher rate of abnormal eating attitudes (as reflected by high EAT-26 score) among adolescents from both Jewish and Arab origins [68, 69].

Adolescent girls from south region of Asia showed a similar trend as that found in the other parts of Asia. Sharma [70] found in his study that consumption of fast food was preferred by more than two-third of the school students aged 9–11 years under the influence of television advertisements. Study also showed that consumption of traditional food items such as pulses, green leafy vegetables, fruits, and milk was found to be low among the study group.

4. The Indian Picture

In India, adolescents (from 10 to 19 years) accounted for 22.8% of the population [71] and they face a series of serious nutritional challenges that are affecting not only their growth and development but also their livelihood as adults. On the other hand, presently Indians are experiencing nutritional and lifestyle transition due to globalisation. Many of the adolescent girls modify their normal dietary pattern and follow disturbed eating behaviours [72] and these also affect their nutritional status [73]. Very few studies have been done in India considering eating behaviour and its impact on nutritional status of adolescent girls.

4.1. Eating Behaviours in Various Regions of India. In north India about 0.4% of college girls, residing in foot hills regions of Himalaya, practiced binge eating (a form of disordered eating behaviour) during festive occasions only to check overeating [74]. In this study, none of the girls reported taking any diet pills, laxatives, or diuretics. Mishra and Mukhopadhyay [72] in their study on Sikkimese adolescent reported that girls often opted for skipping of meals to control their body weight. Some of them reported the habit of snacking between main meals. The same study revealed that girls who remained dissatisfied with their body weight were more inclined to diet. In Delhi, weight concern and dissatisfaction over body weight were prevalent among underweight as well as overweight adolescent girls [73]. Eating behaviours like skipping meals, eating out, and snacking were common among these adolescent girls. Although girls had enough knowledge regarding nutritional deficiency, yet they did not/could not follow normal eating behaviours. As a result their diets remain deficient with energy, protein, iron, niacin, vitamin A, and fibre. The study further revealed that adolescent girls with unhealthy eating behaviours showed lack of interest in their educational assignment than girls with good eating habits. Nutritional disorders among another group of adolescent girls in Delhi indicated that individuals of both high and low socioeconomic groups suffered from anemia [75].

A form of distress and disorder in eating habits and attitude towards the body weight had been reported among the adolescents in Chennai, the southern part of India [76]. Later study by Srinivasan et al. [77] showed that very few adolescents (11%) developed a milder form of eating disorder with the fear of fatness. Augustine and Poojara [78] reported that more than half of the adolescent girls residing in Ernakulam wanted to lose body weight. Results showed that the weight loss plans among the study groups included exercise (21%), followed by meal skipping (20%), starvation (16%), binge eating (6%), and consumption of diet pills (2%), and the most commonly skipped meal was breakfast. Latha et al. [79] studied female adolescent college students (aged 16 to 21 years) at Udipi, Karnataka. The result showed that more than 80% of the girls wanted to become slim because they remain too much busy on thinking about their appearance, body weight, and shape. In this study most of the study participants showed high scores on anxiety, somatic symptoms, and social dysfunction subscales. This indicates that adolescence is the phase of confusion, uncertainties, and

instability. In 2009, two cases of anorexia nervosa (a type of eating disorder) were found by Mendhekar et al. [80]. Both of them were middle class urban adolescent school going girls, who experienced marked weight reduction (BMI > 11.5) and other symptoms of anorexia nervosa. Study showed that factors like parental influence, peer pressure, media habits, and preoccupation with thinness were not the only factors responsible for this disease. The author expressed that clinical symptoms of anorexia nervosa in India may be similar in nature to those in western countries but the psychosocial development and psychodynamic aspects may be different in India.

5. Factors Influencing Eating Behaviours and Body Weight Concerns

5.1. Family Environment and Peer Pressure. Sometimes a child's eating behaviour is influenced by their parents' attitude [8, 9]. Many studies reported that parents, particularly mothers, have a considerable influence on their children's eating and dieting patterns, because of their presumed central role in acting out the nature and importance of thinness and the gender-stereotyped nature of dieting itself [8, 81, 82]. In some cases, parents influence their child to lose weight without imparting the proper knowledge of losing weight. Hence, the children tend to follow unhealthy means while losing weight [83], while other studies showed that the parents did influence their children's eating habits by imparting proper knowledge [84, 85].

Peer influence and group conformity can be considered as important determinants in food acceptability and selection. Baker et al. [11] examined eating behaviours in a sample of 279 adolescents from a midsized catholic girls' school and a large public school of US and showed that adolescents were less likely to have a positive attitude or intention about healthy eating and activity if their parents and peer group do not perceive these behaviours as important in life. Another study carried out among Costa Rican adolescents demonstrated direct impact of peer influence on intake of foods containing saturated fat [10]. Favor [12] found that a teenage girl may eat nothing but a green lettuce salad for lunch following her friend, even though she will become hungry later on.

5.2. Sociocultural and Economic Context. Disordered eating is found among adolescent girls of higher socioeconomic status [7]. On the other hand, Jones et al. [16] observed that socioeconomic status (SES) was not significantly associated with disturbed eating behaviours in a school-based study in Ontario. Similar result has been found by Rogers et al. [86] among another group of adolescents and this study reflected the pervasive influence of the media on all SES groups. The cultural context, especially ethnicity and religion, can also influence the development of disordered eating and body weight concern. Studies indicated that black females had larger body size ideals in both USA [44] and Sub-Saharan Africa [87] than their white counterparts and that they tend to be more satisfied with their actual body size than white females [44]. While an ideal for heavier body image may protect black females from developing anorexic-type eating disorders [88], it may increase their risk of overweight [89]. Abraham and Birmingham [18] found that Muslim adolescent girls and adult women have a higher prevalence of elevated Eating Attitude Test scores compared to non-Muslim.

5.3. Concern over Body Image, Gender, and Age. A person's body image is influenced by his/her belief and attitude as well as societal standards of appearance and attractiveness [79]. Females show greater discrepancy between their perceived body size and their ideal body size compared to males [90]. Moreover, concern over body image is more common among adolescent females than the other age groups [91] and they preferred to be identified as overweight than the males [92].

A report of the 2013 Vermont Youth Risk Behavior Survey [93] has shown that a majority of the students (both male and female) perceived themselves to be normal weight. Females were significantly more likely to consider themselves as overweight compared to males. As a result, two-third of female and one-third of male students seriously tried to lose their body weight.

A good number of studies revealed that girls are less satisfied with their body image and have higher rates of body dissatisfaction over weight than boys [7, 15, 16, 90, 94]. Sometimes society puts pressure on women to conform to the cultural ideal for size and shape [95]. This cultural ideal has changed through mass media towards becoming increasingly thin among females in USA [96]. Many studies revealed that younger girls are significantly less likely to engage in disordered eating behaviour than older ones [16, 19, 53].

5.4. Eating Away from Home. During adolescence teens spend less time with family and more time with friends. This reflects their independent nature at the juncture of boyhood and adulthood. Washi and Ageib [97] showed that most of the adolescents in Jeddah, Saudi Arabia, prefer out-of-home food. Results of their study indicated that more than 80% of the participants depend upon fast food rather than home-made food and 73% of them eat at fast food restaurants. A survey conducted on 379 UK adolescents (11 yrs to 12 yrs of age) revealed that eating outside the home accounted for about 30% of daily energy intake [98]. The study concluded that food consumed at home had better density of micronutrient than food consumed outside. The study also revealed that meals taken during tiffin hours at school are rich in fats but contained less protein, nonstarch polysaccharide, iron, and retinol equivalents.

5.5. Media Habits. Among all factors, media presentation of thin image is a major contributor to current high incidence of body dissatisfaction and eating disorders in women [14, 83, 99, 100]. One naturalistic experiment conducted in Fiji provides strong evidence to support the hypothesis that the media has a significant role in the development of body dissatisfaction and eating disorder symptoms [17]. Fiji was a relatively media-native society with little western mass media influence. In this study, the eating attitudes and behaviours of Fijian adolescent girls were measured prior to the introduction of regional television and after the prolonged exposure to television viewing. The results indicated that following the television exposure, these adolescent girls exhibit a significant increase in disordered eating attitudes and behaviours. Becker et al. [101] showed in their study on Fijian adolescent girls that exposure to social network media was associated with eating pathology among the girls aged 15 to 20 years.

Television advertising and soap operas generally represent the heroine as slim, young, and beautiful. Adolescent girls are very much influenced by watching these advertisements on television and mostly they try to keep their body slim [102]. Fashion magazines have become increasingly popular among majority of the adolescent girls [103]. Some researchers showed significant association between body dissatisfaction among teenage girls and their exposure to thin models in the media [104, 105]. For example, girls who read fashion magazines often compared themselves with the models in the television advertisements and the magazine articles, resulting in more negative feelings about their own body shape [106–109]. Field et al. [13] found in their study that 69% of the girls from US reported that pictures published in magazines influence their idea of perfect body shape and 47% reported losing weight because of these pictures. Study also revealed that females exercise and diet more in response to fashion magazine images. Borzekowski et al. [110] reported that there are many articles available in more than 100 proanorexia websites that not only encourage disordered eating but give specific advice on purging, severe restriction on calorie intake, and excessive exercise. The media (both the printed and the electronic) play significant role in eating behaviours and body image concern of the adolescent girls and it may contribute to the development of eating disorders among them [111].

6. Conclusion

6.1. Main Findings of This Review. Following are the main findings of this review.

(i) The eating behaviours like dieting, fasting, skipping meals, and consumption of fast food are found to be high among adolescent girls both from western and nonwestern countries. This whole range of behaviours may develop physical and mental health risk to the adolescents.

(ii) Adolescents from western countries follow more disturbed eating pattern and show excessive concern over body weight compared to adolescents from nonwestern countries.

(iii) This review identified a good number of factors influencing the body weight concern and eating behaviour of adolescent girls. Studies also identified that mass media, peer pressure, and culture are the main contributors among all.

The cultural context in India has changed in the past few years [77]. A shift towards the concept of thin body image is occurring among girls of urban areas through mass media. A majority of girls are interested in attaining thin body image which sometimes leads to dissatisfaction over body weight. Dissatisfaction over body weight provokes the development of body weight concerns and disordered eating behaviours among these adolescent girls and disordered eating behaviours may induce increased risk of eating disorder during later period. This is further being governed by macrolevel global economic forces. For example, India is passing through a transitional phase in dietary pattern due to influence of economic changes, rapid urbanization, women's participation in workforce, and globalization. This transition is marked by a shift from traditional diet to modern western diet which is usually more varied in nature and more preprocessed food, more food of animal origin, and more added sugar and fat [112, 113]. This kind of dietary practices is found to be high among the adolescents due to its vast availability in the market and another reason may be the market influence of popular fast foods promoted through advertising by mass media [114]. Increase in women's participation in workforce on a large scale restrained working mothers from spending sufficient time with their families. To make up for this gap, they sometimes purchase prepared foods and packet foods from restaurants or grocery stores [115], which can also change the pattern of food consumption among the children. Changes in the dietary pattern might lead to a shift from cereal based diet towards high fat and high sugar rich food items that might lead to obesity and other metabolic disorders.

Therefore, future research should be directed to understanding present eating behaviours and body weight concerns, health risk, and associated factors among adolescent girls in India. Such studies would play an important role in the assessment of current nutritional status of adolescent girls and may help develop meaningful/effective nutritional intervention program by the government.

Conflict of Interests

The authors have no conflict of interests regarding this paper.

Acknowledgment

This research was supported by a grant from the University of Calcutta.

References

[1] M. Story, D. Neumark-Sztainer, and S. French, "Individual and environmental influences on adolescent eating behaviors.," *Journal of the American Dietetic Association*, vol. 102, no. 3, pp. S40–S51, 2002.

[2] H. N. Madanat, R. Lindsay, and T. Campbell, "Young urban women and the nutrition transition in Jordan," *Public Health Nutrition*, vol. 14, no. 4, pp. 599–604, 2011.

[3] American Psychiatric Association, *Diagnostic and Statistical Manual of Mental Disorders: DSM-IV*, American Psychiatric Association, Washington, DC, USA, 4th edition, 1994.

[4] M. Tsai, Y. Chang, P. Lien, and Y. Wong, "Survey on eating disorders related thoughts, behaviors and dietary intake in female junior high school students in Taiwan," *Asia Pacific Journal of Clinical Nutrition*, vol. 20, no. 2, pp. 196–205, 2011.

[5] E. C. Weiss, D. A. Galuska, L. K. Khan, and M. K. Serdula, "Weight-control practices among US adults, 2001-2002," *The American Journal of Preventive Medicine*, vol. 31, no. 1, pp. 18–24, 2006.

[6] C. Costa, E. Ramos, M. Severo, H. Barros, and C. Lopes, "Determinants of eating disorders symptomatology in Portuguese adolescents," *Archives of Pediatrics and Adolescent Medicine*, vol. 162, no. 12, pp. 1126–1132, 2008.

[7] D. Neumark-Sztainer, M. E. Eisenberg, J. A. Fulkerson, M. Story, and N. I. Larson, "Family meals and disordered eating in adolescents: longitudinal findings from Project EAT," *Archives of Pediatrics and Adolescent Medicine*, vol. 162, no. 1, pp. 17–22, 2008.

[8] A. J. Hill and J. A. Franklin, "Mothers, daughters and dieting: investigating the transmission of weight control," *British Journal of Clinical Psychology*, vol. 37, no. 1, pp. 3–13, 1998.

[9] L. Smolak, M. P. Levine, and F. Schermer, "Parental input and weight concerns among elementary school children," *International Journal of Eating Disorders*, vol. 25, pp. 263–271, 1999.

[10] R. Monge-Rojas, H. P. Nuñez, C. Garita, and M. Chen-Mok, "Psychosocial aspects of Costa Rican adolescents' eating and physical activity patterns," *Journal of Adolescent Health*, vol. 31, no. 2, pp. 212–219, 2002.

[11] C. W. Baker, T. D. Little, and K. D. Brownell, "Predicting adolescent eating and activity behaviors: the role of social norms and personal agency," *Health Psychology*, vol. 22, no. 2, pp. 189–198, 2003.

[12] L. J. Favor, *Food as Foe: Nutrition and Eating Disorders*, Courtesy of the National Academic Press, Washington, DC, USA, 2007.

[13] A. E. Field, C. A. Camargo Jr., C. B. Taylor, C. S. Berkey, and G. A. Colditz, "Relation of peer and media influences to the development of purging behaviors among preadolescent and adolescent girls," *Archives of Pediatrics and Adolescent Medicine*, vol. 153, no. 11, pp. 1184–1189, 1999.

[14] T. F. Cash and T. Pruzinsky, *Body Image: A Handbook of Theory, Research and Clinical Practice*, The Guildford Press, London, UK, 1st edition, 2004.

[15] J. Demarest and R. Allen, "Body image: gender, ethnic, and age differences," *Journal of Social Psychology*, vol. 140, no. 4, pp. 465–472, 2000.

[16] J. M. Jones, S. Bennett, M. P. Olmsted, M. L. Lawson, and G. Rodin, "Disordered eating attitudes and behaviours in teenaged girls: a school-based study," *CMAJ*, vol. 165, no. 5, pp. 547–552, 2001.

[17] A. E. Becker, R. A. Burwell, S. E. Gilman, D. B. Herzog, and P. Hamburg, "Eating behaviours and attitudes following prolonged exposure to television among ethnic Fijian adolescent girls," *British Journal of Psychiatry*, vol. 180, pp. 509–514, 2002.

[18] N. K. Abraham and C. L. Birmingham, "Is there evidence that religion is a risk factor for eating disorders?" *Eating and Weight Disorders*, vol. 13, no. 4, pp. e75–e78, 2008.

[19] D. Neumark-Sztainer and P. J. Hannan, "Weight-related behaviors among adolescent girls and boys: results from a national survey," *Archives of Pediatrics and Adolescent Medicine*, vol. 154, no. 6, pp. 569–577, 2000.

[20] J. Wardle and L. Marsland, "Adolescent concerns about weight and eating; a social-developmental perspective," *Journal of Psychosomatic Research*, vol. 34, no. 4, pp. 377–391, 1990.

[21] L. Kann, C. W. Warren, W. A. Harris et al., "Youth Risk Behavior Surveillance—United States, 1995," *Journal of School Health*, vol. 66, no. 10, pp. 365–377, 1996.

[22] J. A. Grunbaum, L. Kann, S. Kinchen et al., "Youth risk behavior surveillance: United States, 2003 (Abridged)," *Journal of School Health*, vol. 74, no. 8, pp. 307–324, 2004.

[23] J. M. Eagles, M. I. Johnston, D. Hunter, M. Lobban, and H. R. Millar, "Increasing incidence of anorexia nervosa in the female population of northeast Scotland," *American Journal of Psychiatry*, vol. 152, no. 9, pp. 1266–1271, 1995.

[24] H. E. Ross and F. Ivis, "Binge eating and substance use among male and female adolescents," *International Journal of Eating Disorders*, vol. 26, pp. 245–260, 1999.

[25] D. Neumark-Sztainer, M. Story, L. B. Dixon, and D. M. Murray, "Adolescents engaging in unhealthy weight control behaviors: are they at risk for other health-comprising behaviors?" *American Journal of Public Health*, vol. 88, no. 6, pp. 952–955, 1998.

[26] H. Crawley and R. Shergill-Bonner, "The nutrient and food intakes of 16-17 year old female dieters in the UK," *Journal of Human Nutrition and Dietetics*, vol. 8, no. 1, pp. 25–34, 1995.

[27] D. Neumark-Sztainer, M. Wall, M. Story, and J. A. Fulkerson, "Are family meal patterns associated with disordered eating behaviors among adolescents?" *Journal of Adolescent Health*, vol. 35, no. 5, pp. 350–359, 2004.

[28] E. Stice, "A prospective test of the dual-pathway model of bulimic pathology: mediating effects of dieting and negative affect," *Journal of Abnormal Psychology*, vol. 110, no. 1, pp. 124–135, 2001.

[29] E. Stice, K. Presnell, L. Groesz, and H. Shaw, "Effects of a weight maintenance diet on bulimic symptoms in adolescent girls: an experimental test of the dietary restraint theory," *Health Psychology*, vol. 24, no. 4, pp. 402–412, 2005.

[30] D. Neumark-Sztainer, S. J. Paxton, P. J. Hannan, J. Haines, and M. Story, "Does Body Satisfaction Matter? Five-year Longitudinal Associations between Body Satisfaction and Health Behaviors in Adolescent Females and Males," *Journal of Adolescent Health*, vol. 39, no. 2, pp. 244–251, 2006.

[31] G. C. Patton, R. Selzer, C. Coffey, J. B. Carlin, and R. Wolfe, "Onset of adolescent eating disorders: population based cohort study over 3 years," *British Medical Journal*, vol. 318, pp. 765–768, 1999.

[32] C. C. Strauss, "Personal and interpersonal characteristics associated with childhood obesity," *Journal of Pediatric Psychology*, vol. 10, no. 3, pp. 337–343, 1985.

[33] J. G. Johnson, P. Cohen, S. Kasen, and J. S. Brook, "Childhood adversities associated with risk for eating disorders or weight problems during adolescence or early adulthood," *The American Journal of Psychiatry*, vol. 159, no. 3, pp. 394–400, 2002.

[34] A. Fagot-Campagna, D. J. Pettitt, M. M. Engelgau et al., "Type 2 diabetes among North American children and adolescents: an epidemiologic review and a public health perspective," *Journal of Pediatrics*, vol. 136, no. 5, pp. 664–672, 2000.

[35] S. Zipfel, B. Löwe, D. L. Reas, H. Deter, and W. Herzog, "Long-term prognosis in anorexia nervosa: lessons from a 21-year follow-up study," *The Lancet*, vol. 355, no. 9205, pp. 721–722, 2000.

[36] R. J. Kuczmarski, C. L. Ogden, S. S. Guo et al., "CDC growth charts for the United States: methods and development," *Vital and Health Statistics*, vol. 11, pp. 1–190, 2002.

[37] C. L. Ogden, K. M. Flegal, M. D. Carroll, and C. L. Johnson, "Prevalence and trends in overweight among US children and adolescents, 1999–2000," *The Journal of the American Medical Association*, vol. 288, no. 14, pp. 1728–1732, 2002.

[38] E. Kjelsås, C. Bjørnstrøm, and K. G. Götestam, "Prevalence of eating disorders in female and male adolescents (14-15 years)," *Eating Behaviors*, vol. 5, no. 1, pp. 13–25, 2004.

[39] M. Yannakoulia, D. Karayiannis, M. Terzidou, A. Kokkevi, and L. S. Sidossis, "Nutrition-related habits of Greek adolescents," *European Journal of Clinical Nutrition*, vol. 58, no. 4, pp. 580–586, 2004.

[40] T. A. Nicklas, L. Myers, C. Reger, B. Beech, and G. S. Berenson, "Impact of breakfast consumption on nutritional adequacy of the diets of young adults in Bogalusa, Louisiana: ethnic and gender contrasts," *Journal of the American Dietetic Association*, vol. 98, no. 12, pp. 1432–1438, 1998.

[41] P. Gleason and C. Suitor, "Children's diets in the mid-1990s: dietary intake and its relationship with school meal participation special nutrition programmes," Report no. CN-01-CD1, US Department of Agriculture, Food and Nutrition Service, Alexandria, Va, USA, 2001.

[42] R. Wahl, "Nutrition in the adolescent," *Pediatric Annals*, vol. 28, no. 2, pp. 107–111, 1999.

[43] I. Attie and J. Brooks-Gunn, "Devolopemental issues in the study of eating problems and disorders," in *The Etiology of Bulimia Nervosa: The Individual and Familial Context*, J. H. Crowther, D. L. Tennenbaum, S. E. Hobfoll, and M. A. P. Stevens, Eds., pp. 35–59, Hemisphere, Washington, DC, USA, 1992.

[44] E. Lynch, K. Liu, B. Spring, A. Hankinson, G. S. Wei, and P. Greenland, "Association of ethnicity and socioeconomic status with judgments of body size: the coronary artery risk development in young Adults (CARDIA) study," *The American Journal of Epidemiology*, vol. 165, no. 9, pp. 1055–1062, 2007.

[45] World Health Organization, "Obesity: Preventing and Managing the Global Epidemic," http://www.who.int/nutrition/publications/obesity/WHO_TRS_894/en/.

[46] M. Grigg, J. Bowman, and S. Redman, "Disordered eating and unhealthy weight reduction practices among adolescent females," *Preventive Medicine*, vol. 25, no. 6, pp. 748–756, 1996.

[47] J. Polivy and C. P. Herman, "Dieting and binging. A causal analysis," *The American Psychologist*, vol. 40, no. 2, pp. 193–201, 1985.

[48] J. D. Killen, C. B. Taylor, M. J. Telch, K. E. Saylor, D. J. Maron, and T. N. Robinson, "Self-induced vomiting and laxative and diuretic use among teenagers. Precursors of the binge-purge syndrome?" *Journal of the American Medical Association*, vol. 255, no. 11, pp. 1447–1449, 1986.

[49] J. Croll, D. Neumark-Sztainer, M. Story, and M. Ireland, "Prevalence and risk and protective factors related to disordered eating behaviors among adolescents: relationship to gender and ethnicity," *Journal of Adolescent Health*, vol. 31, no. 2, pp. 166–175, 2002.

[50] L. Peternel and A. Sujoldžić, "Adolescents eating behavior, body image and psychological well-being," *Collegium Antropologicum*, vol. 33, no. 1, pp. 205–212, 2009.

[51] S. J. Paxton, E. H. Wertheim, K. Gibbons, G. I. Szmukler, L. Hillier, and J. L. Petrovich, "Body image satisfaction, dieting beliefs, and weight loss behaviors in adolescent girls and boys," *Journal of Youth and Adolescence*, vol. 20, no. 3, pp. 361–379, 1991.

[52] E. H. Wertheim, S. J. Paxton, D. Maude, G. I. Szmukler, K. Gibbons, and L. Hiller, "Psychosocial predictors of weight loss behaviors and binge eating in adolescent girls and boys,"

International Journal of Eating Disorders, vol. 12, no. 2, pp. 151–160, 1992.

[53] U. Berger, C. Schilke, and B. Strauß, "Weight concerns and dieting among 8 to 12-year-old children," *PPmP Psychotherapie Psychosomatik Medizinische Psychologie*, vol. 55, no. 7, pp. 331–338, 2005.

[54] A. L. Toselli, S. Villani, A. M. Ferro, A. Verri, L. Cucurullo, and A. Marinoni, "Eating disorders and their correlates in high school adolescents of Northern Italy," *Epidemiologia e Psichiatria Sociale*, vol. 14, no. 2, pp. 91–99, 2005.

[55] J. S. Vander Wal and M. H. Thelen, "Eating and body image concerns among obese and average-weight children," *Addictive Behaviors*, vol. 25, no. 5, pp. 775–778, 2000.

[56] L. Wichstrom, "Social, psychological and physical correlates of eating problems: a study of the general adolescent population in Norway," *Psychological Medicine*, vol. 25, no. 3, pp. 567–579, 1995.

[57] L. L. Farrales and G. E. Chapman, "Filipino women living in Canada: constructing meanings of body, food, and health," *Health Care for Woman International*, vol. 20, no. 2, pp. 179–194, 1999.

[58] P. S. Jennings, D. Forbes, B. McDermott, G. Hulse, and S. Juniper, "Eating disorder attitudes and psychopathology in Caucasian Australian, Asian Australian and Thai university students," *Australian and New Zealand Journal of Psychiatry*, vol. 40, no. 2, pp. 143–149, 2006.

[59] C. R. Lorenzo, P. W. Lavori, and J. D. Lock, "Eating attitudes in high school students in the Philippines: a preliminary study," *Eating and Weight Disorders : EWD*, vol. 7, no. 3, pp. 202–209, 2002.

[60] B. Xie, C. H. Liu, C. P. Chou et al., "Weight perception and psychological factors in Chinese adolescents," *Journal of Adolescent Health*, vol. 33, no. 3, pp. 202–210, 2003.

[61] Y. Luo, W. L. Parish, and E. O. Laumann, "A population-based study of body image concerns among urban Chinese adults," *Body Image*, vol. 2, no. 4, pp. 333–345, 2005.

[62] T. F. Ho, B. C. Tai, E. L. Lee, S. Cheng, and P. H. Liow, "Prevalence and profile of females at risk of eating disorders in Singapore," *Singapore Medical Journal*, vol. 47, no. 6, pp. 499–503, 2006.

[63] L. S. Adair, "Dramatic rise in overweight and obesity in adult Filipino women and risk of hypertension," *Obesity Research*, vol. 12, no. 8, pp. 1335–1341, 2004.

[64] Y. Chang, W. Lin, and Y. Wong, "Survey on eating disorder-related thoughts, behaviors, and their relationship with food intake and nutritional status in female high school students in Taiwan," *Journal of the American College of Nutrition*, vol. 30, no. 1, pp. 39–48, 2011.

[65] V. Eapen, A. A. Mabrouk, and S. Bin-Othman, "Disordered eating attitudes and symptomatology among adolescent girls in the United Arab Emirates," *Eating Behaviors*, vol. 7, no. 1, pp. 53–60, 2006.

[66] A. S. Al-Subaie, "Eating attitudes test in Arabic: Psychometric features and normative data," *Saudi Medical Journal*, vol. 19, no. 6, pp. 769–775, 1998.

[67] S. Al-Adawi, A. S. S. Dorvlo, D. T. Burke, S. Al-Bahlani, R. G. Martin, and S. Al-Ismaily, "Presence and severity of anorexia and bulimia among male and female omani and non-omani adolescents," *Journal of the American Academy of Child and Adolescent Psychiatry*, vol. 41, no. 9, pp. 1124–1130, 2002.

[68] A. Apter, M. Abu Shah, I. Iancu, H. Abramovitch, A. Weizman, and S. Tyano, "Cultural effects on eating attitudes in Israeli subpopulations and hospitalized anorectics," *Genetic, Social, and General Psychology Monographs*, vol. 120, no. 1, pp. 83–99, 1994.

[69] N. R. Maor, S. Sayag, R. Dahan, and D. Hermoni, "Eating attitudes among adolescents," *Israel Medical Association Journal*, vol. 8, no. 9, pp. 627–629, 2006.

[70] I. Sharma, "Trends in the intake of ready-to-eat food among urban school children in Nepal," *SCN News*, vol. 16, pp. 21–22, 1998.

[71] Working group report on Adolescents-of Planning Commission, 2013, http://www.planningcommission.nic.in/aboutus/committee/wrkgrp/wg_adolcnts.pdf.

[72] S. K. Mishra and S. Mukhopadhyay, "Eating and weight concerns among Sikkimese adolescent girls and their biocultural correlates: An exploratory study," *Public Health Nutrition*, vol. 14, no. 5, pp. 853–859, 2010.

[73] R. Chugh and S. Puri, "Affluent adolescent girls of Delhi: eating and weight concerns," *British Journal of Nutrition*, vol. 86, no. 4, pp. 535–542, 2001.

[74] D. Bhugra, K. Bhui, and K. R. Gupta, "Bulimic disorders and sociocentric values in north india," *Social Psychiatry and Psychiatric Epidemiology*, vol. 35, no. 2, pp. 86–93, 2000.

[75] G. Kapoor and S. Aneja, "Nutritional disorders in adolescent girls," *Indian Pediatrics*, vol. 29, no. 8, pp. 969–973, 1992.

[76] T. N. Srinivasan, T. R. Suresh, V. Jayaram et al., "Eating disorders in India," *Indian Journal of Psychiatry*, vol. 37, pp. 26–30, 1995.

[77] T. N. Srinivasan, T. R. Suresh, and V. Jayaram, "Emergence of eating disorders in India. Study of eating distress syndrome and development of a screening questionnaire," *International Journal of Social Psychiatry*, vol. 44, no. 3, pp. 189–198, 1998.

[78] L. F. Augustine and R. H. Poojara, "Prevalane of obesity, weight perceptions and weight control practices among urban college going girls," *Indian Journal of Community Medicine*, vol. 28, no. 4, pp. 187–190, 2003.

[79] K. S. Latha, S. Hegde, S. M. Bhat, P. S. V. N. Sharma, and P. Rai, "Body image, self-esteem and depression in female adolescent college students," *Journal of Indian Association for Child and Adolescent Mental Health*, vol. 2, no. 3, pp. 78–84, 2006.

[80] D. N. Mendhekar, K. Arora, D. Lohia, A. Aggarwal, and R. C. Jiloha, "Anorexia nervosa: an Indian perspective," *National Medical Journal of India*, vol. 22, no. 4, pp. 181–182, 2009.

[81] H. Edmunds and A. J. Hill, "Dieting and the family context of eating in young adolescent children," *International Journal of Eating Disorders*, vol. 25, pp. 435–440, 1999.

[82] S. H. Thompson, A. C. Rafiroiu, and R. G. Sargent, "Examining gender, racial, and age differences in weight concern among third, fifth, eight, and eleven graders," *Eating Behaviors*, vol. 3, no. 4, pp. 307–323, 2003.

[83] A. E. Field, C. A. Camargo Jr., C. B. Taylor, C. S. Berkey, S. B. Roberts, and G. A. Colditz, "Peer, parent, and media influences on the development of weight concerns and frequent dieting among preadolescent and adolescent girls and boys," *Pediatrics*, vol. 107, no. 1, pp. 54–60, 2001.

[84] R. H. Striegel-Moore and A. Kearney-Cooke, "Exploring parents' attitudes and behaviors about their children's physical appearance," *International Journal of Eating Disorders*, vol. 15, no. 4, pp. 377–385, 1994.

[85] M. H. Thelen and J. F. Cormier, "Desire to be thinner and weight control among children and their parents," *Behavior Therapy*, vol. 26, no. 1, pp. 85–99, 1995.

[86] L. Rogers, M. D. Resnick, J. E. Mitchell et al., "The relationship between socioeconomic status and eating-disordered behaviors in a community sample of adolescent girls," *International Journal of Eating Disorders*, vol. 22, pp. 15–23, 1997.

[87] A. A. Caradas, E. V. Lambert, and K. E. Charlton, "An ethnic comparison of eating attitudes and associated body image concerns in adolescent south African school girl," *Journal of Human Nutrition and Dietetics*, vol. 14, pp. 111–120, 2001.

[88] A. D. Powell and A. S. Kahn, "Racial differences in women's desires to be thin," *International Journal of Eating Disorders*, vol. 17, no. 2, pp. 191–195, 1995.

[89] K. J. Flynn and M. Fitzgibbon, "Body images and obesity risk among black females: a review of the literature," *Annals of Behavioral Medicine*, vol. 20, no. 1, pp. 13–24, 1998.

[90] R. M. Gardner, B. N. Friedman, and N. A. Jackson, "Body size estimations, body dissatisfaction, and ideal size preferences in children six through thirteen," *Journal of Youth and Adolescence*, vol. 28, no. 5, pp. 603–618, 1999.

[91] H. Bruch, "Developmental considerations on anorexia nervosa and obesity," *Canadian Journal of Psychiatry*, vol. 26, no. 4, pp. 212–217, 1981.

[92] L. Kann, S. A. Kinchen, B. I. Williams et al., "Youth risk behavior Surveillance-United States, 1997," *Journal of School Health*, vol. 68, no. 9, pp. 355–369, 1998.

[93] "The 2013 Vermont Youth Risk Behavior Survey," http://healthvermont.gov/research/yrbs/2013/documents/2013_yrbs_full_report.pdf.

[94] A. M. Gustafson-Larson and R. D. Terry, "Weight-related behaviors and concerns of fourth-grade children," *Journal of the American Dietetic Association*, vol. 92, no. 7, pp. 818–822, 1992.

[95] L. J. Heinberg, "Theories of body image disturbance: perceptual, developmental and sociocultural models," in *Body Image, Eating Disorders and Obesity*, K. Thompson, Ed., pp. 27–47, American Psychological Association, Washington, DC, USA, 1996.

[96] C. V. Wiseman, J. J. Gray, J. E. Mosimann, and A. H. Ahrens, "Cultural expectations of thinness in women: an update," *International Journal of Eating Disorders*, vol. 11, no. 1, pp. 85–89, 1992.

[97] S. A. Washi and M. B. Ageib, "Poor diet quality and food habits are related to impaired nutritional status in 13- to 18-year-old adolescents in Jeddah," *Nutrition Research*, vol. 30, no. 8, pp. 527–534, 2010.

[98] R. C. Adamson, N. Crombie, and T. Kirk, "A critique of the effects of snacking on body weight status," *European Journal of Clinical Nutrition*, vol. 50, no. 12, pp. 779–783, 1996.

[99] M. P. Levine and K. Harrison, "The role of mass media in the perpetuation and prevention of negative body image and disordered eating," in *Handbook of Eating Disorders and Obesity*, J. K. Thompson, Ed., pp. 695–717, John Wiley, New York, NY, USA, 2003.

[100] A. Nishina, N. Y. Ammon, A. D. Bellmore, and S. Graham, "Body dissatisfaction and physical development among ethnic minority adolescents," *Journal of Youth and Adolescence*, vol. 35, no. 2, pp. 179–191, 2006.

[101] A. E. Becker, K. E. Fay, J. Agnew-Blais, A. N. Khan, R. H. Striegel-Moore, and S. E. Gilman, "Social network media exposure and adolescent eating pathology in Fiji," *British Journal of Psychiatry*, vol. 198, no. 1, pp. 43–50, 2011.

[102] M. Tiggemann and A. S. Pickering, "Role of television in adolescent women's body dissatisfaction and drive for thinness," *International Journal of Eating Disorders*, vol. 20, no. 2, pp. 199–203, 1996.

[103] K. Harrison, "Ourselves, our bodies: thin-ideal media, self-discrepancies, and eating disorder symptomatology in adolescents," *Journal of Social and Clinical Psychology*, vol. 20, no. 3, pp. 289–323, 2001.

[104] G. Cafri, Y. Yamamiya, M. Brannick, and J. K. Thompson, "The influence of sociocultural factors on body image: a meta-analysis," *Clinical Psychology: Science and Practice*, vol. 12, no. 4, pp. 421–433, 2005.

[105] H. A. Hausenblas, A. Campbell, J. E. Menzel, J. Doughty, M. Levine, and J. K. Thompson, "Media effects of experimental presentation of the ideal physique on eating disorder symptoms: a meta-analysis of laboratory studies," *Clinical Psychology Review*, vol. 33, no. 1, pp. 168–181, 2013.

[106] D. Clay, V. L. Vignoles, and H. Dittmar, "Body image and self-esteem among adolescent girls: testing the influence of sociocultural factors," *Journal of Research on Adolescence*, vol. 15, no. 4, pp. 451–477, 2005.

[107] A. E. Field, S. B. Austin, C. A. Camargo Jr. et al., "Exposure to the mass media, body shape concerns, and use of supplements to improve weight and shape among male and female adolescents," *Pediatrics*, vol. 116, no. 2, pp. e214–e220, 2005.

[108] L. J. Hofschire and B. S. Greenberg, "Media's impact on adolescents' body dissatisfaction," in *Sexual Teens, Sexual Media*, J. D. Brown, J. R. Steele, and K. Walsh-Childers, Eds., pp. 125–149, Lawrence Erlbaum, Mahwah, NJ, USA, 2001.

[109] D. C. Jones, T. H. Vigfusdottir, and Y. Lee, "Body image and the appearance culture among adolescent girls and boys: an examination of friend conversations, peer criticism, appearance magazines, and the internalization of appearance ideals," *Journal of Adolescent Research*, vol. 19, no. 3, pp. 323–339, 2004.

[110] D. L. G. Borzekowski, S. Schenk, J. L. Wilson, and R. Peebles, "E-Ana and e-Mia: a content analysis of pro-eating disorder web sites," *The American Journal of Public Health*, vol. 100, no. 8, pp. 1526–1534, 2010.

[111] "Obesity, eating disorders, and the media," in *Children, Adolescents and the Media*, V. C. Strasburger, B. J. Wilson, and A. B. Jordon, Eds., pp. 337–400, Sage, Thousand Oaks, Calif, USA, 2013.

[112] P. Pingali, "Westernisation of Asian Diets and the Transformation of Food Systems: Implications for Research and Policy," 2004, http://www.abengoa.es/export/sites/abengoa_corp/resources/pdf/biofuels/Food_prices/1_P_Pingali.pdf.

[113] B. M. Popkin, L. S. Adair, and S. W. Ng, "Global nutrition transition and the pandemic of obesity in developing countries," *Nutrition Reviews*, vol. 70, no. 1, pp. 3–21, 2012.

[114] N. Vaida, "Prevalence of fast food intake among urban adolescent students," *The International Journal of Engineering and Science*, vol. 2, pp. 353–359, 2013.

[115] "Working moms spend less time daily on kids' diet, exercise," http://www.sciencedaily.com/releases/2012/08/120827162011.htm.

18

Diabetic Complications among Adult Diabetic Patients of a Tertiary Hospital in Northeast Ethiopia

Asrat Agalu Abejew,[1] Abebe Zeleke Belay,[1] and Mirkuzie Woldie Kerie[2]

[1]Department of Pharmacy, College of Medicine and Health Sciences, Wollo University, P.O. Box 1145, Dessie, Ethiopia
[2]Department of Health Services Management, College of Public Health and Medical Sciences, Jimma University, P.O. Box 1637, Jimma, Ethiopia

Correspondence should be addressed to Asrat Agalu Abejew; asratagl@yahoo.com

Academic Editor: Guang-Hui Dong

Background. The diabetic complications are becoming common community problems. The outcomes of diabetic complications are increased hospitalization, increased direct patient costs, and mortality. In Dessie, the prevalence of the diabetic complications is not well studied so far. Thus, the aim of this study is to assess prevalence of diabetic complications and associated factors among adult diabetic patients of Dessie Referral Hospital, Northeast Ethiopia. *Methods*. Cross-sectional study was conducted in the diabetic clinic of Dessie Referral Hospital from April to May 31, 2013. All diabetic patients who visited the clinic during the study period were included. Data was collected using interview guided self-administered questionnaire. Presence of complications and the type of medications the patient was on were identified through review of patient records. Data were cleaned, coded, and entered into SPSS for Windows version 17.0. Descriptive statistics and chi-square tests were carried out to meet the stated objective. *The Results*. Overall 129 (59.7%) of the patients were found to have been affected by one or more of the diabetic complications. Complications were identified mainly among type II diabetic patients. The age of patients (*P* value-0.048), type of diabetes (*P* value-0.00), and medication (*P* value-0.00) were strongly associated with the occurrence of diabetic complication but self-reported adherence, attitude, and knowledge level of patients and the family history were not associated with the presence of complication. *Conclusion*. The prevalence of complications among diabetic patients in Dessie Referral Hospital was high. Targeted counseling and health information provision to the patients by the clinical staff will be helpful in reducing avoidable morbidity and mortality in the patients.

1. Introduction

Diabetes mellitus (DM) is a group of common metabolic disorders that share the phenotype of hyperglycemia, which are caused by a complex interaction of genetics and environmental factors. It is the leading cause of end-stage renal disease (ESRD), traumatic lower extremity amputations, and adult blindness. It also predisposes to cardiovascular diseases. With an increasing incidence worldwide, DM will be a leading cause of morbidity and mortality in the foreseeable future. The goal of treatment for DM is to prevent mortality and complications by normalizing blood glucose level. But blood glucose level might be increased despite appropriate therapy resulting in complications, such as disturbances in fat metabolism, nerve damage, and eye disease [1–5].

Different studies, in fact, of different methodological quality [6] have documented the complications of diabetes in different setups including hospitals and the community [7–9] including its contributing factors like poor attitude [10–13] and adherence [14–17]. These all affect the treatment outcome and may lead to complications and thus to death [18, 19].

Studies have reported that diabetes and its complications are among the common reasons for inpatient admissions, accounting for about 4.4% [18] of total admissions leading to about 3.4% [20] to 32.5% [19] total deaths. The prevalence of chronic complications varies from 52.0% to 74.2% [7,

TABLE 1: Characteristics of the diabetic patients in Dessie Referral Hospital, 2013.

Variable	Frequency (%)
Sex	
Male	125 (57.9)
Female	91 (42.1)
Total	**216 (100)**
Age	
≤30	53 (24.5)
31–45	51 (29.6)
≥45	112 (51.9)
Total	**216 (100)**
Religion	
Muslim	157 (72.7)
Orthodox	58 (26.9)
Protestant	1 (0.5)
Total	**126 (100)**
Ethnicity	
Amhara	204 (94.4)
Oromo	6 (2.8)
Tigrie	3 (1.4)
Others	3 (1.4)
Total	**216 (100)**
Educational status	
Illiterate	99 (45.8)
1–8	63 (29.2)
9–12	31 (14.4)
Higher education	23 (10.6)
Total	**160 (100)**
Marital status	
Never married	94 (43.5)
Married	93 (43.1)
Divorced	11 (5.1)
Widowed	18 (8.3)
Total	**216 (100)**
Current Job	
Gov't employee	17 (11.8)
Merchant	11 (7.6)
Farmer	43 (29.9)
Retired	12 (8.3)
Housewife	23 (16.0)
Others**	38 (26.4)
Total	**144 (100)**
Duration since diagnosed	
<5	93 (43.1)
5–9	79 (36.6)
10–14	24 (11.1)
15–19	8 (3.7)
≥20	12 (5.6)
Total	**216 (100)**
Monthly income	
<100 birr	185 (85.6)
100–199 birr	6 (2.8)
200–299 birr	4 (1.9)

TABLE 1: Continued.

Variable	Frequency (%)
300–499 birr	12 (5.6)
>500 birr	9 (4.2)
Total	**216 (100)**

Others: **student, mechanic, daily laborer.*

TABLE 2: The regimen and specific drugs used to manage types I and II diabetes in Dessie Referral Hospital, 2013 ($n = 216$).

	Frequency (%)
Regimen	
Oral hypoglycemic agents	111 (51.4)
Insulin only	102 (47.2)
Oral hypoglycemic agents and insulin	3 (1.4)
Specific drugs	
NPH** insulin	102 (47.2)
Glibenclamide and metformin	62 (28.7)
Metformin	31 (14.4)
Glibenclamide	18 (8.3)
Metformin and NPH insulin	3 (1.4)
Total	**216 (100)**

NPH** *neutral protamine Hagedorn.*

8, 21, 22]. The most common chronic complications were erectile dysfunction (64%) [23], visual disturbance (33.8%) [7], and cardiovascular disorders (30.1%) [22], though hypertension alone was (68%) [24], neuropathy (29.5%) [7], and nephropathy (15.7%) [7]. Likewise acute complications had similar trend which ranges 30.5% among which diabetic ketoacidosis (DKA) was 71%, followed by hypoglycemia (19.4%) but hyperosmolar hyperglycemic state (HHS) was insignificant [7]. The common risk factors for occurrence of complications were gender [10], long duration with diabetes [21], poor and inadequate glycemic control [9], negative attitude towards diabetes [9, 11, 25, 26], poor treatment adherence [14, 27, 28], and poor knowledge about the disease and its management [9, 11]. Thus, better understanding of perceptions and attitudes among both patients and providers is needed to guide initiatives to improve the management of diabetes [6, 16].

Hence, the common causes of diabetic complications are poor control of diabetes either due to nonadherence, poor attitude towards the disease and its complications, unhealthy diet, and insufficient physical activity, and due to poor management by the health care professionals [10, 18, 29, 30]. On top of these complications diabetes can predispose the patient for different infections [7, 19, 21, 31, 32]. The final outcome of diabetes is a disability, and/or death [19, 21, 29, 32], and of course has great economic impact which is direct (medical and treatment costs) and indirect (costs of hospitalizations, loss of vision, lower extremity amputations, kidney failure, and cardiovascular events) [33, 34]. Thus, prevention is most cost effective than treatment and management of diabetic complications [35, 36].

Most of the studies cited above are from the developed countries [30, 35, 37]; to our knowledge such studies are

TABLE 3: Distribution of variables based on the type of diabetes in Dessie Referral Hospital, 2013 ($n = 216$).

S. no.	Variables	Type of diabetes		Total
		Type I (%)	Type II (%)	
1	Is there complication?			
	Yes	24 (35.8)	105 (70.5)	129 (59.7)
	No	43 (64.2)	44 (29.5)	87 (40.3)
	Total	**67 (100)**	**149 (100)**	**216 (100)**
2	Sex of patients			
	Male	41 (61.2)	84 (56.4)	125 (57.9)
	Female	26 (48.8)	65 (43.6)	91 (42.1)
	Total	**67 (100%)**	**149 (100)**	**216 (100)**
3	Age category			
	<30	31 (46.3)	22 (14.8)	53 (24.5)
	31–45	24 (35.8)	27 (18.1)	51 (23.6)
	>45	12 (17.9)	100 (67.1)	112 (51.9)
	Total	**67 (100)**	**149 (100)**	**216 (100)**
4	Family history of patients			
	Present	17 (25.4)	16 (10.7)	33 (15.3)
	No family history	47 (70.1)	124 (83.2)	171 (79.2)
	I don't know	3 (4.5)	9 (6.0)	12 (5.6)
	Total	**67 (100)**	**149 (100)**	**216 (100)**
5	Category of duration (in years)			
	<5	21 (31.3)	72 (48.32)	93 (43.1)
	5–9	37 (55.2)	42 (28.2)	79 (36.6)
	10–14	7 (10.4)	17 (11.4)	24 (11.1)
	15–19	0	8 (5.4)	8 (3.7)
	>20	2 (3)	10 (6.7)	12 (5.6)
	Total	**67 (100)**	**149 (100)**	**216 (100)**
6	Overall knowledge scores			
	Good	37 (55.2)	71 (47.7)	108 (50)
	Negative/poor	30 (44.8)	78 (52.3)	108 (50)
	Total	**67 (100)**	**149 (100)**	**216 (100)**
7	Self-reported adherence			
	Good	19 (28.4)	47 (31.5)	66 (30.6)
	Poor	48 (71.6)	102 (68.5)	150 (69.4)
	Total	**67 (100)**	**149 (100)**	**216 (100)**
9	Overall attitude scores			
	Good	37 (55.2)	75 (50.3)	112 (51.9)
	Negative/bad	30 (44.8)	74 (49.7)	104 (48.1)
	Total	**67 (100)**	**149 (100)**	**216 (100)**

lacking in Ethiopia and other similar settings. Thus, this study is aimed at determining the prevalence of diabetes related complications and associated risk factors among diabetic patients of a referral hospital in Northeastern Ethiopia.

2. Methods and Materials

2.1. Study Setting. A cross sectional study was conducted from April to May 31, 2013, in the diabetic clinic of Dessie Referral Hospital, located in Dessie town, northeast Ethiopia, 400 km from Addis Ababa. This hospital is the only referral hospital in the Northeastern part of Ethiopia. There are 165 health professionals working in the hospital. In the hospital

there are different clinics among which the diabetic followup clinic is the one serving for treatment and followup of diabetic patients coming to the hospital. The service is provided in the clinic twice a week on every Tuesday and Thursday.

2.2. Study Participants. All diabetic patients visited the adult diabetic clinic of the hospital during the study period. Since all diabetic patients were included in the study, sample size determination and sampling techniques were not used.

2.3. Data Collection Process. Pretested data was collected by four nurses trained for the purpose of the data collection. All

TABLE 4: Distribution of chronic diabetic complications in Dessie Referral Hospital, April–June, 2013.

S. no.	Complications	Frequency (%)
1	Hypertension	39 (43.3)
2	Visual disturbance	26 (28.9)
3	Neuropathy	13 (14.4)
4	Foot ulceration	4 (4.4)
5	Foot ulceration	4 (4.4)
6	Nephropathy	2 (2.2)
7	Impotence	2 (2.2)
8	Total	**90 (100)**

patients visiting the hospital during the three-month period of data collection period were given the self-administered questionnaires and get interviewed if they do not read and write. Patients who visited the hospital for the second time were excluded from study and the first visit's data was taken. The questionnaire contains 18 knowledge, 19 attitude, and 16 practice related questions in addition to 16 general and sociodemographic questions. In addition the last one-month adherence was assessed based on the patients report. Diagnosis of diabetic complications was done by physician and complications and laboratory results were taken from patient cards. The collected data were cleared and checked every day for completeness and consistency before processing.

2.4. Data Processing and Analysis. Collected data were edited, coded, and entered into SPSS for Windows version 17. Descriptive statistics was computed to determine frequency, means, and standard deviations whereas chi-square tests were carried out to determine the association between variables.

2.5. Ethical Consideration. Prior to the study ethical approval was obtained from the ethical review board of Wollo University. The management of the Hospital was requested for cooperation with a formal letter from Wollo University (WU). During and after the data collection process all hospitals and patient-related data were kept confidential. Each study participant signed written consent to participate in the study.

2.6. Operational Definition and Terms

(i) *Good self-reported adherence*: patients who answered correctly more than or equal to mean score.

(ii) *Poor self-reported adherence*: patients who answered below the mean score.

(iii) *Good attitude*: patients who answered correctly more than mean score.

(iv) *Poor/negative attitude*: patients who answered below the mean score.

(v) *Good knowledge*: patients who answered correctly more than mean score.

(vi) *Poor knowledge*: patients who answered below the mean score.

(vii) *Acute complications*: including diabetic ketoacidosis and hyperosmolar hyperglycemic.

(viii) *Chronic complications*: including vascular (microvascular and macrovascular) and nonvascular complications of diabetes.

3. Results

3.1. Sociodemographic Characteristics of Diabetic Patients. Two hundred and sixteen (216) diabetic patients who came to the followup clinic during the 2-month period of data collection were included in the study. The majority of the patients (57.4%) were males, Amhara by ethnic group (94.4%) and Muslims by religion (72.7%). The median age of the patients was 45 (±17.677) and they were known diabetic patients for the mean duration of 5.00 (±5.70) years (Table 1).

The majority of the patients, 145 (67.1%), were of type II with the remaining 71 (32.9%) being type I patients. The medications used for the treatment of diabetes were oral hypoglycemic agents, 111 (51.39%), either in combination or alone. But it was noted that insulin was used for both type I and II diabetics to manage the complications (Table 2).

3.2. Prevalence of Diabetic Complications among Diabetic Patients. The overall complications were 129 (59.7%) of which 105 (48.6%) were from type II patients. When we see the type specific complications, 105 (70.5%) and 24 (35.8%) were among types II and I diabetes, respectively. Attitude 37 (55.2%) and knowledge levels 37 (55.2%) are better among the type I diabetic patients when compared to type II patients (Table 3).

More than half, 129 (59.7%), of the patients have experienced at least one complication. About 90 (58.8%) and 63 (41.2%) of patients have experienced chronic and acute complications, respectively. Hypertension 39 (43.3%), visual disturbance 26 (28.9%), and neuropathy 13 (14.4%) were the three most common chronic complications in the diabetic clinic (Table 4), whereas the three most common acute diabetic complications were DKA 43 (68.3%), hypoglycemia 15 (28.3.7%), and HHS 5 (7.9%).

3.3. Factors Associated with Diabetic Complications. The age of patients, type of diabetes, the regimen, and specific medications the patient is taking were strongly associated with the presence of complication but it has to be noted that self-reported adherence, attitude and knowledge level of patients, as well as the average blood glucose level, and the family history, were not associated with the presence of complication (Table 5). Close to nine in ten, 183 (86.11%), the three-month average blood glucose level is still elevated.

4. Discussion

This study examines diabetic complications in the diabetic clinic in referral hospital. It is highlighted that diabetic complications are common in the Ward in which the majority were among type II patients and around 41% of patients have

Table 5: Association of specific factors with presence of complications among diabetic patients in Dessie Referral Hospital, 2013 ($n = 216$).

Variables	Is there complication?			P value
	Yes	No	Total	
Age of patients				
<30	25	28	53	
31–45	29	22	51	0.048
>45	75	37	112	
Sex				
Male	75	50	125	0.517
Female	54	37	91	
Type of diabetes				
Type I	24	43	67	0.00
Type II	105	44	149	
The regimen the patient is taking				
Oral hypoglycemic agents	78	33	111	
Insulin only	48	54	102	0.001
Oral hypoglycemic agents and insulin	2	1		
Specific drugs				
Glibenclamide	17	1	18	
Metformin	29	2	31	
Glibenclamide and metformin	39	23	62	0.00
NPH insulin	42	60	108	
Metformin and NPH	2	1	3	
Self-reported adherence				
Good	36	30	66	0.303
Poor	93	57	150	
Overall attitude scores				
Good	65	47	216	0.35
Negative/bad	64	40	104	
Overall knowledge scores				
Good	61	47	108	0.203
Poor	68	40	108	

microvascular complications alone or with other macrovascular complications. It is indicated that different factors have been implicated as risks for occurrence of the complications.

In this study, 59.7% of diabetic patients had at least one diabetic complication. This was lower than the finding reported from Jimma, Ethiopia, where 83.00% of the patients had complications [7]. The majority of the complications (48.6%) in this study were among type II patients, which is similar to another study in Jimma (52.5%) and Taiwan (52.6%) [7, 38]. The fact that a diagnosis of complications was made by general practitioners, the sociocultural differences in health seeking behavior and disclosing complications like sexual problems might result in the differences.

In this study, 70.5% of type II patients have at least one complication. This was similar to other studies in Libya (68.7%), Iran (74.2%), and Russia (70.7%) [8, 21, 39]. But it was higher than another study in China (52.0%) [22]. The difference might lie at the level of practice and the attitude and knowledge gap between the patients.

Acute complications occurred in 28.24% of the patients of which 61.71% had diabetic ketoacidosis as a complication

at least once. Similar findings were reported by an earlier study in Jimma, Ethiopia [7]. Moreover, diabetic ketoacidosis occurred in both types of diabetic patients [7, 40, 41]. This indicated that diabetic ketoacidosis is the problem of both types I and II diabetes. Hyperosmolar hyperglycemic state occurred in 7.9% of patients in this study. This is high when compared with other studies in different studies which was insignificant or none [7, 8, 22]. The reason might be due to the type of medications to control the blood glucose level and poor integrated effort in the management of patients on top of poor knowledge and attitude of patients.

In this study, chronic complication occurred in more than a third of the patients (58.8%). This is almost comparable with other reports in Jimma (52.5%) and China (52%) [7, 22] but it was lower than reports in Iran (75%) and Libya (68.7%) [8, 22]. Hypertension (43.3%), visual disturbance (25.68%), and neuropathy (14.4%) were the commonest chronic complications in this study. Except hypertension this was similar with the study in Ethiopia (visual disturbance (33.8%), neuropathy (29.5%), and hypertension (24.9%)) but its pattern is totally different than in China [7, 22]. The difference in management practitioners and the screening practices in different hospitals might have contributed to differences in occurrences of complications doubling with medication selection, poor knowledge, and attitude of patients.

In this study, age of patients, type of diabetes, antidiabetic drugs, and type of diabetes were significantly associated with the occurrences of diabetic complications in the clinic. This was similar with other studies in Ethiopia, Jordan, Libya, and Taiwan, [7, 9, 21, 38].

As limitation of study, it must be noted that this study did not determine severity of complications, and outcomes of the complications. Protein concentration, HbA1c, and direct ophthalmoscopy to detect retinal changes were not performed. Moreover, clinical findings and questionnaire based approaches were used to determine complications and the factors that could affect their occurrences.

In Conclusion. Diabetic complications in Dessie Referral Hospital were prevalent. Type II patients were more prone to complications in the hospital. The contributing factors for occurrences of complications were multiple. There should be training on the management of the diabetic patients and of course screening of complications should soon be starting. Thus, integrated effort should be in place to prevent the development of complications and manage the disease progression.

Conflict of Interests

The authors declare that they have no conflict of interests.

Authors' Contribution

Asrat Agalu Abejew was involved in the design of the study, data analysis, and interpretation of the findings, report writing, review of the report, and paper preparation. Abebe Zeleke Belay was involved in the data analysis and interpretation of the findings, and writing and review of the report. Mirkuzie Woldie Kerie was involved in the review of the final paper. All authors read and approved the final paper.

Acknowledgments

The authors are thankful to the Wollo University for funding and Dessie Referral Hospital for permission they obtained to conduct this study.

References

[1] A. S. Fauci, D. L. Kasper, D. L. Longo et al., *Harrison's: Principles of Internal Medicine*, McGraw-Hill, New York, NY, USA, 17th edition, 2008.

[2] M. von Korff, W. Katon, E. H. B. Lin et al., "Potentially modifiable factors associated with disability among people with diabetes," *Psychosomatic Medicine*, vol. 67, no. 2, pp. 233–240, 2005.

[3] E. B. Rimm, J. Chan, M. J. Stampfer, G. A. Colditz, W. C. Willett, and R. E. Laporte, "Prospective study of cigarette smoking, alcohol use, and the risk of diabetes in men," *British Medical Journal*, vol. 310, no. 6979, pp. 555–559, 1995.

[4] P. H. Wise, F. M. Edwardes, R. J. Craig et al., "Diabetes and associated variables in the South Australia Aboriginal," *Australian & New Zealand Journal of Medicine*, vol. 6, no. 3, pp. 1991–1996, 1976.

[5] N. V. Emanuele, T. F. Swade, and M. A. Emanuele, "Consequences of alcohol use in diabetics," *Alcohol Research & Health*, vol. 22, no. 3, pp. 211–219, 1998.

[6] E. Vermeire, P. van Royen, S. Coenen, J. Wens, and J. Denekens, "The adherence of type 2 diabetes patients to their therapeutic regimens: a qualitative study from the patient's perspective," *Practical Diabetes International*, vol. 20, no. 6, pp. 209–214, 2003.

[7] D. Worku, L. Hamza, and K. Woldemichael, "Patterns of diabetic complications at Jimma University Specialized Hospital, Southwest Ethiopia," *Ethiopian Journal of Health Sciences*, vol. 20, no. 1, pp. 33–39, 2010.

[8] M. H. Khazai, B. Khazai, Z. Zargaran, Z. Moosavi, and F. K. Zand, "Diabetic complications and risk factors in recently diagnosed type II diabetes: a case-control study," *ARYA Journal*, vol. 2, no. 2, pp. 9–83, 2006.

[9] M. Khattab, Y. S. Khader, A. Al-Khawaldeh, and K. Ajlouni, "Factors associated with poor glycemic control among patients with Type 2 diabetes," *Journal of Diabetes and Its Complications*, vol. 24, no. 2, pp. 84–89, 2010.

[10] J. T. Fitzgerald, R. M. Anderson, and W. K. Davis, "Gender differences in diabetes attitudes and adherence," *The Diabetes Educator*, vol. 21, no. 6, pp. 523–529, 1995.

[11] N. Gul, "Knowledge, attitudes and practices of type 2 diabetic patients," *Journal of Ayub Medical College, Abbottabad*, vol. 22, no. 3, pp. 128–131, 2010.

[12] A. H. Eldarrat, "Diabetic patients: their knowledge and perception of oral health," *Libyan Journal of Medicine*, vol. 6, no. 1, pp. 1–5, 2011.

[13] R. M. Anderson, M. B. Donnelly, and R. F. Dedrick, "Measuring the attitudes of patients towards diabetes and its treatment," *Patient Education and Counseling*, vol. 16, no. 3, pp. 231–245, 1990.

[14] M. Clark, "Adherence to treatment in patients with type 2 diabetes," *Journal of Diabetes Nursing*, vol. 8, no. 10, pp. 389–391, 2004.

[15] N. Hermanns, M. Mahr, B. Kulzer, S. E. Skovlund, and T. Haak, "Barriers towards insulin therapy in type 2 diabetic patients: results of an observational longitudinal study," *Health and Quality of Life Outcomes*, vol. 8, article 113, 2010.

[16] M. Peyrot, R. R. Rubin, T. Lauritzen, F. J. Snoek, D. R. Matthews, and S. E. Skovlund, "Psychosocial problems and barriers to improved diabetes management: results of the Cross-National Diabetes Attitudes, Wishes and Needs (DAWN) Study," *Diabetic Medicine*, vol. 22, no. 10, pp. 1379–1385, 2005.

[17] E. H. B. Lin, M. von Korff, P. Ciechanowski et al., "Treatment adjustment and medication adherence for complex patients with diabetes, heart disease, and depression: a randomized controlled trial," *Annals of Family Medicine*, vol. 10, no. 1, pp. 6–14, 2012.

[18] E. A. Ajayi and A. O. Ajayi, "Pattern and outcome of diabetic admissions at a federal medical center: a 5-year review," *Annals of African Medicine*, vol. 8, no. 4, pp. 271–275, 2009.

[19] A. Chijioke, A. N. Adamu, and A. M. Makusidi, "Mortality patterns among type 2 diabetes mellitus patients in Ilorin, Nigeria," *Journal of Endocrinology, Metabolism and Diabetes of South Africa*, vol. 15, no. 2, pp. 79–82, 2010.

[20] D. Bradshaw, V. Pillay-Van Wyk, R. Laubscher et al., *Cause of Death Statistics for South Africa: Challenges and Possibilities for Improvement*, South Africa Burden of Disease Research Unit, 2010.

[21] R. B. Roaeid and A. A. Kablan, "Diabetes mortality and causes of death in Benghazi: a 5-year retrospective analysis of death certificates," *Eastern Mediterranean Health Journal*, vol. 16, no. 1, pp. 65–69, 2010.

[22] Z. Liu, C. Fu, W. Wang, and B. Xu, "Prevalence of chronic complications of type 2 diabetes mellitus in outpatients—a cross-sectional hospital based survey in urban China," *Health and Quality of Life Outcomes*, vol. 8, article no. 62, 2010.

[23] J. Peter, C. K. Riley, B. Layne, K. Miller, and L. Walker, "Prevalence and risk factors associated with erectile dysfunction in diabetic men attending clinics in Kingston, Jamaica," *Journal of Diabetology*, vol. 2, article 2, 2012.

[24] A. Raval, E. Dhanaraj, A. Bhansali, S. Grover, and P. Tiwari, "Prevalence & determinants of depression in type 2 diabetes patients in a tertiary care centre," *Indian Journal of Medical Research*, vol. 132, no. 8, pp. 195–200, 2010.

[25] P. Mukhopadhyay, B. Paul, D. Das, N. Sengupta, and R. Majumder, "Perceptions and practices of type 2 diabetics: a cross-sectional study in a tertiary care hospital in Kolkata," *International Journal of Diabetes in Developing Countries*, vol. 30, no. 3, pp. 143–149, 2010.

[26] R. I. Ekore, I. O. Ajayi, A. Arije, and J. O. Ekore, "Attitude, diabetic foot care, education, knowledge: type 2 diabetes mellitus," *African Journal of Primary Health Care & Family Medicine*, vol. 2, p. 10, 2010.

[27] J. N. Kalyango, E. Owino, and A. P. Nambuya, "Non-adherence to diabetes treatment at mulago hospital in Uganda: prevalence and associated factors," *African Health Sciences*, vol. 8, no. 2, pp. 67–73, 2008.

[28] A. R. Khan, Z. N. Al-Abdul Lateef, M. A. Al Aithan, M. A. Bu-Khamseen, I. Al Ibrahim, and S. A. Khan, "Factors contributing to non-compliance among diabetics attending primary health centers in the Al Hasa district of Saudi Arabia," *Journal of Family and Community Medicine*, vol. 19, no. 1, pp. 26–32, 2012.

[29] Institute for Clinical Systems Improvement, *Health Care Guideline: Diagnosis and Management of Type 2 Diabetes Mellitus in Adults*, 2012, https://www.icsi.org/.

[30] R. Sharma, V. L. Grover, and S. Chaturvedi, "Recipe for diabetes disaster: a study of dietary behaviors among adolescent students in south Delhi, India," *International Journal of Diabetes in Developing Countries*, vol. 31, no. 1, pp. 4–8, 2011.

[31] R. Yadav, P. Tiwari, and E. Dhanaraj, "Risk factors and complications of type 2 diabetes in Asians," *CRIPS*, vol. 9, no. 2, pp. 8–12, 2008.

[32] J. J. Holewski, K. M. Moss, R. M. Stess, P. M. Graf, and C. Grunfeld, "Prevalence of foot pathology and lower extremity complications in a diabetic outpatient clinic," *Journal of Rehabilitation Research and Development*, vol. 26, no. 3, pp. 35–44, 1989.

[33] C. L. Triplitt, C. A. Reasner, and W. L. Isley, *Pharmacotherapy: A Pathophysiologic Approach*, edited by J. T. Dipiro, R. L. Talbert, G. C. Yee, McGraw-Hill, New York, NY, USA, 7th edition, 2008.

[34] P. H. Rayappa, K. N. M. Raju, A. Kapur, S. Bjork, C. Sylvest, and K. M. D. Kumar, "Economic cost of diabetes care the bangalore urban district diabetes study," *International Journal of Diabetes in Developing Countries*, vol. 19, pp. 87–97, 1999.

[35] P. Urbansk, A. Wolf, and W. Herman, Cost-effectiveness Issues of Diabetes Prevention and Treatment, https://dpg-storage.s3.amazonaws.com/dce/resources/cost_effective.pdf.

[36] D. F. Williamson, F. Vinicor, and B. A. Bowman, "Primary prevention of type 2 diabetes mellitus by lifestyle intervention: implications for health policy," *Annals of Internal Medicine*, vol. 140, no. 11, pp. 951–957, 2004.

[37] S. E. Skovlund and M. Peyrot, "The diabetes attitudes, wishes, and needs (DAWN) program: a new approach to improving outcomes of diabetes care," *Diabetes Spectrum*, vol. 18, no. 3, pp. 136–142, 2005.

[38] G. D. Chen, C. N. Huang, Y. S. Yang, and C. Y. Lew-Ting, "Patient perception of understanding health education and instructions has moderating effect on glycemic control," *BMC Public Health*, vol. 14, no. 1, article 683, 2014.

[39] L. Litwak, S.-Y. Goh, Z. Hussein, R. Malek, V. Prusty, and M. E. Khamseh, "Prevalence of diabetes complications in people with type 2 diabetes mellitus and its association with baseline characteristics in the multinational A1chieve study," *Diabetology and Metabolic Syndrome*, vol. 5, no. 1, article 57, 2013.

[40] American Diabetes Association, "Standards of medical care in diabetes—2013," *Diabetes Care*, vol. 36, supplement 1, pp. S11–S66, 2013.

[41] A. E. Kitabchi, G. E. Umpierrez, J. M. Miles, and J. N. Fisher, "Hyperglycemic crises in adult patients with diabetes," *Diabetes Care*, vol. 32, no. 7, pp. 1335–1343, 2009.

19

Rural-Urban Differences in Health Care Expenditures: Empirical Data from US Households

Wei-Chen Lee,[1] Luohua Jiang,[2] Charles D. Phillips,[3] and Robert L. Ohsfeldt[3]

[1] *Center to Eliminate Health Disparities, University of Texas Medical Branch, Galveston, TX, USA*
[2] *Department of Epidemiology and Biostatistics, School of Rural Public Health, Texas A&M Health Science Center, College Station, TX, USA*
[3] *Department of Health Policy and Management, School of Rural Public Health, Texas A&M Health Science Center, College Station, TX, USA*

Correspondence should be addressed to Robert L. Ohsfeldt; rohsfeldt@sph.tamhsc.edu

Academic Editor: Shenying Fang

Purpose. To estimate the rural-urban differences in expenditures of outpatient care, hospital inpatient care, hospital emergency room services, medications, and total services. *Methods.* This cross-sectional study used data from the 2010 Medical Expenditure Panel Survey. The overall sample size for the study was 22,772. Weighted frequencies, means, or percentages were estimated to illustrate the distribution of each variable. Five two-part utilization models were then fit to determine the likelihood of having nonzero expenses and to identify how residence in a rural versus urban area affected expenditures in our five expense categories. Quantile regressions were estimated to further explore relationships between residence and each quantile of nonzero expenditure. *Results.* The results of two-part model suggest that rural populations spent more on medications, while urban populations spent more on emergency care. However, no rural-urban difference was found in total health expenditures. The results of quantile regressions suggest that the highest users (at the upper quantiles) of medication and total expenditure experienced the strongest positive effects of living in rural areas. *Conclusions.* Total health expenditures do not seem to vary significantly across urban and rural areas. However, rurality does have important effects on those who make the most use of outpatient care and prescription medications. Reviewing total health expenditures for urban and rural populations is not enough. Policymakers should monitor the effects of geographic differences, especially in the highest expenditure quantiles, for specific types of health expenditures. Differences in the influence of rurality across this distribution of health expenditures may provide important guidance for interventions.

1. Introduction

The Center for Medicare & Medicaid Services (CMS) reported that national health expenditures grew dramatically from $1493.3 billion in 2001 to $2700.7 billion in 2011 [1]. National health expenditures are now projected to reach $4,781.0 billion in 2021 [2]. Hospital care, professional services, and prescription drugs are the three categories of health expenditures with the highest per capita figures [1]. On average, individuals spent $2,734 on hospital care, $1,740 on physician services (excluding dental services), and $845 on prescription drugs in 2011.

The growth of healthcare expenditures is of particular concern to rural populations whose incomes are significantly lower than their urban counterparts [3]. This research examines rural-urban differences in total health care expenditures, as well as expenditures for different types of health services (i.e., outpatient care, hospital inpatient care, hospital emergency room services, and prescription drugs).

Data for health expenditures for individuals residing in urban or rural areas were obtained from the Medical Expenditure Panel Survey (MEPS). As a nationally representative data source, MEPS data are particularly well suited for the task of estimating rural-urban differences in health care expenditures [4]. Among prior studies using MEPS data, findings about differences in health expenditures between rural and urban populations have been quite mixed. Ziller and colleagues concluded that residents in rural areas had higher out-of-pocket spending on healthcare than those living in urban areas [5]. However, expenditures for dental care for older adults living in large metropolitan areas were higher than those in small metropolitan and nonmetropolitan areas [6]. On the other hand, Chevarley and colleagues pointed out that there were no geographic differences in healthcare expenditures for children [7]. Another study about veterans' healthcare expenditures concluded that rural veterans (VA) younger than 65 years spent $1,100 less on average than urban VA users, but the average rural VA user aged 65 and older spent $250 more than urban veterans [8].

This study extends existing research in two important ways. First, the study focuses on urban-rural differences in health spending for the four most costly categories. Second, in addition to using traditional two-part models to examine the relationship between the urban-rural residency and health expenditures, exploratory quantile regression models were used to assess the extent to which urban-rural differences vary across quantiles of the expenditure distribution. The latter may be important because a number of studies have reported an extraordinarily high concentration of healthcare costs and utilization among small segments of the population [9–12]. For example, 64 percent of total healthcare expenditures were accumulated by only 15 percent of patients [12].

2. Methods

2.1. Data Source. The cross-sectional data used in this study were drawn from a subsample of the 2010 Medical Expenditure Panel Survey (MEPS), a nationally representative survey of the US civilian noninstitutionalized population [13]. The subsample of individual household members consisted of households in the 2010 MEPS sample who also participated in the National Health Interview Survey (NHIS) in 2008 or 2009. The sampling plan of the NHIS followed a multistage area probability design but oversampled households with Blacks, Hispanics, Asians, and low income families to improve the precision of estimates for these selected subgroups [14]. People who were in the military, born abroad, institutionalized, or who died during the reference period were not eligible for this survey.

Like NHIS, the AHRQ used a multistage stratified sampling design [15]. The first stage consisted of a sample of 428 PSUs drawn from 1,900 geographically defined PSUs nationwide [16]. Each PSU contained a county, a small group of contiguous counties, or a metropolitan statistical area (MSA). The second stage sampling used either area segments or permit segments to draw survey samples. An area segment comprised about eight, twelve, or sixteen addresses. A permit segment covered housing units built after the 2000 census, which generally included four addresses.

This 2010 file contains the household component (HC) and the medical provider component (MPC). Individual characteristics such as gender were collected through computer assisted personal interviewing (CAPI) technology in the HC [13]. With permission from the household survey respondents, the MPC collected data about visits, diagnosis, charges, and payments from the healthcare providers of household members. The MPC data supplemented the MEPS household reported information on health expenditures.

Households selected through the stratified sampling approach were interviewed 5 times across two years. Data for the year 2010 came from rounds 3–5 of panel 14 (a subsample of the 2008 NHIS responding households) and rounds 1–3 of panel 15 (a subsample of the 2009 NHIS responding households) [15]. The response rate of panel 14 was 85.2% and 84.0% for panel 15. The public use dataset pooled 18,398 families with 31,228 valid cases.

This study sample was limited to adults 18 years or older who completed health-related questions such as disease diagnoses. The final sample included 22,772 ($= n$) adults that after the application of appropriate sampling weights represented 229,857,784 ($= N$) adults in the US.

2.2. Dependent Variables: Healthcare Expenditures. Unlike the NHIS, the MEPS contained the healthcare expenditures reported by household members and medical providers served as dependent variables in this study [15]. Expenditures are the sum of out-of-pocket payments and payments by private insurance, Medicaid, Medicare, TRICARE, and other sources. In addition to total health expenditures, expenditures for four types of health services were chosen for this study: (1) expenses for outpatient care (for both hospital-based and office-based providers of outpatient services), (2) expenditures for hospital inpatient care, (3) expenditures for hospital emergency room services, and (4) prescription drugs expenses.

Outpatient care data were provided by doctors practicing in either private clinics or hospital-based outpatient departments. Expenditures of hospital inpatient care and hospital emergency room services included both hospital facility expenses and payments for physicians whose inpatient services delivered in hospital settings. Expenditures for prescription medicines were obtained through both household interviews and pharmacy component surveys. Only prescription forms with valid fields for national drug code, medication name, strength of medicine (amount and unit), quantity (package size and amount), and payments by source were treated as valid cases. The last type of expenditure covered all services, including dental services and all other health services not included in our four subcategories of expenditures.

A traditional two-part model was used for expenditure data analysis. The first part of the two-part model focused on a dichotomous dependent variable indicating whether individuals had any expenditures in a particular service category (expenditure = $0 or >$0). The second part of the two-part model focused on the level of expenditures for individuals with nonzero expenditures in each of the service categories. Given skew in the distribution of expenditures, the level of nonzero health expenditures was transformed to the logarithmic scale for all of the expenditure categories.

AHRQ uses a hot-deck imputation process for missing data when both HC and MPC components were not collected or incomplete [15]. Regression models based on medical events with complete information were used to predict total expenses. Variables with known values such as total charge and provider type were used as predictors to form groups of donor events on expenditures. Then, a donor event with the closest predicted payment pattern was used to impute the missing values, taking into account the sampling weights associated with the MEPS complex survey design. Unfortunately, there is no variable in the MEPS data to flag which expenditure values were imputed, making it impossible to compare expenditures with and without imputation.

2.3. Independent Variables: Geographic Factor. The main independent variable of interest is an individual's place of residence (0 = rural, 1 = urban). Based on the 2000 report of Office of Management and Budget (OMB), urban areas in the MEPS refer to a metropolitan core based statistical area (CBSA), an area comprising at least one urbanized area that has a population of at least 50,000 [17]. The Office of Rural Health Policy (ORHP) defined all other areas as rural [18].

2.4. Covariates: Individual Characteristics. According to Andersen's model for individual use of health care [19, 20], this study used self-reported measures: (1) predisposing characteristics—age 18–44, 45–64, 65, and older, gender (female or male), race/ethnicity Hispanic, African American, White, or other, and highest level of education degree when the respondent first entered the study (degree lower than high school, high school, or higher than high school); (2) enabling resources—poverty status (poor or near poor, low income, middle income, or high income) and health insurance held (any private insurance, only public insurance, or uninsured); and (3) healthcare needs—the average perceived health status (very good or excellent, good, poor, or fair), average perceived mental health status (very good or excellent, good, poor, or fair), limitation in physical functioning (no limitation or any limitation), and presence of chronic diseases with relatively high prevalence (high blood pressure, heart diseases, stroke, emphysema, chronic bronchitis, high cholesterol, cancer, diabetes, joint pain, arthritis, and asthma). The functional limitation variable summarized whether a person had any activities of daily living (ADL), instrumental activities of daily living (IADL), or sensory limitations during any of the survey rounds [15].

2.5. Statistical Analyses. To reflect the complex survey design, the AHRQ used the Taylor-series linearization method to produce person-level variables for analysis, including *perwt10f* for sampling weight, *varstr* for strata, and *varpsu* for PSU [15]. Weighted frequencies, means, or percentages were estimated to illustrate the distribution of each variable. Correlations among independent variables were low enough ($r < 0.75$) to rule out multicollinearity.

Five two-part models were fit to the expenditure variables. In the first part, logistic regression models were used to determine the impact of urban-rural residency status on the likelihood of having nonzero expenditures (>\$0) in 2010 for each of the five expenditure categories. In the second part, regression models were used to assess the impact of urban-rural residency status on the natural logarithm of positive expenditure among individuals with positive healthcare

expenditures for each of the five expenditure categories. In both parts, the models adjusted for the personal characteristics described in detail above: age, gender, race/ethnicity, educational attainment, poverty status, insurance status, perceived physical health status, perceived mental health status, limited physical activity, and a count of comorbid conditions.

Quantile regression models were then estimated to explore the relationships between urban or rural residency (for individuals with nonzero expenditures) at various quantiles of the nonzero expenditure distribution, adjusting for personal characteristics covariates. Taking into account the survey design, the bootstrapping method was used to draw an alternative sampling weight as well as to obtain standard errors without assumption. The regression coefficient at a given quantile indicates the effect of residence (i.e., rural or urban) on a unit change in that expenditure variable, assuming that the other variables are fixed, with 95% confidence interval bands. Two-tailed P values less than or equal to 0.05 were considered statistically significant. The goodness of fit was first examined by fitting the design-based model (i.e., takes the survey design structure into account), then estimating the corresponding probabilities, and subsequently using independently and identically distributed- (i.i.d.-) based tests. All data analyses were performed using Stata 13 using the "svy" procedure to incorporate survey sampling weights [21].

3. Results

Table 1 provides descriptive comparisons of weighted mean healthcare expenditures for persons living in rural or urban areas, as well as standard errors (SE), percentage with zero expenditures, and P values for bivariate tests for any urban/rural differences. Overall, 15.8% of the weighted sample was from rural areas.

Rural populations spent more money on prescription drugs than urban populations (urban: \$1061.4; rural: \$1278.3; $P = 0.007$). After excluding zero users, urban populations (\$1636.4) spent more than rural populations (\$1167.4) on emergency room services ($P = 0.0011$). Next, there were higher proportions of zero users in rural areas than in urban areas in terms of emergency care, prescription drugs, and all services received ($P < 0.052$).

Focusing on the cumulative distribution of nonzero expenditures, the results indicate that in both urban and rural areas a small percentage of people accounted for a relatively large percentage of healthcare expenditures. For instance, less than 2% of rural or urban populations accounted for half of hospital inpatient care and emergency room service expenditures. In these two areas, expenditures were slightly more concentrated in urban versus rural areas.

Table 2 provides the weighted percentages and P values for the personal characteristic covariates across rural and urban populations. Due to the large sample size, P values for hypothesis tests of the null of no difference in means or proportions tend to be small even when the absolute differences in point estimates means or proportions are not large. On average, rural populations are more likely to be old

TABLE 1: Comparisons of weighted individual expenditure distributions by residence and type of service, MEPS 2010.

Weighted mean (SE) or percentage	Urban (N = 19,561)	Rural (N = 3,211)	P value
Outpatient care			
Include zero ($)	1252.7 (43.3)	1306.2 (62.2)	0.4826
Exclude zero ($)	1852.5 (60.7)	1893.5 (81.6)	0.6854
Zero users (%)	32.4%	31.0%	0.5458
Lower half of cumulative sum (%)	63.1%	64.2%	
Higher half of cumulative sum (%)	4.5%	4.8%	
Hospital inpatient care			
Include zero ($)	1602.8 (90.8)	1574.7 (160.4)	0.8775
Exclude zero ($)	18838.5 (853.9)	15747.0 (1293.7)	0.0538
Zero users (%)	91.5%	90.0%	0.0853
Lower half of cumulative sum (%)	7.3%	8.3%	
Higher half of cumulative sum (%)	1.2%	1.7%	
Hospital emergency room			
Include zero ($)	187.1 (9.8)	163.4 (19.1)	0.2870
Exclude zero ($)	1636.4 (76.4)	1167.4 (113.0)	0.0011
Zero users (%)	88.6%	86.0%	0.0087
Lower half of cumulative sum (%)	10.4%	12.5%	
Higher half of cumulative sum (%)	1.1%	1.5%	
Prescription drugs			
Include zero ($)	1061.4 (31.0)	1278.3 (71.7)	0.0073
Exclude zero ($)	1611.5 (43.8)	1741.7 (93.6)	0.2187
Zero users (%)	34.1%	26.6%	<0.0001
Lower half of cumulative sum (%)	60.9%	66.3%	
Higher half of cumulative sum (%)	4.9%	7.0%	
Total expenditures			
Include zero ($)	4929.5 (123.1)	5172.3 (269.2)	0.4136
Exclude zero ($)	5867.1 (143.2)	6007.2 (307.6)	0.6788
Zero users (%)	16.0%	13.9%	0.0521
Lower half of cumulative sum (%)	78.3%	79.3%	
Higher half of cumulative sum (%)	5.7%	6.8%	

Note: the last item "total expenditures" is not the sum of the above four services but the overall healthcare expenditure of each individual who might also use other services such as dental care.

$(P < 0.0001)$, white $(P < 0.0001)$, less educated $(P < 0.0001)$, and poor $(P < 0.0001)$, more likely to rely on public insurance $(P = 0.004)$, to perceive poorer physical $(P < 0.0001)$ and mental health status $(P = 0.002)$, to have physical limitations $(P < 0.0001)$, and to have multiple chronic diseases $(P < 0.0001)$.

Table 3 reports the results of two-part models by weighted coefficients for the urban (versus rural) residency variable, and the associated confidence intervals and P values. The tests of goodness-of-fit suggest no evidence of lack of fit. In these logistic regression models that serve as the first part of the two-part model, urban residents were less likely to have zero expenditure for prescription drugs, compared to rural residents $(P = 0.012)$. The estimated odds-ratio is 0.80, which indicates that urban residents were 20% less likely to have zero prescription drug expenditure. Results for the residency variable in the other models indicate very small differences that do not approach statistical significance.

In the linear regression models that constitute the second part of the two-part model, urban residents displayed higher levels of expenditures for emergency services $(P = 0.011)$. The estimated impact of urban residency is a 0.22 increase in conditional log-emergency-care-expenditure $(\beta = 0.22)$, compared to rural populations.

Quantile regression models facilitate analysis of the full conditional distributional characteristics of the outcomes variables and yield estimates for the 5 conditional quantiles of expenditure given rurality (Figures 1, 2, 3, 4, and 5). In each figure, the solid line represents the estimated median effect and the dashed lines represent the associated confidence interval for the residency (urban) coefficient from the second part of the two-part model (reported in Table 3). If the solid line stays going down, it means living in rural areas is associated with the high expenditures. For example, the solid line descends toward increasing dollar values beginning around the 75th quantile in both Figures 4 and 5, though

TABLE 2: Weighted description of personal characteristics by residence, MEPS 2010.

Weighted percentage	Urban (N = 19,561)	Rural (N = 3,211)	P value
Predisposing			
Age			
18–44	49.0	43.0	
45–64	34.8	36.7	0.0003
65 and older	16.2	20.3	
Gender (% of women)	51.5	51.9	0.6206
Race/ethnicity			
Others	7.3	3.3	
Hispanic	15.4	6.4	<0.0001
Non-Hispanic black	12.2	7.6	
Non-Hispanic white	65.1	82.6	
Education level			
Lower than high school	16.5	22.8	
Equal to high school	53.3	58.0	<0.0001
Higher than high school	30.2	19.2	
Enabling			
Poverty			
Poor or near poor	16.5	20.4	
Low income	13.0	15.3	<0.0001
Middle income	29.5	34.5	
High income	41.0	29.8	
Health insurance status			
Any private insurance	68.0	63.9	
Only public insurance	16.6	21.0	0.0039
Uninsured	15.4	15.1	
Care needs			
Perceived physical health status			
Very good or excellent	59.1	53.2	
Good	27.0	29.1	0.0001
Poor or fair	13.9	17.7	
Perceived mental health status			
Very good or excellent	70.0	65.0	
Good	22.9	26.6	0.0023
Poor or fair	7.1	8.3	
Any limitation on functions (% of having any limitation)	25.3	33.3	<0.0001
Number of chronic diseases			
No chronic disease	35.7	30.3	
1 chronic disease	21.9	19.3	<0.0001
2 and more chronic diseases	42.4	50.4	

the effect is not statistically significant. By contrast, rural residents had less expenditure on emergency room and the effect is statistically different from zero at very high quantiles (Figure 3). The coefficient for rurality grows from $318.0 at the 0.75th quantile to $1682.6 at the 0.95th quantile ($P < 0.05$).

4. Discussion

4.1. Comparisons of Healthcare Expenditures between Rural and Urban Areas. This study compared urban and rural populations with respect to their medical expenditures. To deal with high frequencies of zero expenditure, this study used

TABLE 3: Two-part model estimated of impact of urban (versus rural) residency, weighted data adjusted for personal characteristics covariates, MEPS 2010.

	O.R. (95% C.I.)	P value
First-part (logistic regression)		
Outpatient care	1.086 (0.944, 1.249)	0.246
Hospital inpatient care	0.943 (0.783, 1.138)	0.542
Hospital emergency room	0.933 (0.787, 1.106)	0.422
Prescription drugs	0.801 (0.673, 0.953)	0.012
Total expenditures	1.020 (0.830, 1.252)	0.853
	β (95% C.I.)	P value
Second part (linear regression)		
Outpatient care	0.027 (−0.056~0.111)	0.521
Hospital inpatient care	0.050 (−0.174~0.274)	0.659
Hospital emergency room	0.217 (0.050~0.385)	0.011
Prescription drugs	0.023 (−0.087~.133)	0.678
Total expenditures	0.018 (−0.058~0.095)	0.634

Note: C.I.—confidence interval. Personal characteristics covariates: age, gender, race/ethnicity, educational attainment, poverty status, insurance status, perceived physical health status, perceived mental health status, functional limitations, and a count of comorbid conditions.

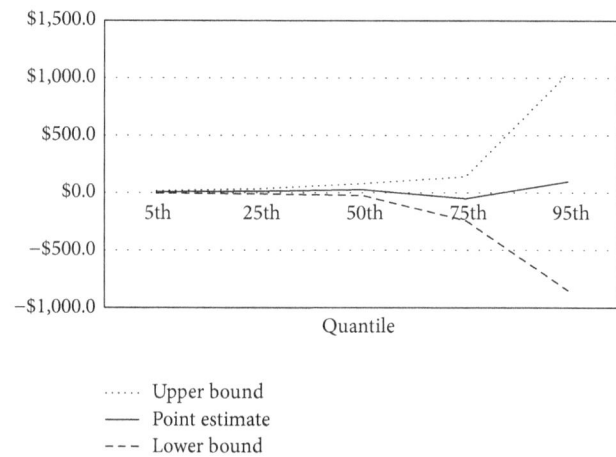

...... Upper bound
—— Point estimate
--- Lower bound

FIGURE 1: Weighted relationship between residence and nonzero expenditure of outpatient care, adjusted by 10 covariates.

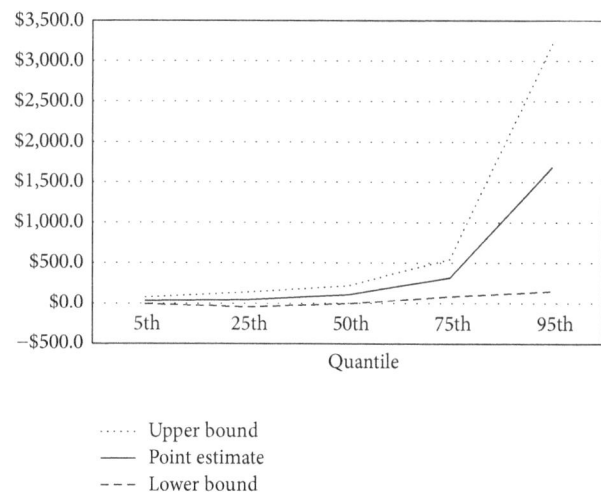

...... Upper bound
—— Point estimate
--- Lower bound

FIGURE 2: Weighted relationships between residence and nonzero expenditure of hospital inpatient care, adjusted by 10 covariates.

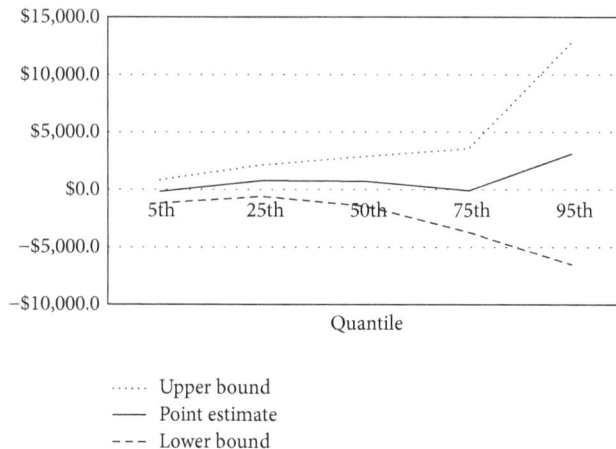

...... Upper bound
—— Point estimate
--- Lower bound

FIGURE 3: Weighted relationships between residence and nonzero expenditure of hospital emergency room service, adjusted by 10 covariates.

both two-part models and quantile regression models with adjustment for differences in a variety of personal characteristics for rural and urban residents. The statistical procedures yielded population-weighted estimates and demonstrated the distributions of demographics and healthcare needs, enabling factors for those dwelling in urban or in rural areas.

We hypothesized that expenditures would be higher for rural populations than for urban populations, possibly due to a greater prevalence of poor health status in rural populations [22], or due to inferior access to (or quality of) preventative care in rural areas [23]. Based on the findings of two-part models, there was no difference in total health expenditures (including or excluding zero users) between rural-urban residents. Although a higher proportion of urban residents had zero total health expenditures, after adjusting

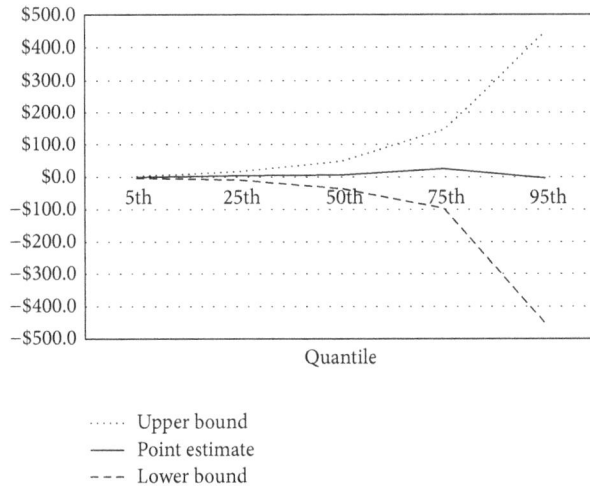

FIGURE 4: Weighted relationships between residence and nonzero expenditure of prescription drug, adjusted by 10 covariates.

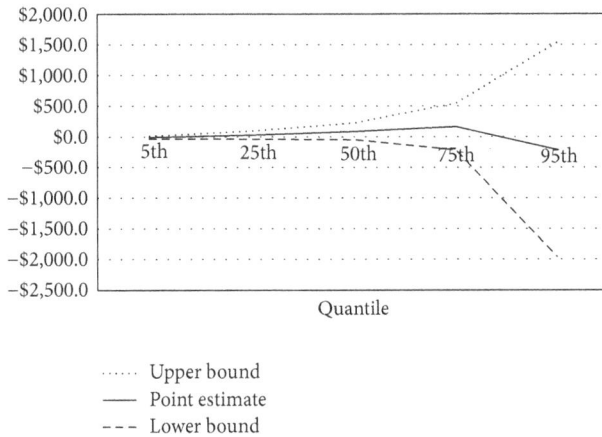

FIGURE 5: Weighted relationships between residence and nonzero total expenditure, adjusted by 10 covariates.

for personal characteristics of rural and urban residents, there was no significant rural-urban difference in the likelihood of zero total expenditure. It suggests that policy makers should look beyond total expenditure when comparing rural-urban differences in health care expenditure.

Expenditures of four different types of health expenditures were also compared between rural and urban populations. Higher proportions of rural dwellers were likely to exhibit expenditures (versus no expenditures) for hospital emergency room services and prescription drugs, though only the prescription drugs differential was statistically significant after adjusting for personal characteristics. However, the urban residents using emergency care services had higher emergency care expenditures than the rural residents who used emergency services.

Rural residents had significantly higher expenditures for prescription medications than their urban counterparts. The MEPS only provides the overall payment information rather

than identifying whether pharmacies prescribe and/or fill the prescriptions. However, this result probably is consistent with findings in previous studies that rural residents heavily rely on local pharmacies for keeping them healthy [3, 24, 25]. Since rural adults aged 18 and older in this study were generally older and less educated, had loser income, and were more reliant on public insurance and in poorer health, the rural populations were found to have higher out-of-pocket expenditures on prescription medications [5, 25, 26].

Employing the quantile regression model is the major extension of previous work. The quantile regression results suggested that the impact of urban-rural residency status might be more pronounced at the highest expenditure quantiles. The trend toward a positive impact of rural residency on expenditures for prescription drugs at higher expenditure quantiles is consistent with the findings of two-part models as well as past studies [27]. These results imply that even looking beyond subcategories of health expenditures may not tell the entire story of differences in expenditures between those dwelling in urban and rural areas. Using methods that allow the investigator to compare these different areas among residents with different levels of health care expenditures may also be enlightening.

4.2. Limitations. Selecting MEPS as the data source had several limitations for addressing our research questions. First of all, Franco pointed out that one-quarter of rural home care users were served by an urban agency and 3% of urban residents were served by a rural agency [28]. Nevertheless, the MEPS did not identify location of providers or the distances between users' homes and providers. Likewise, detailed information about physicians' referral patterns, hospital characteristics, and county characteristics were found to influence choice of healthcare providers [29, 30]. But the MEPS data set provides no information to assess the associations of these factors with health care expenditures. Further studies are needed to address these issues.

Second, this study only focuses on healthcare expenditures of four types of services used by noninstitutionalized adults aged 18 and older. It is inappropriate to employ the research findings to interpret other kinds of health services (e.g., dental care) and other age groups (e.g., newborns). Research about healthcare utilization/expenditures has gathered increasing attention in recent years [31]. More comparative studies using the MEPS to analyze other types of healthcare expenses and to include other age groups are highly recommended.

Conflict of Interests

The authors declare that there is no conflict of interests regarding the publication of this paper.

References

[1] Center for Medicare & Medicaid Services (CMS), "National health expenditures; aggregate and per capita amounts, annual percent change and percent distribution: selected calendar

year 1960–2011," 2012, http://www.cms.gov/Research-Statistics-Data-and-Systems/Statistics-Trends-and-Reports/NationalHealthExpendData/Downloads/tables.pdf.

[2] CMS, "National health expenditure projections 2011–2021," 2012, http://www.cms.gov/Research-Statistics-Data-and-systems/Statistics-Trends-and-Reports/NationalHealthExpendData/Downloads/Proj2011PDF.pdf.

[3] W. Hawk, "Expenditures of urban and rural households in 2011," 2013, http://www.bls.gov/opub/btn/volume-2/expenditures-of-urban-and-rural-households-in-2011.htm.

[4] J. W. Cohen, A. C. Monheit, K. M. Beauregard et al., "The medical expenditure panel survey: a national health information resource," *Inquiry*, vol. 33, no. 4, pp. 373–389, 1996.

[5] E. C. Ziller, A. F. Coburn, and A. E. Yousefian, "Out-of-pocket health spending and the rural underinsured," *Health Affairs*, vol. 25, no. 6, pp. 1688–1699, 2006.

[6] R. J. Manski, H. S. Goodman, B. C. Reid, and M. D. Macek, "Dental insurance visits and expenditures among older adults," *American Journal of Public Health*, vol. 94, no. 5, pp. 759–764, 2004.

[7] F. M. Chevarley, P. L. Owens, M. W. Zodet, L. A. Simpson, M. C. McCormick, and D. Dougherty, "Health care for children and youth in the United States: annual report on patterns of coverage, utilization, quality, and expenditures by a county level of urban influence," *Ambulatory Pediatrics*, vol. 6, no. 5, pp. 241–264, 2006.

[8] A. N. West and W. B. Weeks, "Health care expenditures for urban and rural veterans in veterans health administration care," *Health Services Research*, vol. 44, no. 5, pp. 1718–1734, 2009.

[9] K. D. Bertakis, R. Azari, L. J. Helms, E. J. Callahan, and J. A. Robbins, "Gender differences in the utilization of health care services," *Journal of Family Practice*, vol. 49, no. 2, pp. 147–152, 2000.

[10] P. Diehr, D. Yanez, A. Ash, M. Hornbrook, and D. Y. Lin, "Methods for analyzing health care utilization and costs," *Annual Review of Public Health*, vol. 20, pp. 125–144, 1999.

[11] J. Pasic, J. Russo, and P. Roy-Byrne, "High utilizers of psychiatric emergency services," *Psychiatric Services*, vol. 56, no. 6, pp. 678–684, 2005.

[12] M. von Korff, J. Ormel, W. Katon, and E. H. B. Lin, "Disability and depression among high utilizers of health care: a longitudinal analysis," *Archives of General Psychiatry*, vol. 49, no. 2, pp. 91–100, 1992.

[13] Agency for Healthcare Research and Quality (AHRQ), MEPS-HC Panel Design and Data Collection Process, 2013, http://meps.ahrq.gov/mepsweb/survey_comp/hc_data_collection.jsp.

[14] Center for Disease Control and Prevention (CDC), 2010 National Healthcare Quality and Disparities Reports, 2011, http://www.ahrq.gov/research/findings/nhqrdr/nhqrdr10/datasources/cdc.html.

[15] AHRQ, MEPS HC-138: 2010 Full Year Consolidated Data File, Published 2012. Accessed April 26, 2013, http://meps.ahrq.gov/data_stats/download_data_files_detail.jsp?cboPufNumber=HC-138.

[16] CDC, "About the National Health Interview Survey," 2013, http://www.cdc.gov/nchs/nhis/about_nhis.htm.

[17] J. T. Spotila, "Standards for defining metropolitan and micropolitan areas: notice," 2000, http://www.whitehouse.gov/sites/default/files/omb/fedreg/metroareas122700.pdf.

[18] Office of Rural Health Policy (ORHP), "Definition of Rural," 2012, http://www.hrsa.gov/ruralhealth/policy/definition_of_rural.html.

[19] R. M. Andersen, "Revisiting the behavioral model and access to medical care: does it matter?" *Journal of Health and Social Behavior*, vol. 36, no. 1, pp. 1–10, 1995.

[20] R. Andersen and J. F. Newman, "Societal and individual determinants of medical care utilization in the United States," *Milbank Memorial Fund Quarterly. Health & Society*, vol. 51, no. 1, pp. 95–124, 1973.

[21] StataCorp, *Stata Statistical Software: Release 12*, StataCorp LP, Station, Tex, USA, 2011.

[22] R. A. Crosby, M. L. Wendel, R. C. Vanderpool, and B. R. Casey, *Rural Populations and Health*, John Wiley & Sons, San Francisco, Calif, USA, 2012.

[23] J. N. Laditka, S. B. Laditka, B. Olatosi, and K. T. Elder, "The health trade-off of rural residence for impaired older adults: longer life, more impairment," *Journal of Rural Health*, vol. 23, no. 2, pp. 124–132, 2007.

[24] T. D. McBride, "Why are health care expenditures increasing and is there a rural differential?" *Rural Policy Brief*, vol. 10, no. 7, pp. 1–8, 2005.

[25] National Economic Council, "Prescription drug coverage & rural Medicare beneficiaries: a critical unmet need," 2005, http://clinton4.nara.gov/media/pdf/rural_report_6-13.pdf.

[26] C. Caplan and N. Brangan, "Prescription drug spending and coverage among rural Medicare beneficiaries in 2003," 2004, http://assets.aarp.org/rgcenter/post-import/dd106_rx_spending.pdf.

[27] UnitedHealth Group, "Modernizing rural health care: coverage, quality and innovation," 2011, http://www.unitedhealthgroup.com/Error/PageNotFound.aspx.

[28] S. J. Franco, *Medicare Home Health Care in Rural America. Policy Analysis Brief (No. 1)*, NORC Walsh Center for Rural Health Analysis, Bethesda, Md, USA, 2004.

[29] M. J. Hall, J. Marsteller, and M. Owings, "Factors influencing rural residents' utilization of urban hospitals," *National health statistics reports*, vol. 18, no. 31, pp. 1–12, 2010.

[30] M. J. Hall, M. F. Owings, and J. A. Shinogle, "Inpatient care in rural hospitals at the beginning of the 21st century," *Journal of Rural Health*, vol. 22, no. 4, pp. 331–338, 2006.

[31] Federal Trade Commission and the Department of Justice, "Improving health care: a dose of competition," 2004, https://www.ftc.gov/reports/healthcare/040723healthcarerpt.pdf.

20

Perspectives on Employment Integration, Mental Illness and Disability, and Workplace Health

Nene Ernest Khalema[1,2,3] **and Janki Shankar**[4]

[1] *Human Sciences Research Council, Private Bag X41, Pretoria 0001, South Africa*
[2] *School of Public Health, University of Alberta, Edmonton, AB, Canada T6G 2R3*
[3] *School of Built Environment and Development Studies, University of KwaZulu-Natal, Durban 4041, South Africa*
[4] *Faculty of Social Work, University of Calgary, No. 444, 11044-82 Avenue, Edmonton, AB, Canada T6G OT2*

Correspondence should be addressed to Nene Ernest Khalema; ekhalema@hsrc.ac.za

Academic Editor: John Godleski

This paper reviews the literature on the interplay between employment integration and retention of individuals diagnosed with mental health and related disability (MHRD). Specifically, the paper addresses the importance of an integrative approach, utilizing a social epidemiological approach to assess various factors that are related to the employment integration of individuals diagnosed with severe mental illness. Our approach to the review incorporates a research methodology that is multilayered, mixed, and contextual. The review examines the literature that aims to unpack employers' understanding of mental illness and their attitudes, beliefs, and practices about employing workers with mental illness. Additionally we offer a conceptual framework entrenched within the social determinants of the mental health (SDOMH) literature as a way to contextualize the review conclusions. This approach contributes to a holistic understanding of workplace mental health conceptually and methodologically particularly as practitioners and policy makers alike are grappling with better ways to integrate employees who are diagnosed with mental health and disabilities into to the workplace.

1. Introduction

Employment is an important social determinant of health and participation in employment can enhance health and wellbeing. Unfortunately, the majority of individuals with serious mental illness are unemployed [1–5]. For those with mental illness who are employed there is increasing evidence that current workplace environments are contributing to the development and/or exacerbation of mental illness and disability [6, 7]. Limited mental health literacy among employers has been identified as a major barrier to people diagnosed with mental health and related disability (MHRD), making a successful return to work or sustaining employment difficult [8]. Although there is a considerable body of the clinical literature on the experiences of individuals with severe mental health illness in the workplace, much less has been written about an epidemiological approach to understanding employers' perspectives on hiring workers who experience mental illness and related disability and the kinds of support they need for reintegrating these workers in the workplace. A research approach proposed in this paper makes it possible to assess employers' perspectives on employing workers with mental illness and related disability, their attitudes and concerns about employing workers with these conditions, and the kinds of information and support they need to facilitate the worker's return to work. Possible findings will advance the understanding about the kinds of resources and support employers need to promote and how to manage mental health issues in the workplace. They will also contribute to an emerging conceptual framework [9] on employment integration of people with mental illness and the role of employers within this framework.

2. Mental Illness, Employment Integration, and Workplace Health

Unemployment rates among people with serious mental illness range between 80% and 90% [8–11], making this group one of the most recipients of social security in Canada and the United States [12, 13]. This is unfortunate because most people with the illness desire and can work [5, 14–16], but they are excluded from the workforce because of stigma of the illness. For those with mental illness who are in the workforce, there are issues related to sustaining their capacity for productive work. Health Canada estimates that the loss of productivity resulting from mental illness and "disability" costs the Canadian economy $14.4 billion annually [17]. According to the Diagnostic and Statistical Manual (DSM V), disability relevant to mental illness refers to "impairment in one or more areas of functioning as a result of mental illnesses. These may include the person's thought processes, perceptions of reality, emotions or judgments and may lead to disturbed behavior." Mental illness for the purposes of this study will include all disorders included in the DSM V. Not all individuals who are affected by mental illness may experience disability. However, a significant number of affected individuals are known to experience difficulties that interfere with their ability to learn and thus function effectively in their worker role. Mental illness can affect cognitive functioning, particularly attention, concentration, memory, thinking, reasoning, and problem solving [18]. These can be compounded by medication side effects, which may include restlessness, fatigue, drowsiness and lethargy, and memory lapses. All these factors can make it difficult for the affected employee to cope with the demands of work. Currently, mental illness and addiction account for 60–65% of all disability insurance claims among Canadian and American employers [8]. Therefore, the issue of improving employment outcomes for people with mental illness has become a priority for employers and provincial governments in Canada.

Research to improve employment outcomes for this population initially focused on understanding who respond best to vocational interventions on the basis of individual, demographic, clinical, and social variables. However, few strong associations were found between these variables and employment success defined variously in terms of job attainment, job retention, or number of hours worked [1, 2, 19]. Contemporary conceptualizations have moved beyond individually focused models to understand employment of people with mental illness as a dynamic process of interaction among several factors like the strengths, competencies, and needs of the worker, the nature of the job, and the demands of the work environment [20]. Attention is now directed to also studying factors in the work environment particularly the role of employers in assisting people with mental illness to gain and/or sustain employment and maintain productivity, health, and well-being.

3. Research on Employer Concerns and Beliefs about Employees with Mental Illness and Disability

Mental illness creates several barriers to employment. While the disability associated with the illness may create problems as discussed above, factors, such as poor educational achievements, stigma, lack of adequate vocational and clinical services, policy disincentives to employment, limitations of current disability support management services, legislation, and policy direction related to hiring and accommodating persons with mental health related disabilities, all add to the barriers that workers with mental health illness face [13, 21, 22]. One of the greatest barriers however is employer stigma and discrimination at the workplace. Surveys conducted in the US show that approximately 70% of employers are reluctant to hire someone with a history of substance abuse or someone currently taking antipsychotic medication [23], while almost a quarter would dismiss someone who had not disclosed a mental illness [24]. Also employees with mental illness are among the first employees to be retrenched in times of economic downturn [25]. The literature on employer attitudes shows that employers express a wide range of negative beliefs regarding hiring individuals with mental illness. These include concerns such as poor quantity and quality of work, brief tenure, absenteeism, and low flexibility. Employers also express concerns about the work personality of people with mental illness and these include beliefs about the need for excessive supervision, taking little pride in work, low acceptance of work role, difficulty following instructions, poor social competence, and low work persistence [26]. Employers report negative beliefs about people with mental illness with respect to factors such as motivation to work, work quantity, likelihood of injury, difficulties following directions, making friends, and becoming angry [27]. A Canadian study on stigma of mental illness defined 5 distinct assumptions held within the workplace that contribute to the disposition towards acting in a discriminatory manner: the assumption of incompetence, the assumption of dangerousness and unpredictability, the belief that mental illness is not a legitimate illness, the belief that working is unhealthy for people with mental illness, and the assumption that employing people with mental illness represents an act of charity inconsistent with workplace needs [9].

Employees with mental health problems report that once their mental illness becomes known, they experience discrimination from coworkers, feel socially marginalized, have to cope with negative comments from workmates, and have to return to positions of reduced responsibility [25, 28, 29]. Consequently, half of the competitive jobs acquired by people with mental illness end unsatisfactorily as a result of problems that occur once the job is in progress and largely as a result of interpersonal difficulties [30]. While clearly the lack of mental health literacy among employers, employees, managers, and supervisors is a prime reason for these beliefs and attitudes, there are few Canadian studies that have examined what employers know about mental illness and disability and how they deal with mental health issues in the workplace. Mental health literacy among employers will have to be addressed as a priority if people with mental illness are to be hired and retained as valued employees. This not only will help to reduce stigma, but also can enhance the likelihood of speedy identification and resolution of mental health problems in the workplace [8].

4. Employer Diversity in Hiring Practices

Different employers in different work environments often accommodate the needs of workers with mental illness differently. Research suggests that employers with previous experience of employing people diagnosed with mental health and related disability (MHRD) and employers in social service and nonprofit sector may be more willing than others to employ workers with mental illness [26, 31–33]. But there is little information on what support sectors like retail, transport, police force, and so forth need if they are to employ these workers. There is evidence that cultural backgrounds of employers influence hiring practices and willingness to accommodate the needs of workers with mental illness [34]. Company size is another factor that may influence hiring. Smaller employers may not hire workers with mental health disabilities because of concerns that they may not fit in with the physically intimate and generalist nature of small business [35]. However, much of this empirical literature comes from the United States or United Kingdom. As highlighted by Stuart [36], attempting to understand the perspectives, attitudes, concerns, and support needs of Canadian employers from data collected in social and economic systems with fundamentally different philosophical positions on work, economics, health, social welfare, workplace disability, and mental health care is fraught with difficulty as all these can impact workplace environments. There is a critical need for information on the perspectives and concerns of a range of Canadian employer groups in order to design intervention programs that target the needs of different groups and work environments.

5. Supporting Employees with Mental Illness: Needs of Employers

Only a small body of published information has focused on the support needs of employers [33, 37–41]. Employers may be more willing to employ if they have greater clarity about their roles and responsibilities when they hire a worker with mental illness and understand legislative requirements and the kinds of accommodations these workers may require. A recent pilot study conducted by the authors showed that employers want guidance and timely support from qualified persons like doctors or mental health workers to deal with specific issues like mental health crisis in the workplace, discussing performance issues with a worker diagnosed with mental illness, maintaining confidentiality with coworkers, and creating supportive work environments. This study also suggested that some workers with mental illness do not welcome interactions between their employers and treatment providers due to the risk of discrimination [40, 41]. Canadian studies show that employers who are affiliated with an employment program within a mental health agency or who are associated with projects offering employment support to people with mental illness have more positive attitudes towards hiring these individuals [20, 37]. Access to support and consultation from employment support providers can serve as an incentive to employers to employ and retain employees with mental illness. Overall, the findings suggest that direct and positive contact with workers with mental health disabilities and access to timely consultation from employment support or treatment providers can encourage positive beliefs among employers about the work capacity of

people diagnosed with MHRD that may positively influence hiring decisions. Finally, there is evidence that during times of economic downturn labor force participation of people with disabilities goes down at a rate that is greater than the general population [42, 43]. Yet there is little information on employers' experience during periods of economic downturn and the impact of this on their decision to employ or retain workers with mental illness.

6. Policies and Program Initiatives to Improve Hiring and Retention of Workers Mental Health Related Disabilities

Canada like Australia, the United States, United Kingdom, and many developed OECD countries has legislation that aims to reduce discrimination against people with disabilities in all areas including employment. While countries like Australia, the United States, United Kingdom, and some OECD countries have national disability legislation that protects the rights of workers with disabilities, in Canada discrimination against these workers is governed by the number of federal acts like the Canadian Human Rights Act (CHRA) (1977), the Charter of Rights and Freedoms (CRF) (1982), and the Employment Equity Act (EEA) (1986). Under these legislations, employers cannot discriminate against workers with disabilites and also have a legal duty to provide reasonable accommodations for these workers if and when they disclose their disability. A review of the legislation in these countries however shows that these are far from sufficient to promote employment for workers with disabilities. Policy instruments that are additionally required include supported employment programs, employer education, and financial incentives for employers [44].

Many countries now offer tax credits and other financial incentives to employers to employ workers with disabilities. In the United States, the Disabled Access Credit program [45] provides a nonrefundable credit for small businesses that incur expenditures for the purpose of providing access to persons with disabilities. There is also a Work Opportunity Credit program [45] that provides eligible employers with a tax credit up to 40 percent of the first $6,000 of first-year wages of a new employee if the employee has a recognized disability. The credit is available to the employer once the employee has worked for at least 120 hours or 90 days. The Canadian Government has introduced several funding grants for small business in Ontario to improve workplace accessibility and hire skilled persons with disabilities. Many of these programs are part of Canada's Economic Action Plan to help improve the labor market opportunities and conditions for Canadians with disabilities. The Opportunities Fund for People with Disabilities, for example, provides individuals and local organizations with business funding grants to support unemployed or underemployed people with disabilities [46]. The Alberta Employment First Strategy in particular aims to increase hiring and retention of workers with disabilities by providing resources and supports for employers and enhanced employment support for people with disabilities, including youth and mental health clients [47]. Under the Australian Disability Works program, an employer who employs workers with disability can receive financial assistance to purchase a range of work-related modifications and services for people who are about to start a job or who are currently working. For workers with mental health conditions, the employer may be provided with mental health first aid training [48]. The Disabilities Act in Austria actively promotes the employment of severely disabled individuals by requiring employers to hire one severely disabled worker per 25 nondisabled workers. Failure to adhere to this rule can result in the employer having to pay a noncompliance tax. A review of this policy shows that the hiring obligation of the Disabilities Act in Austria has generated a positive impact on the employment of disabled workers [49].

Many of Russia's regional governments, including the administration of Moscow, have developed programs to assist disabled people in finding jobs. In conjunction with these programs, the state compensates employers for the worker's salary for one year. Due to an increase in the number of people with disabilities who gained employment due to this program, it has been implemented in many regions across of Russia. Although these are significant improvements worldwide, there is little information on whether these financial incentives for employers have led to an increase in the number of workers with mental health related disabilities gaining and sustaining employment (http://www.disabilityworld.org/04-05_02/employment/russia.shtml).

In terms of programs for people with mental health related disabilities, the United States, Canada, Australia, and many other OECD countries have supported employment (SE) programs that offer individualized and intensive support to these workers as well as assisting employers in providing workplace accommodations thereby increasing the likelihood of successful employment outcomes. SE programs provide a combination of mental health and vocational support and have been shown to be the most effective one for getting people with mental illness, specifically those with serious mental health conditions into the workforce [50]. While SE programs are more costly than mainstream employment services, long-term cost savings to the health care and social assistance system have made them a desired form of employment assistance [51]. SE programs are articulated through specific models of employment services. Individual placement support (IPS) is one of the models with the most research to support its widespread use.

Since IPS has a well-established evidence base, service providers in many countries have adopted this approach in their agencies with some modifications depending on their local context. The goal of IPS is to place people in competitive employment as soon as possible without any preemployment training by assisting them to find jobs of their choice. Postemployment support is also provided to ensure long-term job tenure [52]. Researchers and mental health services are now looking to better understand the essential components of IPS so that adaptations can be made to respond to the needs of specific job seekers and local settings [53]. Hybrid models that include adding clinical interventions such as motivational interviewing and cognitive remediation have shown promise [54]. However, ongoing research and practice in the field are needed to evaluate the potential of these approaches.

Two components of the IPS approach that are of increasing concern are the lack of preemployment training and postemployment support.

A Canadian study has found that 40 percent of supported employment participants who have severe mental illness did not obtain jobs. The same study also found that job tenure was typically found to be less than five months [55]. While the IPS SE model has shown much success in creating job opportunities, the low job retention rates and quality of employment have created mixed opinions regarding its overall success. This could be because funding mechanisms for most employment support programs do not provide sufficient time to provide the full range of essential activities specified by the IPS model. A factor that has been repeatedly highlighted as a key to the success of IPS SE is the availability of long-term unlimited support. Many service providers however are able to offer only time-limited supports.

SE employment programs based on the IPS model largely address the needs of people with severe mental disorders (SMDs). According to a recent OECD study typically three-fourths of those who experience mental health related disabilities have mental disorders like depression, anxiety, and substance abuse disorders, often referred to as "common mental disorders" (CMDs). Yet there is a dearth for programs and policies that address the needs of these workers. Despite being less disabling than mental disorders like schizophrenia, any of these conditions can evolve to become so severe that they could be classified as SMDs [56]. Lately there has been some increase in programs, training workshops, and online resources that aim at educating employers about their responsibilities as supervisors and provide skills to frontline supervisors/managers on dealing with performance issues of workers and crisis situations arising from mental health issues of workers. Noteworthy among these programs in Canada are Mental Health Works (http://www.mentalhealthworks.ca/) and Workplace Strategies for Mental Health initiated by Great-West Life Centre for Mental Health in the Workplace (http://www.workplacestrategiesformentalhealth.com/). However, little is known about the extent to which front line managers are able to access these programs due to time and resource constraints.

7. Filling the Knowledge Gaps in the Literature

Despite the existence of legislation and programs to increase hiring and retention of workers with mental health disabilities, many studies have consistently shown that there is little change in employers' attitudes towards hiring or accommodating these workers [44], suggesting that there are several gaps in our understanding of the role of employers in facilitating the reintegration of workers with mental illness into the workforce.

First, as discussed above, much of our understanding about employers' perspectives, attitudes, and concerns is based on research conducted in countries other than Canada. By highlighting the perspectives of employers and their understanding of mental illness, a significant contribution to the small body of the literature on mental health literacy and concerns of employers will be advanced. This will lead to interventions to counter employer stigma and discrimination. This approach will also help vocational rehabilitation and employment support providers to target industries that have low levels of concern about mental illness and disability for the purposes of job development, job matching, and placement.

Second, there is a dire need to educate employers on the value of employing and retaining people with mental illness as well as the need to promote and encourage workplace accommodations. Currently, funding mechanisms for most employment support programs do not provide sufficient time to provide these essential activities. Employers are also often unwilling to take a chance on including people with mental illnesses in their workforce. If employment prospects for people with mental health are to be improved, the attitudes held by employers and coworkers need to be challenged.

Third, only a small body of the published literature has explored the challenges that employers, especially front line managers, face when dealing with mental health issues in the workplace and the kinds of information and support they need to facilitate the worker's reentry and integration into the work environment. Allan [57] highlights that "from the perspective of the employer the critical issue related to health is productivity. Protecting productivity, managing risks to productivity, restoring lost productivity and maximizing productivity are all key issues for employers." Thus, the proposed research must illuminate how employers balance these perspectives with the needs of workers who experience mental illness and disability, especially in times of economic downturn and global recession and what supports they need to incorporate best practice. Current research that has attempted to examine these issues is based on small samples of employers who are affiliated with mental health agencies or supported employment programs.

8. Conclusion

The review of the literature provided in this paper highlights the interplay between employment integration and retention of individuals diagnosed with mental health and related disability (MHRD). The paper stressed the importance of an integrative approach, utilizing a social epidemiological approach to assess various factors that are related to the employment integration of individuals diagnosed with severe mental illness. From the review, it is clear that assessing employers' perspectives (i.e., their attitudes and concerns) on employing workers with mental illness and related disabilities and the kinds of information and support employers need to facilitate the worker retention are critical in understanding workplace mental health. Further, the review suggests that integrating quantitative and qualitative research methods can lend depth and clarity to understanding not only mental health literacy of employers, but also resources needed to support employees with severe mental health issues in the workplace. As such, research on employment integration of mentally ill workers and workplace health requires research and conceptual protocols tailored for these special populations.

The goal here is to use research approaches, frameworks, and appropriate tools to meet these objectives. Valuable information about employers' understanding of mental health and related disability (MHRD), therefore, requires a deeper understanding of concerns about why employers employ people with MHRD and the resources they need if they are to do so. Equally important is utilizing diverse methodologies and approaches to assist not only mental health epidemiologists and occupational health researchers, but also employees with MHRD, service providers, policy and decision-making bodies, teachers, academia, and the local community in finding possible interventions. It is our hope that further research in this area will yield valuable information that may lead to programs/interventions aimed at enhancing public awareness about the work capacity of people with MHRD and the supports they and their employers need if these individuals are to be successful at work. Enhanced awareness among employers and all sectors of the community will help to reduce the stigma and discrimination associated with mental illness.

At the policy level, we hope that the research will facilitate discussions around the need for healthy public policy that supports the involvement of employers and the business community in education, advocacy, and workforce development efforts that meet the needs of job seekers and the organizations employing them. Furthermore, we hope that by assessing employers' perspectives policy leaders would examine policy initiatives that support employers when they employ people with MHRD and provide appropriate workplace accommodations. Additionally, we hope that resources would be developed to support the development of intersectoral partnerships between the industry, the treatment system, and providers of vocational and employment support services; these can enhance awareness among clinicians about employment needs of consumers, encourage early referral to vocational services, and return to work (or gain employment) for individuals with MHRD. This research approach has the potential to inform the limited knowledge that currently exists in the social epidemiological field where there is increasing acknowledgement by scholars for the need for research around employment integration, workplace health, and responsive practice.

In conclusion, our review linking supportive employment, mental illness and disability, and workplace health has potential to inform epidemiological studies on mental illness and disability, specifically understanding employer perspectives on mental illness and disability, their attitudes and concerns about hiring workers with these conditions, and resources and support required to integrate and retain individuals diagnosed with mental illness and disability. Throughout our review, we have argued for an integrative approach that takes into consideration broader determinants of mental health (SDOMH). As researchers working on integrating supportive employment, mental health epidemiology, and workplace health, we grapple with how to move forward this research agenda and our review of the literature offers a unique and integrative approach to assess the interplay between employment integration and retention of individuals diagnosed with mental illness and disability. We hope that this approach will pave a way for collaborative demonstration projects between mental health rehabilitation, social epidemiologists, social workers, employment support providers, and the business industry.

Conflict of Interests

The authors declare that there is no conflict of interests regarding the publication of this paper.

References

[1] W. A. Anthony, "Characteristics of people with psychiatric disabilities that are predictive of entry into the rehabilitation process and successful employment outcomes," *Psychosocial Rehabilitation Journal*, vol. 17, pp. 3–14, 1994.

[2] P. G. Arns and J. A. Linney, "Work , self and life satisfaction for persons with severe and persistent mental disorders," *Psychosocial Rehabilitation Journal*, vol. 17, pp. 63–80, 1993.

[3] G. R. Bond, R. E. Drake, K. T. Mueser, and D. R. Becker, "An update on supported employment for people with severe menial illness," *Psychiatric Services*, vol. 48, no. 3, pp. 335–346, 1997.

[4] R. Bland, "Mental Health in Alberta: updates of interest," in *Proceedings of the CMHA Annual Meeting*, 2006.

[5] G. R. Bond, R. E. Drake, and D. R. Becker, "An update on randomized controlled trials of evidence-based supported employment," *Psychiatric Rehabilitation Journal*, vol. 31, no. 4, pp. 280–290, 2008.

[6] National Mental Health Association, "Supported employment for persons with psychiatric disabilities: a review of effective services," July 2005, http://nmha.org/pedu/adult/supported_employment.pdf.

[7] J. H. Noble, R. S. Honberg, L. Lee Hall, and L. M. Flynn, "Nami executive summary," *Journal of Disability Policy Studies*, vol. 10, no. 1, pp. 10–17, 1999.

[8] M. Kirby, "Out of the shadows at last-transforming mental health, mental illness and addiction services in Canada," Final Report of the Standing Senate Committee on Social Affairs, Science and Technology, 2006.

[9] T. Krupa, B. Kirsh, L. Cockburn, and R. Gewurtz, "A model of stigma of mental illness in employment," *Work*, vol. 33, no. 4, pp. 413–425, 2009.

[10] D. Gilbride, R. Stensrud, C. Ehlers, E. Evans, and C. Peterson, "Employers' attitudes toward hiring persons with disabilities and vocational rehabilitation services," *Journal of Rehabilitation*, vol. 66, no. 4, pp. 17–23, 2000.

[11] M. McQuilken, J. H. Zahniser, J. Novak, R. D. Starks, A. Olmos, and G. R. Bond, "The work project survey: consumer perspective on work," *Journal of Vocational Rehabilitation*, vol. 18, no. 1, pp. 59–68, 2003.

[12] K. Sanderson and G. Andrews, "Common mental disorders in the workforce: recent findings from descriptive and social epidemiology," *Canadian Journal of Psychiatry*, vol. 51, no. 2, pp. 63–75, 2006.

[13] A. A. Murphy, M. G. Mullen, and B. Spagnolo, "Enhancing individual placement and support: promoting job tenure by integrating natural supports and supported education," *The American Journal of Psychiatric Rehabilitation*, vol. 8, pp. 37–61, 2005.

[14] K. W. D. Liu, V. Hollis, S. Warren, and D. L. Williamson, "Supported-employment program processes and outcomes: experiences of people with Schizophrenia," *The American Journal of Occupational Therapy*, vol. 61, no. 5, pp. 543–554, 2007.

[15] C. Macias, L. T. DeCarlo, Q. Wang, J. Frey, and P. Barreira, "Work interest as a predictor of competitive employment: policy implications for psychiatric rehabilitation," *Administration and Policy in Mental Health*, vol. 28, no. 4, pp. 279–297, 2001.

[16] G. Morgan, "We want to be able to work," *Mental Health Today*, pp. 32–34, 2005.

[17] T. Stephens and N. Joubert, "The economic cost of mental health problems in Canada," *Chronic Diseases in Canada*, vol. 22, pp. 18–23, 2001, http://www.phac-aspc.gc.ca/publicat/cdic-mcc/22-1/d_e.html.

[18] W. Spaulding and M. Sullivan, "From laboratory to clinic: psychological methods and principles in psychiatric rehabilitation," in *Handbook of Psychiatric Rehabilitation*, R. P. Liberman, Ed., vol. 166, pp. 30–55, 1992.

[19] S. R. McGurk, K. T. Mueser, P. D. Harvey, R. LaPuglia, and J. Marder, "Cognitive and symptom predictors of work outcomes for clients with schizophrenia in supported employment," *Psychiatric Services*, vol. 54, no. 8, pp. 1129–1135, 2003.

[20] B. Kirsh, T. Krupa, L. Cockburn, and R. Gewurtz, "Work initiatives for persons with severe mental illnesses in Canada: a decade of development," *Canadian Journal of Community Mental Health*, vol. 25, no. 2, pp. 173–191, 2006.

[21] J. A. Cook, "Employment barriers for persons with psychiatric disabilities: update of a report for the president's commission," *Psychiatric Services*, vol. 57, no. 10, pp. 1391–1405, 2006.

[22] L. Cockburn, T. Krupa, J. Bickenbach et al., "Work and psychiatric disability in Canadian disability policy," *Canadian Public Policy*, vol. 32, no. 2, pp. 197–211, 2006.

[23] T. L. Scheid, "Employment of individuals with mental disabilities: business response to the ADA's challenge," *Behavioral Sciences & the Law*, vol. 17, pp. 73–91, 1999.

[24] N. Sartorius and H. Schulze, *Reducing Stigma due to Mental Illness: A Report from a Global Program of the World Psychiatric Association*, Cambridge University Press, 2005.

[25] H. Stuart, "Mental illness and employment discrimination," *Current Opinion in Psychiatry*, vol. 19, no. 5, pp. 522–526, 2006.

[26] E. Diksa and E. S. Rogers, "Employer concerns about hiring persons with psychiatric disability: results of the employer attitude questionnaire," *Rehabilitation Counseling Bulletin*, vol. 40, no. 1, pp. 31–44, 1997.

[27] J. A. Cook, L. A. Razzano, D. M. Straiton, and Y. Ross, "Cultivation and maintenance of relationships with employers of people with psychiatric disabilities," *Psychosocial Rehabilitation Journal*, vol. 17, no. 3, pp. 103–116, 1994.

[28] O. F. Wahl, "Mental health consumers' experience of stigma," *Schizophrenia Bulletin*, vol. 25, no. 3, pp. 467–478, 1999.

[29] B. Schulze and M. C. Angermeyer, "Subjective experiences of stigma. A focus group study of schizophrenic patients, their relatives and mental health professionals," *Social Science and Medicine*, vol. 56, no. 2, pp. 299–312, 2003.

[30] D. R. Becker, R. E. Drake, G. R. Bond, H. Xie, B. J. Dain, and K. Harrison, "Job terminations among persons with severe mental illness participating in supported employment," *Community Mental Health Journal*, vol. 34, no. 1, pp. 71–82, 1998.

[31] N. E. Khalema and N. Eshkakogan, *Recruitment and Retention of Human Service Personnel in the Human Service Sector: A Research Report*, Government of Alberta Children and Youth Services Branch and MacEwan Institute for Research on Family & Youth, 2008.

[32] J. M. Levy, D. J. Jessop, A. Rimmerman, and P. H. Levy, "Employment of persons with severe disabilities in large businesses in the United States," *International Journal of Rehabilitation Research*, vol. 14, no. 4, pp. 323–332, 1991.

[33] C. Hand and J. Tryssenaar, "Small business employers' views on hiring individuals with mental illness," *Psychiatric Rehabilitation Journal*, vol. 29, no. 3, pp. 166–173, 2006.

[34] H. W. H. Tsang, B. Angell, P. W. Corrigan et al., "A cross-cultural study of employers' concerns about hiring people with psychotic disorder: implications for recovery," *Social Psychiatry and Psychiatric Epidemiology*, vol. 42, no. 9, pp. 723–733, 2007.

[35] B. Angell, M. Spitzmueller, and P. Corrigan, "Stigma in the hiring process: employer perceptions of mental illness and substance abuse," in *Work and Well-being Research and Evaluation Program*, Centre for Addiction and Mental Health, 2009.

[36] H. Stuart, "Stigma and work," *Health Papers*, vol. 5, pp. 100–111, 2004.

[37] C. Mizzoni and B. Kirsh, "Employer perspectives on supervising individuals with mental health problems," *Canadian Journal of Community Mental Health*, vol. 25, no. 2, pp. 193–206, 2006.

[38] M. L. Kirzner, R. Baron, and I. Rutman, *Employer Participation in Supported and Transitional Employment for Persons with Long Term Mental Illness*, Matrix Research Institute, Philadelphia, Pa, USA, 1992.

[39] L. Cockburn, B. Kirsh, T. Krupa, and R. Gewurt, "Mental health in the workplace: why businesses are paying attention," *Occupational Therapy Now*, vol. 6, no. 5, 2004.

[40] J. Shankar and F. Collyer, "Support needs of people with mental illness in vocational rehabilitation programs: the role of the social network," *International Journal of Psychosocial Rehabilitation*, vol. 7, pp. 15–28, 2003.

[41] J. Shankar, "The role of ongoing support in improving job tenure for people who experience psychiatric disability," Fourth Annual Mental Health Showcase, Alberta, Canada, 2008.

[42] R. Warner, *Recovery from Schizophrenia: Psychiatry and Political Economy*, Routledge, London, UK, 1994.

[43] E. Yelin, "The impact of labor market trends on the employment of persons with disabilities," *American Rehabilitation*, vol. 26, pp. 21–33, 2001.

[44] M. J. Prince, "What about a disability rights act for Canada? Practices and lessons from America, Australia and United Kingdom," *Canadian Public Policy*, vol. 36, no. 2, pp. 199–214, 2010.

[45] Internal Revenue Service IRS, 2013, http://www.irs.gov/Businesses/Small-Businesses-&-Self-Employed/Tax-Benefits-for-Businesses-Who-Have-Employees-with-Disabilities.

[46] Service Canada, 2013, http://www.servicecanada.gc.ca/eng/of/index.shtml?utm_source=Opportunities+Fund+for+Persons+with+Disabilities&utm_medium=Link&utm_campaign=Action_Plan_Skills_Fall_2013.

[47] Alberta Human Services, "Employment First Strategy. Making Progress," 2014, http://humanservices.alberta.ca/disability-services/employment-first.html.

[48] Australian Disability Employment Services, 2014, http://www.humanservices.gov.au/customer/services/centrelink/disability-employment-services.

[49] *Disabilities Act in Austria*, 2014, http://www.ohchr.org/Documents/Issues/Disability/SubmissionWorkEmployment/Response-Austria.pdf.

[50] M. Corbière, N. Lanctôt, T. Lecomte et al., "A pan-canadian evaluation of supported employment programs dedicated to people with severe mental disorders," *Community Mental Health Journal*, vol. 46, no. 1, pp. 44–55, 2010.

[51] E. Latimer, "An effective intervention delivered at sub-therapeutic dose becomes an ineffective intervention," *The British Journal of Psychiatry*, vol. 196, no. 5, pp. 341–342, 2010.

[52] G. R. Bond, R. E. Drake, and D. R. Becker, "An update on randomized controlled trials of evidence-based supported employment," *Psychiatric Rehabilitation Journal*, vol. 31, no. 4, pp. 280–290, 2008.

[53] M. P. Salyers, A. B. McGuire, G. R. Bond et al., "What makes the difference? Practitioner views of success and failure in two effective psychiatric rehabilitation approaches," *Journal of Vocational Rehabilitation*, vol. 28, no. 2, pp. 105–114, 2008.

[54] S. R. McGurk, K. T. Mueser, K. Feldman, R. Wolfe, and A. Pascaris, "Cognitive training for supported employment: 2-3 year outcomes of a randomized controlled trial," *The American Journal of Psychiatry*, vol. 164, no. 3, pp. 437–441, 2007.

[55] M. Corbière, N. Lanctôt, T. Lecomte et al., "A pan-canadian evaluation of supported employment programs dedicated to people with severe mental disorders," *Community Mental Health Journal*, vol. 46, no. 1, pp. 44–55, 2010.

[56] OECD Mental Health Work Project, *Sick on the Job? Myths and Realities about Mental Health and Work*, 2011.

[57] P. Allan, "For employer productivity is critical," *Health Care Papers*, vol. 5, no. 2, pp. 95–97, 2005.

21

Reducing Colorectal Cancer Incidence and Disparities: Performance and Outcomes of a Screening Colonoscopy Program in South Carolina

Sudha Xirasagar,[1] Yi-Jhen Li,[1] James B. Burch,[2,3,4] Virginie G. Daguisé,[5] Thomas G. Hurley,[2] and James R. Hébert[2,3]

[1] Department of Health Services Policy and Management, University of South Carolina, Arnold School of Public Health, 915 Greene Street, Columbia, SC 29208, USA

[2] South Carolina Statewide Cancer Prevention & Control Program, University of South Carolina, 915 Greene Street, Columbia, SC 29208, USA

[3] Department of Epidemiology and Biostatistics, University of South Carolina, Arnold School of Public Health, 915 Greene Street, Columbia, SC 29208, USA

[4] WJB Dorn Department of Veterans Affairs Medical Center, 6439 Garners Ferry Road, Columbia, SC 29209-1639, USA

[5] Division of Cancer Prevention and Control, South Carolina Department of Health and Environmental Control, 2100 Bull Street, Columbia, SC 29201, USA

Correspondence should be addressed to Sudha Xirasagar; sxirasagar@sc.edu

Academic Editor: Haiying Chen

This study evaluated the efficiency, effectiveness, and racial disparities reduction potential of Screening Colonoscopies for People Everywhere in South Carolina (SCOPE SC), a state-funded program for indigent persons aged 50–64 years (45–64 years for African American (AA)) with a medical home in community health centers. Patients were referred to existing referral network providers, and the centers were compensated for patient navigation. Data on procedures and patient demographics were analyzed. Of 782 individuals recruited (71.2% AA), 85% (665) completed the procedure (71.1% AA). The adenoma detection rate was 27.8% (males 34.6% and females 25.1%), advanced neoplasm rate 7.7% (including 3 cancers), cecum intubation rate 98.9%, inadequate bowel preparation rate 7.9%, and adverse event rate 0.9%. All indicators met the national quality benchmarks. The adenoma rate of 26.0% among AAs aged 45–49 years was similar to that of older Whites and AAs. We found that patient navigation and a medical home setting resulted in a successful and high-quality screening program. The observed high adenoma rate among younger AAs calls for more research with larger cohorts to evaluate the appropriateness of the current screening guidelines for AAs, given that they suffer 47% higher colorectal cancer mortality than Whites.

1. Introduction

There is wide variation across population subgroups in cancer incidence, mortality, or both. Nationally in the United States of America, African Americans (AAs) have ≈17% higher colorectal cancer (CRC) incidence and ≈47% higher mortality than Whites [1]. AAs also are diagnosed at younger ages, on average and with later-stage disease, have a higher incidence before the recommended screening age of 50 years, and tend to have worse prognoses even after accounting for other factors [2, 3]. These disparities tend to be much larger in South Carolina (SC) than in the US average [4, 5].

The majority of CRCs in average-risk individuals arise from the polyp-to-cancer pathway, which translates into an opportunity to prevent cancers by removing polyps detected through screening age-appropriate adults. Of all cancer screening tests, colonoscopy is the most effective both for early detection and, more importantly, for primary prevention of CRC because it enables removal of precancerous polyps before they turn cancerous. Colonoscopy has some disadvantages, however. It requires specially trained physicians and is expensive and invasive, requiring a well-equipped and well-staffed facility for safe, high-quality performance. Consequently, health insurance remains a key determinant of colonoscopy screening completion, which currently stands at 19.1% among working-age uninsured adults in the 2010 National Health Interview Survey Data, compared to 56.7% among those privately insured [6]. Despite many uninsured individuals having primary care access through the ambulatory care safety net, mainly federally qualified health centers (FQHC), the colonoscopy rate among this subgroup is low, about 24% [7], because FQHCs cannot obtain adequate volumes of charity colonoscopy care.

SC has the 16th highest percentage of uninsured adults in the USA [8] and has a higher proportion of AA population (30%) than the national average. The program, Screening Colonoscopies for People Everywhere in South Carolina (SCOPE SC), was designed to leverage the medical home relationship of FQHCs with uninsured individuals. A sum of $1 million was authorized by the South Carolina Legislature for the Department of Health and Environmental Control (SCDHEC) to cover screening colonoscopy of average-risk established FQHC patients ≥50 years old (≥45 years for AAs) with income ≤200% of poverty and without private or Medicaid insurance. Based on studies showing that patient navigation improves colonoscopy completion rates [9, 10], the program asked participating FQHCs to use their existing colonoscopy referral channels and funded patient navigation services to maximize screening completion and other facilitation services. The SCDHEC program office organized referrals and follow-up care for individuals who experienced a complication or were diagnosed with cancer.

About 800 screening procedures were targeted, based on an average cost of $1,000 each (covering provider reimbursement at Medicare rates, patient navigation, and program evaluation). Provider reimbursements were contingent upon reporting to the program, thus allowing for monitoring of procedure quality and completeness. At the end of year 1, SCDHEC assigned the program performance evaluation to an external academic research team, the results of which are presented in this paper.

2. Methods

Four FQHC sites participated in the SCOPE SC program, having been identified based on elevated CRC incidence, mortality, and late-stage CRC rates; resources and infrastructure; and a geographic distribution pattern providing for statewide representation. The program was promoted via direct notification of FQHC staff and outreach workers through promotional materials (postcards and posters) and by including the program on the American Cancer Society's toll-free telephone hotline. Eligible individuals included current FQHC patients with current SC residency, US citizenship (established with the social security number), no health insurance, income ≤200% of the federal poverty limit, age eligible (50–64 years for Whites without a CRC family history, 45–49 years for Whites with CRC family history, and 45–64

years for AAs regardless of family history), no gastrointestinal symptoms, and not being up to date with CRC screening per published guidelines (Figure 1). All beneficiaries were referred to by their primary care physician at a participating FQHC. If not a current FQHC patient, they were required to enroll as patients for purposes of adequate care and referral for complications, cancer diagnosis and/or follow-up surveillance.

Each FQHC had at least one navigator dedicated to the program. Eligible patients were identified by the primary physician and referred to the navigator for obtaining preauthorization from SCDHEC program staff. The patient then received a bowel preparation kit that included written instructions, and the procedure was scheduled. Navigators included FQHC nurses or administrative staff who routinely interacted with patients. FQHCs were compensated for navigation, $25 for the initial referral and associated paperwork and $75 for successful completion of the procedure. SCOPE SC program staff provided one-on-one training to navigators and FQHC staff administering the program. The training consisted of several hours of instruction emphasizing the importance of an adequate bowel preparation including detailed instructions for patients, methods to help patients plan for their procedure (e.g., obtaining transportation and other care-related advice), and details on program administration, referrals, and other resources.

As a condition of reimbursement, participating FQHCs, endoscopy clinics, FQHCs, and laboratory service providers submitted standard forms on all eligible individuals referred for colonoscopy. Data collected included demographic, relevant family and personal medical history (submitted by FQHCs), clinical procedure and polyp information (by colonoscopy providers), and polyp histopathology features (by laboratory service providers). SCDHEC established a medical quality assurance committee consisting of community-based, SCDHEC, and academic physicians that monitored procedure quality throughout the year by periodically reviewing the clinical and pathology data for all cases submitted by providers. When suboptimal outcomes were identified (low polyp detection rate, poor bowel preparation rate, or placing multiple polyps from different colorectal segments in a single jar), potential causes were discussed by the committee and feedback communicated to providers through the SCOPE SC program manager.

The study sample consisted of year I data on all screening colonoscopies provided during fiscal year 2009-10 (July 1 through June 30). The study team systematically reviewed the data files compiled from the patient referral, screening, and laboratory forms together against the original patient forms for accuracy and entered missing/discrepant data. Data entry was completed onsite within the SCDHEC data system. Files were linked, deidentified, and extracted in Excel format into University of South Carolina (USC) computers. The study was approved by the USC and SCDHEC Institutional Review Boards.

Univariate statistics (and chi-square tests where applicable) are used to present the program's efficiency (in outreach and procedure completion), beneficiary demographics, disparity populations reached, procedure effectiveness (cecum

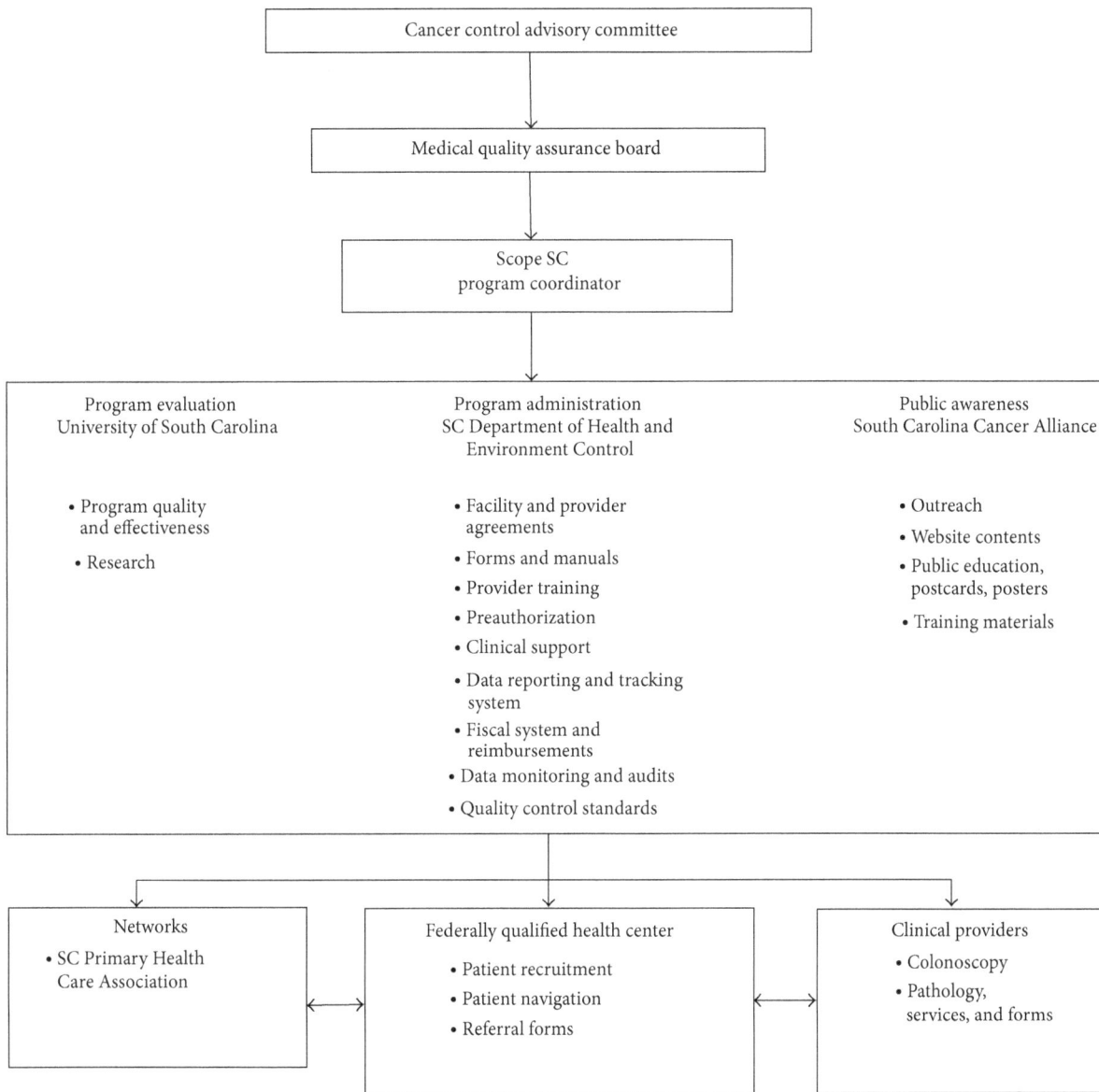

FIGURE 1: SCOPE SC program organization chart.

intubation, polyp detection and retrieval, adenoma, advanced neoplasm, and cancer detection rates), bowel preparation quality, and patient safety (adverse event rate). SAS version 9.2 was used.

3. Results

Table 1 summarizes the SCOPE SC year 1 program performance on efficiency, effectiveness, and patient safety. Of 782 eligible beneficiaries identified by the four participating FQHCs, 665 (85%) completed the procedure. The unadjusted cecum intubation rate was 98.1% (the US Multisociety Task Force (USMSTF), adjusted cecal intubation rate was 98.6%, excluding unintubated cases due to poor bowel preparation) [11], and the circumstance-adjusted cecum intubation rate was 98.9% (excluding unintubated cases due to poor bowel

preparation and medical reasons requiring procedure termination) [12]. All rates, including the unadjusted rate, exceeded the USMSTF benchmark of 95% [11].

The polyp detection rate was 56.4% (proportion of screened persons with ≥1 polyp detected). The adenoma detection rate (having any polyp with an adenomatous or carcinomatous histology, excluding hyperplastic polyps and normoplastic or lymphoid tissue) was 27.8% overall, 34.6% for men and 25.1% for women. Both rates exceed the USMSTF minimum standards of >25% for men and >15% for women [11]. The advanced neoplasm detection rate (adenomas ≥ 10 mm, villous/tubulovillous adenomas, high-grade dysplasia, or cancer) was 7.7% overall, 9.9% in men and 6.8% among women. Three cancer cases were found, 0.4% of those were screened. No benchmark exists for advanced neoplasm detection [11], although the USMSTF notes a documented

TABLE 1: SCOPE SC program performance in year 1: efficiency of patient recruitment, effectiveness of procedure performance, and patient safety.

Performance indicator	Number/%
Program efficiency	
Program target number of colonoscopy screenings (funding available)	800
Number of eligible beneficiaries identified	782
Number of who completed colonoscopy	665
% of eligible beneficiaries navigated through procedure completion	85%
Number of performing physicians	32
Bowel preparation status documented (benchmark 100%) [12]	98.5%
Patient safety: adverse event rate (benchmark 2%, all event types) [12]	0.9%*
Procedure performance quality	
Cecal intubation rate (benchmark 95%) [12]	98.9%
Bowel preparation status rated fair, good, or excellent	92.1%
Proportion of screened persons with polyp(s)	56.4%
Proportion of polyps completely removed	93.1%**
Proportion of polyps retrieved for pathology exam (benchmark 95%) [11]	99.9%
Polyp, adenoma, and cancer detection	
Proportion of screened persons with polyp(s)	56.4%**
Proportion of screened persons with hyperplastic polyp(s)	34.6%**
Proportion of screened persons with adenoma(s) found (ADR) (benchmark 15% for women and 25% for men) [12]	27.8%
Proportion with advanced neoplasm removed (cancer and polyps at imminent risk of cancer)	7.7%**
Diagnosed with colorectal cancer	3 (0.45%)
Total number of polyps removed	917
Total number of adenomas removed	338
Total number of advanced neoplasms removed	58

Advanced neoplasms include adenomas ≥10 mm in diameter, adenomas with villous or tubule villous features or high-grade dysplasia, and cancer or carcinoid tumor.
*n = 6 (1) bleeding, (2) incomplete colonoscopy due to torsion, and (3) unspecified but having good bowel preparation and the procedure was completed, no perforations.
**No national quality benchmarks exist for these indicators.

range of 3–10% [11] in US colonoscopy cohorts. The SCOPE SC rate is close to the upper end of the documented range.

Adverse events were documented in 0.9% of procedures, within the benchmark limit (n = 6 cases, (1) bleeding, (2) incomplete colonoscopy due to torsion, and (3) unspecified but having good bowel preparation and the procedure was completed, no perforations). The USMSTF benchmarks are <1/300 case of sedation-related complications requiring endotracheal intubation or mask ventilation, <1 bowel perforation per 1000 procedures, and <1/100 major postpolypectomy bleeding [11]. Documentation of bowel preparation status was available for 98.5% of recipients (655 out of 665), slightly lower than the benchmark of 100% [11]. Bowel preparation status is important for maximizing polyp detection [13, 14], and poor bowel preparation may trigger cancellation of the procedure. Therefore adequate bowel contributes to the cancer protection effectiveness of colonoscopy [15]. Bowel preparation status was good or excellent in 69.3%, fair in 22.7%, and poor in 7.9% of the patients. The nationwide rate of poor preparation is 25% [14]. There are no USMSTF benchmarks for rates of good/poor bowel preparation although a benchmark exists for the rate of documentation of bowel preparation status (100%).

Of a total of 917 polyps found, 916 (99.9%) were retrieved for pathological examination (benchmark 95%) [11]. A total of 338 adenomas (including advanced neoplasms) were removed among the 665 patients, for an average of 0.51 adenomas per subject screened. Of these, 58 (0.09 per subject screened) were advanced neoplasms. There are no benchmarks established for the mean number of adenomas per screened subject. Three cancer cases were found at colonoscopy, two cancers located in the rectum and one in the sigmoid colon. Of 55 advanced adenomas, 76.4% were 10 mm or more in diameter, 16.4% had villous or tubulovillous features, and 5.5% showed high grade dysplasia. Additionally, there were 8 serrated adenomas. Among the 45–49-year-old AAs, 6 had advanced adenomas.

Table 2 shows the demographic characteristics of beneficiaries, the adenoma rate, and advanced neoplasm rate among the demographic subgroups. Most beneficiaries were female (71.1%), African American (71.1%), and lived in the Midlands region of SC (75.3%). The mean age was 55.2 (SD = 4.9) years, and majority (64.4%) were aged 50–59 years. The adenoma detection rate among males was 34.6%, and among females 25.1% (P = 0.01). The rate was 26.0% among those 45–49 years old (all AA), 28.4% in the 50–59 year age

TABLE 2: SCOPE SC beneficiary demographics and corresponding adenoma detection rates ($n = 665$).

	Number of beneficiaries	Adenoma detection rate	Advanced neoplasm detection rate
Geographic region			
Upstate	142 (21.5%)	38/141 (27.0%)	16/141 (11.3%)
Midlands	501 (75.3%)	140/498 (28.1%)	33/498 (6.6%)
Low country	22 (3.3%)	6/22 (27.3%)	2/22 (9.1%)
Patients			
Gender			
Male	192 (28.9%)	66/191 (34.6%)	19/191 (9.9%)
Female	473 (71.1%)	118/470 (25.1%)	32/470 (6.8%)
Race*			
White	164 (24.9%)	51/163 (31.3%)	17/163 (10.4%)
Black	468 (71.1%)	123/465 (26.5%)	31/465 (6.7%)
Other	26 (4.0%)	5/26 (19.2%)	2/26 (7.7%)
Age (years)**			
45–49***	77 (11.6%)	20/77 (26%)	6/77 (7.8%)
50–59	426 (64.4%)	120/423 (28.4%)	35/423 (8.3%)
60–64	159 (24.0%)	43/158 (27.2%)	9/158 (5.7%)
Family history			
Yes	85 (12.8%)	25/85 (29.4%)	9/85 (10.6%)
No or missing****	580 (87.2%)	159/576 (27.6%)	42/576 (7.3%)

Note: denominators for adenoma and advanced neoplasm detection rate vary due to missing data.
* Race information was missing for 7 patients.
** Age information was missing for 1 patient.
*** Includes 14 Whites screened due to a family history of colorectal cancer.
**** Question design did not permit distinction between absence of family history and nonresponse.

group, and 27.2% in the 60–64 age group ($P = 0.89$). When examined by race, 31.3% of Whites, 26.5% of AAs, and 19.2% of other race/ethnicities had ≥1 adenoma ($P = 0.31$). There was no significant difference in adenoma rates by geographic region. AAs aged 45–49 years were as likely as older Whites and AAs (aged over 50 years) to have an adenoma after controlling for gender ($P = 0.56$).

Table 3 presents the performance of SCOPE SC in addressing racial disparities in CRC. Of screening-eligible beneficiaries recruited at the FQHCs, 71.2% were AA. Among those who completed colonoscopies, 71.1% were AA. The adenoma detection and advanced neoplasm detection rates are also presented.

4. Discussion

There is little documentation of state-funded CRC screening programs for the indigent, particularly statewide programs emphasizing colonoscopy as the primary screening test. One study documented the program design and beneficiary profile of Louisiana's state-funded screening program that offered fecal immunochemical testing (FIT) to the medically indigent attending FQHCs followed by colonoscopy for those with abnormal FIT tests [16]. The State of Delaware has implemented a colonoscopy-based screening program for the uninsured since 2002. Its performance and outcomes up to

2009 are documented [17]. By 2009 the program had wiped out racial disparities in screening (74% of AAs and Whites being up to date with CRC screening in the BRFSS 2009 data, of which 85% was accounted for by colonoscopy screening in both racial groups). Similar to the Delaware program the SCOPE SC program chose to fund primary colonoscopy screening in view of low (per test) sensitivity of FIT for CRC prevention [18]. In the SC program 85% of 782 persons who were recruited completed the screening colonoscopy procedure compared to 66% of 975 persons recruited for the FIT procedure in Louisiana, despite the significantly invasive and therefore potentially intimidating nature of colonoscopy relative to FIT.

The design and performance of the SCOPE SC program in year 1 were consistent with the US Healthy People 2020 goal of "health equity, elimination of disparities and improving the health of all groups" by "facilitating high-quality, longer lives, free of preventable disease, disability, injury and premature death" [19]. The Healthy People 2010 goal of reducing CRC mortality to 13.9/100,000 [19] remained far beyond reach (current rate 21.9/100,000) [1], partly due to disproportionately high CRC mortality among AAs [20] (47% higher than among Whites). In the SCOPE SC program 71% of beneficiaries were AA, and the mean beneficiary age was 55.2 years. All of these features are encouraging. Considering the potential for cumulative cancer mortality gain, the mean

TABLE 3: SCOPE SC performance in addressing racial disparities in colorectal cancer.

Race/ethnicity	Eligible beneficiaries recruited	Percent completed colonoscopy	Percent with adenomas found	Percent with advanced neoplasms
African American	493	468 (95.0%)	123 (26.3%)	31 (6.6%)
White	172	164 (95.3%)	51 (31.1%)	17 (10.4%)
Other/missing	117	33 (28.2%)	10 (30.3%)	3 (9.1%)
Total	782	665 (85.0%)	184 (27.7%)	51 (7.7%)

beneficiary age was close to the recommended screening commencement age of 50 years, indicating that SCOPE SC gave the beneficiary cohort an early start for optimal preventive benefit, with more potential life years saved than would be the case if the mean age were higher. A high proportion of AA among beneficiaries served (71% compared to the state's overall AA population of 29%) indicates that SCOPE SC succeeded in focusing more resources on this high-disparity group. Equal proportions of screening-eligible AAs and Whites recruited actually completed the procedure. Of the AA population in SC 51.3% live below 200% of poverty compared to 31.4% of Whites [21]. The screening coverage advantage that was achieved for AAs relative to Whites is consistent with the performance of Delaware's statewide screening program for the medically indigent implemented from 2002 to 2011. The Delaware program achieved a 100% reduction in colonoscopy screening disparities between AAs and Whites [17]. One study limitation is the lack of information on the reasons/barriers for completion of the procedure among those who did not complete the procedure.

Almost 12% of beneficiaries were AAs aged 45–49 years. Unexpectedly, we found that the adenoma rate and advanced neoplasm rate in this age group were similar to the rates found among older Whites and AA. A study limitation is that potential recruitment bias favoring those with a family history among younger AAs cannot be ruled out. Although the patient referral form had a question on family history, the design was such that nonresponse could not be distinguished from those without a family history. However the frequency of adenomas was not different among those with a family history of CRC (Table 2).

Our finding suggests that SCOPE SC's innovation of extending coverage to AAs aged 45–49 years is justified and is consistent with the American College of Gastroenterology recommendations [22], earlier than the American Cancer Society's recommended screening age of 50 years uniformly for all racial groups [23]. Currently almost no insurance plan covers screening prior to 50 years of age. Our findings emphasize the need for further research with larger cohorts to verify the evidence for changing the screening eligibility age for AAs. On another note, the preponderance of women (71%) among SCOPE SC beneficiaries indicates that more focused efforts to recruit males are needed.

Provider engagement and influence on patients' decisions to undergo elaborate colon preparation are facilitated by an established doctor-patient relationship, usually not an option for uninsured patients relying on episodic charity care received from sporadically available providers in emergency

rooms and free clinics. Because FQHCs serve as a primary care medical home for the uninsured, they present an opportune setting for colonoscopy screening programs targeting the medically indigent. The SCOPE SC program chose to deploy FQHCs as the patient recruiting sites and provided funds to cover colonoscopy costs and patient navigation, which yielded highly encouraging results: rapid accrual of targeted beneficiaries, very high procedure completion rate of 85.0%, and high rates of acceptable bowel preparation. The critical role of patient navigation in improving bowel preparation and adenoma detection is well documented [24–26]. The procedure completion rate of 85% exceeds the documented rate of 66% following structured patient navigation efforts in New York City [9] and is similar to a recently documented rate of 91% colonoscopy completion following a comprehensive patient navigator program in New York City [27].

Despite meeting or exceeding the USMSTF benchmark rates for cecum intubation, polyp retrieval, and adenoma detection, the cohort had a suboptimal bowel preparation rate (considering fair and poor preparation) of 30.6%, which is consistent with the 34% rate achieved in a Medicaid primary care clientele in New York City by implementing comprehensive patient navigation services [27]. The cohort's 7.9% rate of poor bowel preparation (which causes cancellation of the procedure and sometimes termed as "inadequate preparation" [27]) is much lower than the national average of 25% [14]. The higher rate of adequate bowel preparation for the cohort is attributable, at least in part, to the detailed data collection system coupled with ongoing quality monitoring and feedback by an expert panel, instead of the widely prevalent practice of after-the-fact program evaluation typical of most programs. Three cancer cases were detected and referred for treatment. All were asymptomatic patients. Cancer stage information is not available.

In conclusion, year 1 of the SCOPE SC program served as a successful pilot validation of the program's innovative design elements: leveraging the medical home relationships of the uninsured with FQHCs, purposive funding of patient navigation, and extending coverage to AA aged 45–49 years. Results show that high completion rates can be achieved within an *ad hoc* program's fiscal year timeline. The program design enabled scarce dollars to selectively reach out to populations with the greatest need, thereby maximizing the program's potential contribution to the healthy people 2020 goal for reducing overall CRC mortality. Expansion of earmarked appropriations for colonoscopy screening of the medically indigent in SC makes sound economic sense as the state and federal governments stand to reap Medicaid and Medicare cost savings on CRC treatment in later years. Appropriations should be linked to a structured quality management system via establishment of provider accountability systems that track performance against quality indicators.

The relatively high rate of adenomas and advanced neoplasms among AAs aged 45–49 years is both intriguing and potentially very important. Given the increased probability of more aggressive disease at younger ages [28], this has major implications for policy and practice aimed at reducing racial disparities in CRC incidence and mortality. This result calls for further investigation with larger screening cohorts.

Abbreviations

CRC: Colorectal cancer
FIT: Fecal immunochemical testing
FQHC: Federally qualified health centers
SC: South Carolina
SCDHEC: South Carolina Department of Health and Environmental Control
SCOPE SC: Screening Colonoscopies for People Everywhere in South Carolina
US: United States
USC: University of South Carolina
USMSTF: US Multisociety Task Force.

Disclosure

The content is solely the responsibility of the authors and does not necessarily represent the official view of the National Cancer Institute or the National Institutes of Health.

Conflict of Interests

The authors declare that there is no conflict of interests regarding the publication of this paper.

Acknowledgments

The authors acknowledge Sonya Younger, MBA, Program Manager of the SCOPE SC Program, for her role in program management and data collection. This work was supported by four Grants, Contract no. CY-11-032 SCOPE SC Colonoscopies-Quality Indicators and Equity of Participant Referrals (PI: S Xirasagar) from the South Carolina Department of Health and Environmental Control, Grant no. 1R15CA156098-01 (PI: S Xirasagar) awarded by the National Cancer Institute, Grant no. 3U48DP001936, South Carolina Cancer Prevention and Control Research Network (JR Hebert, P.I.) from the Centers for Disease Prevention and Control, and K05 CA136975, an Established Investigator Award in Cancer Prevention and Control from the Cancer Training Branch of the National Cancer Institute to JR Hébert.

References

[1] B. K. Edwards, E. Ward, B. A. Kohler et al., "Annual report to the nation on the status of cancer, 1975–2006, featuring colorectal cancer trends and impact of interventions (risk factors, screening, and treatment) to reduce future rates," *Cancer*, vol. 116, no. 3, pp. 544–573, 2010.

[2] J. J. Fenton, D. J. Tancredi, P. Green, P. Franks, and L.-M. Baldwin, "Persistent racial and ethnic disparities in up-to-date colorectal cancer testing in medicare enrollees," *Journal of the American Geriatrics Society*, vol. 57, no. 3, pp. 412–418, 2009.

[3] US Cancer Statistics Working Group 2011, http://apps.nccd.cdc.gov/uscs/.

[4] V. G. Daguise, J. B. Burch, M.-J. Horner et al., "Colorectal cancer disparities in South Carolina: descriptive epidemiology, screening, special programs, and future direction," *Journal of the South Carolina Medical Association*, vol. 102, no. 7, pp. 212–220, 2006.

[5] J. R. Hébert, V. G. Daguise, D. M. Hurley et al., "Mapping cancer mortality-to-incidence ratios to illustrate racial and sex disparities in a high-risk population," *Cancer*, vol. 115, no. 11, pp. 2539–2552, 2009.

[6] J. A. Shapiro, C. N. Klabunde, T. D. Thompson, M. R. Nadel, L. C. Seeff, and A. White, "Patterns of colorectal cancer test use, including CT colonography, in the 2010 National Health Interview Survey," *Cancer Epidemiology Biomarkers and Prevention*, vol. 21, no. 6, pp. 895–904, 2012.

[7] M. Lopez-Class, G. Luta, A.-M. Noone et al., "Patient and provider factors associated with colorectal cancer screening in safety net clinics serving low-income, urban immigrant Latinos," *Journal of Health Care for the Poor and Underserved*, vol. 23, no. 3, pp. 1011–1019, 2012.

[8] U.S. Census Bureau 2010, http://www2.census.gov/library/publications/2008/demo/p60-235/p60no235_table8.pdf.

[9] L. A. Chen, S. Santos, L. Jandorf et al., "A program to enhance completion of screening colonoscopy among urban minorities," *Clinical Gastroenterology and Hepatology*, vol. 6, no. 4, pp. 443–450, 2008.

[10] J. Christie, S. Itzkowitz, I. Lihau-Nkanza, A. Castillo, W. Redd, and L. Jandorf, "A randomized controlled trial using patient navigation to increase colonoscopy screening among low-income minorities," *The Journal of the National Medical Association*, vol. 100, no. 3, pp. 278–284, 2008.

[11] D. K. Rex, J. H. Bond, S. Winawer et al., "Quality in the technical performance of colonoscopy and the continuous quality improvement process for colonoscopy: recommendations of the U.S. Multi-Society Task Force on Colorectal Cancer," *The American Journal of Gastroenterology*, vol. 97, no. 6, pp. 1296–1308, 2002.

[12] F. Aslinia, L. Uradomo, A. Steele, B. D. Greenwald, and J.-P. Raufman, "Quality assessment of colonoscopic cecal intubation: an analysis of 6 years of continuous practice at a University hospital," *The American Journal of Gastroenterology*, vol. 101, no. 4, pp. 721–731, 2006.

[13] F. Froehlich, V. Wietlisbach, J.-J. Gonvers, B. Burnand, and J.-P. Vader, "Impact of colonic cleansing on quality and diagnostic yield of colonoscopy: The European Panel of Appropriateness of Gastrointestinal Endoscopy European Multicenter Study," *Gastrointestinal Endoscopy*, vol. 61, no. 3, pp. 378–384, 2005.

[14] G. C. Harewood, V. K. Sharma, and P. de Garmo, "Impact of colonoscopy preparation quality on detection of suspected

colonic neoplasia," *Gastrointestinal Endoscopy*, vol. 58, no. 1, pp. 76–79, 2003.

[15] C. A. Burke and J. M. Church, "Enhancing the quality of colonoscopy: the importance of bowel purgatives," *Gastrointestinal Endoscopy*, vol. 66, no. 3, pp. 565–573, 2007.

[16] H. J. Nuss, D. L. Williams, J. Hayden, and C. R. Huard, "Applying the social ecological model to evaluate a demonstration colorectal cancer screening program in Louisiana," *Journal of Health Care for the Poor and Underserved*, vol. 23, no. 3, pp. 1026–1035, 2012.

[17] S. S. Grubbs, B. N. Polite, J. Carney Jr. et al., "Eliminating racial disparities in colorectal cancer in the real world: it took a village," *Journal of Clinical Oncology*, vol. 31, no. 16, pp. 1928–1930, 2013.

[18] J. A. Wilschut, J. D. F. Habbema, M. E. van Leerdam et al., "Fecal occult blood testing when colonoscopy capacity is limited," *Journal of the National Cancer Institute*, vol. 103, no. 23, pp. 1741–1751, 2011.

[19] US Department of Health and Human Services 2010, http://healthypeople.gov/2020/about/disparitiesAbout.aspx.

[20] S. Agrawal, A. Bhupinderjit, M. S. Bhutani et al., "Colorectal cancer in African Americans," *The American Journal of Gastroenterology*, vol. 100, no. 3, pp. 515–524, 2005.

[21] US Census Bureau 2012, http://www.census.gov/.

[22] O. G. Dominic, T. McGarrity, M. Dignan, and E. J. Lengerich, "American College of Gastroenterology guidelines for colorectal cancer screening 2008," *The American Journal of Gastroenterology*, vol. 104, no. 10, pp. 2626–2627, 2009.

[23] American Cancer Society 2013, http://www.cancer.org/cancer/colonandrectumcancer/moreinformation/colonandrectumcancerearlydetection/colorectal-cancer-early-detection-acs-recommendations.

[24] G. Abuksis, M. Mor, N. Segal et al., "A patient education program is cost-effective for preventing failure of endoscopic procedures in a gastroenterology department," *The American Journal of Gastroenterology*, vol. 96, no. 6, pp. 1786–1790, 2001.

[25] A. Kakkar and B. C. Jacobson, "Failure of an internet-based health care intervention for colonoscopy preparation: a caveat for investigators," *JAMA Internal Medicine*, vol. 173, no. 14, pp. 1374–1376, 2013.

[26] X. Liu, H. Luo, L. Zhang et al., "Telephone-based re-education on the day before colonoscopy improves the quality of bowel preparation and the polyp detection rate: a prospective, colonoscopist-blinded, randomised, controlled study," *Gut*, vol. 63, no. 1, pp. 125–130, 2014.

[27] B. Lebwohl, A. I. Neugut, E. Stavsky et al., "Effect of a patient navigator program on the volume and quality of colonoscopy," *Journal of Clinical Gastroenterology*, vol. 45, no. 5, pp. e47–e53, 2011.

[28] US Cancer Statistics Working Group 2013, Accessed at U.S. Department of Health and Human Services Centers for Disease Control and Prevention and National Cancer Institute, http://apps.nccd.cdc.gov/uscs/.

22

Clinical and Microbiologic Efficacy of a Water Filter Program in a Rural Honduran Community

Jaclyn Arquiette,[1,2] Michael P. Stevens,[1] Jean M. Rabb,[1] Kakotan Sanogo,[1] Patrick Mason,[3] and Gonzalo M. L. Bearman[1]

[1] Virginia Commonwealth University Medical Center, Richmond, VA 23284, USA
[2] Virginia Commonwealth University, School of Medicine, Richmond, VA 23284, USA
[3] Quest Diagnostics Nichols Institute, Chantilly, VA 20153, USA

Correspondence should be addressed to Jaclyn Arquiette; jaclyn.arquiette@gmail.com

Academic Editor: Gudlavalleti Venkata Murthy

Water purification in the rural Honduras is a focus of the nonprofit organization Honduras Outreach Medical Brigade Relief Effort (HOMBRE). We assessed water filter use and tested filter microbiologic and clinical efficacy. A 22-item questionnaire assessed water sources, obtainment/storage, purification, and incidence of gastrointestinal disease. Samples from home clay-based filters in La Hicaca were obtained and paired with surveys from the same home. We counted bacterial colonies of four bacterial classifications from each sample. Sixty-five surveys were completed. Forty-five (69%) individuals used a filter. Fifteen respondents reported diarrhea in their home in the last 30 days; this incidence was higher in homes not using a filter. Thirty-three paired water samples and surveys were available. Twenty-eight samples (85%) demonstrated bacterial growth. A control sample was obtained from the local river, the principal water source; number and bacterial colony types were innumerable within 24 hours. Access to clean water, the use of filters, and other treatment methods differed within a geographically proximal region. Although the majority of the water samples failed to achieve bacterial eradication, water filters may sufficiently reduce bacterial coliform counts to levels below infectious inoculation. Clay water filters may be sustainable water treatment measures in resource poor settings.

1. Introduction

Worldwide, over 1 billion people lack access to improved sources of drinking water. The lack of potable water greatly contributes to the presence of water-related illness, especially in developing countries [1].

Many communities in Honduras lack access to clean water. This is especially true in rural areas; approximately ninety-nine percent of the country's urban population has access to improved water compared to eighty-two percent of the country's rural population [2]. As much as ninety percent of rural water supplies in Honduras come from intermittent or unreliable sources [3], and water purification efforts reach sixty percent of the country's total population, yet only fifty percent of the country's rural communities [3].

Worldwide, diarrhea is among the leading causes of mortality in children under the age of five. Availability of clean water has previously been associated with lower mortality and a lower risk of child diarrhea [4]. The lack of clean drinking water in rural Honduran communities results in a large potential for the development of waterborne illnesses and potential death in infants and young children. Diarrhea accounted for seven percent of deaths in children under five in Honduras in 2010 [5]. A discrepancy exists in the infant mortality rate in children younger than five between urban Honduran communities (twenty-nine percent) and rural Honduras (forty-three percent) [5] and may be partly consistent with the differences in access to clean drinking water as well as other differences between the two communities.

Point-of-use (POU) technologies are interventions that provide clean water to homes where public water treatment is unavailable. Household based clay water filters are a POU mechanism with the potential to reduce diarrheal illness.

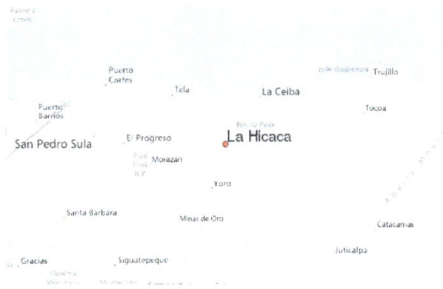

FIGURE 1: La Hicaca, Northern Honduras.

Beginning in the late 1980s and early 1990s, ceramic filters began to appear in poor communities in developing countries as a means of providing clean drinking water [6]. These devices reduce the levels of turbidity and bacteria in water by ninety-nine percent [7]. Water flows through the filter, impregnated with colloidal silver, at a flow rate of one to two liters per hour. As the water flows through the pores in the clay, bacteria and other turbidities become trapped and the antimicrobial properties of the silver impede the growth and replication of bacteria [8]. Previous field studies demonstrated decreased risk and incidence of gastrointestinal disease following implementation of water filter use, though further testing was necessary for conclusive results [9].

The Virginia Commonwealth University Global Health and Health Disparities Program (GH2DP) and the Honduras Outreach Medical Brigade Relief Effort (HOMBRE), a university affiliated medical relief program, began the distribution of water filters in 2008 in the rural Honduran town of La Hicaca (Figure 1) [10]. These filters are made in country by local artisans following Potters for Peace guidelines. For approximately twenty-five dollars per filter, a family has access to clean drinking water for a minimum of two years. Previous work by HOMBRE missions revealed that, among those without access to clean or filtered water, water treatment and nutrition were the main health concerns [11]. Surveys administered by the 2011 brigade in La Hicaca reported the use of a home water filter by forty percent of respondents [12]. However, the clinical and microbiologic efficacy of the filters provided by HOMBRE is unknown.

2. Objectives

The purpose of this study was to assess drinking water sources, methods of water treatment, water filter use, and self-reported incidence of diarrhea in the rural Honduran community La Hicaca as well as in 17 geographically proximal villages with a total population of approximately 2000. Additionally, microbiologic testing of water filters was completed to assess their effectiveness in the eradication of microorganisms.

3. Methods

3.1. Survey and Interviewing. The VCU Institutional Review Board approved a 22-item questionnaire. The questionnaire

was administered in Spanish at the HOMBRE clinic site of La Hicaca in June 2012. Eligible subjects were any Spanish-speaking individual over the age of 18 seeking care at the HOMBRE clinic in La Hicaca during June 2012. The questionnaire addressed four areas pertinent to water use. Four questions addressed water sources and their frequency of use. These questions employed multiple-choice answers. Seven multiple-choice questions addressed water obtainment and storage. Seven questions addressed water purification, including the use of a water filter as well as additional methods of treatment. Of these seven questions, five were multiple-choice and the remaining two used a Likert scale to identify the frequency of use of a particular treatment method as "always," "most of the time," "some of the time," "hardly ever," or "never." The final four questions addressed the incidence of gastrointestinal disease within the preceding thirty days in the home of the survey respondent: three were multiple choice questions and the final used a Likert scale to assess the degree of agreement that using a water filter resulted in less diarrhea in the home within the last year. Diarrhea was defined as three or more loose stools in a period of twenty-four hours [13].

The study was completed over five clinical encounter days. The author (Jaclyn Arquiette) conducted each interview, assisted during several interviews by trained, bilingual team members. Interviews were conducted using convenience-sampling methodology. Each survey was administered as a structured individual interview. Survey responses were collected on paper.

3.2. Statistical Analysis. Survey responses were analyzed using SAS statistical software (version 9.2, SAS Institute, Inc., Cary, NC). A descriptive analysis of the data was conducted using mean values, frequency counts, and percent response where applicable. A 2-way chi-squared test of significance was employed to determine a difference in response across homes with and without water filters as well as across homes from La Hicaca and the other villages.

3.3. Water Filter Sampling. All water samples were tested for the presence of coliform bacteria using Coliscan Easygel kits [14]. Samples were collected over a period of three days. Five milliliters from each sample was added to the Coliscan gel. The mixture was shaken by hand and poured into individual plates. Each sample incubated for the same amount of time (24 hours) at room temperature before being read. At the time of reading, four types of bacterial colonies were counted and the results were recorded on site.

A sample was collected from the local river/stream and a public spigot to serve as controls. After incubation, the number of bacterial colonies on each plate was counted and recorded. For standardization purposes, innumerable colonies were recorded as "innumerable," "too many to count," or "too smeared to count." The controls collected from the public spigot and the local stream both had innumerable bacterial colonies growing at the time of recording. In subsequent analysis these counts were recorded as greater than the highest countable number of colonies. Following the instructions provided in the Coliscan kit, [14] colony counts were converted to the number of colony forming units (CFU) per one hundred milliliters (CFU/100 mL) by dividing 100 by the number of milliliters of the sample (5) and multiplying that result by the number of colonies detected on the plate. The number of samples growing each type of colony was recorded ($n = x$) below the specific classification of bacteria. Samples with an individual colony type that had an innumerable number of colonies growing are noted as 10000+.

3.4. Linkage of Water Filter Sampling and Surveys. HOMBRE maintains records of distributed household based clay water filters. These records contribute to an organized system for present and future filter distribution. For the purposes of water filter sampling, a registry of homes in La Hicaca that received a water filter in 2010 or 2011 was utilized to identify homes from which a sample could be obtained. Each sample received an identification number. Concurrently, the survey obtained from the same home received the same identification number for future analysis.

3.5. Ethical Approval. The study was approved by the VCU IRB, Office of Research Subjects Protection; the approval number was HM14199.

Prior to the June trip, physician leaders of the brigade met with both the local Ministry of Health and local community leaders to discuss the plans for the clinical and research aspects of the year's trip. The goals of this trip were to prioritize a formal assessment of the previously implemented water filter program, to assess new concerns of local leaders, and to provide local leaders with updates on prior years work.

4. Results

4.1. Population Characteristics. Sixty-five surveys were collected. Fifty-seven percent ($n = 37$) came from La Hicaca, and forty-three percent ($n = 28$) came from other villages visiting the clinic. Twelve home villages were reported. Table 1 lists the distribution of surveys by village.

4.2. Access to Clean Water and Water Sources. Eighty percent ($n = 52$) of individuals surveyed stated that they had access to clean water, while twenty percent ($n = 13$) did not. One hundred percent of respondents from La Hicaca ($n = 37$) indicated that they had access to clean water compared to 54% ($n = 15$), $P < 0.0001$, of respondents from the surrounding villages. Respondents reported use of a variety of different primary drinking water sources, summarized in Table 2. Twenty-five percent ($n = 16$) of all respondents used a public faucet as their main water source, 46% ($n = 30$) used a private faucet, 11% ($n = 7$) used a well, 6% ($n = 4$) used a river or stream directly, and 12% ($n = 8$) used another source as their main water source.

The results of survey questions examining water sources are summarized in Table 2. Comparisons between La Hicaca and the other villages are also provided.

TABLE 1: Distribution of surveys by village.

Village	Number of surveys
Agua Caliente	2
Agua Sarca	3
El Chorro	3
El Urraco	2
La Culata	3
La Esperanza	3
La Florida	4
La Hicaca	37
La Vega	1
Lomitas	2
San Felix	1
Santa Maria	4

Thirty-seven (57%) of the surveys were from La Hicaca and 28 (43%) were from surrounding villages.

4.3. Water Obtainment and Storage. Ninety-five percent ($n = 62$) of respondents obtained their water on foot and 5% ($n = 3$) "were not sure" which method of transportation they used to obtain water. The types of containers utilized for both water transportation and water storage in the home were assessed, the use of a lid to cover containers, methods of cleaning water containers, and hand hygiene (washing with soap and water) prior to cleaning containers.

Ninety-one percent ($n = 59$) used a plastic container to store water in their home, 5% ($n = 3$) used a glass container, and 5% ($n = 3$) were not sure about the make of the container for water storage. Table 2 lists responses to questions regarding water obtainment and storage.

4.4. Water Treatment. Sixty-nine percent ($n = 45$) of all survey respondents used a filter to clean their water. All of these individuals received filters from the HOMBRE medical team except for one, which had a filter from an unknown source.

A comparison of water treatment methods between La Hicaca and the surrounding villages is summarized in Table 2. Differences existed between these groups regarding the methods of water treatment employed. There was one respondent from a surrounding village who indicated filter use but not if it was used exclusively or in conjunction with another treatment method.

Data was collected on the use of other forms of water treatment including boiling of water, use of bottled water, and use of chlorine tablets. These methods were not used at a frequency similar to that of water filters.

4.5. Microbiologic Testing of Water Filters. Of the thirty-seven homes surveyed in La Hicaca, thirty-three water filter samples were obtained and paired with the survey of an individual living in the same home. At the time of collection, the year the family received the filter was recorded. Eleven of the sampled filters were from 2010, fourteen from 2011, one from 2012 (from a home that did not receive a filter in 2010), and seven from an unknown year. These results are listed in

TABLE 2: Results.

Self-reported sources of water			
	All respondents	La Hicaca	Surrounding villages
Public faucet	16/65 (25%)	15/37 (41%)	1/28 (4%)
Private faucet	30/65 (46%)	22/37 (60%)	8/28 (29%)
Well	7/65 (11%)	0	7/28 (25%)
River/stream	4/65 (6%)	0	4/28 (14%)
Other	8/65 (12%)	0	8/28 (29%)
Water obtainment and storage, all respondents % (N)			
Use of plastic container for water transport			60/65 (92%)
Use of plastic container for water storage			59/65 (91%)
Clean water transport container with soap and water			58/65 (89%)
Clean water storage container with soap and water			59/65 (91%)
Wash hands with soap and water before filling water containers			59/65 (91%)
Use lid for containers for water transport and storage			41/65 (63%)
Use lid for containers for water transport only			1/65 (2%)
Use lid for containers for water storage only			12/65 (19%)
Do not use a lid for water transport or storage			10/65 (15%)
Employed methods of water treatment, % (N)			
		La Hicaca	Other villages
Water filter only		17/37 (46%)	1/28 (3.5%)
Other methods only		0	8/28 (28.5%)
Water filter and other methods		19/37 (51%)	7/28 (25%)
None		1/37 (3%)	12/28 (43%)

TABLE 3: Mean bacterial colony count (CFU/100 mL) by bacterial type and year of filter distribution.

Year of filter distribution (number of samples)	Colony type and mean number CFU/100 mL			
	Enterobacter/ Citrobacter/Klebsiella (SD)	Proteus/ Salmonella (SD)	E. coli (SD)	Noncoliform bacteria (SD)
2012 (5)	0	256.2 (572.3)	0	0
2011 (14)	765.7 (2183.2)	552.9 (1124.5)	140 (495.8)	0
2010 (11)	3434.5 (3763.9)	1734.5 (1845.6)	16.4 (29.4)	120 (311.8)

The number of colony forming units was obtained by counting the number of colonies of each type on the sample plate. This was converted into number of CFU/100 mL dividing 100 by the number of mL of the sample (5 mL) and multiplying that number by the number of colonies counted on the plate.

Table 3 and demonstrate low numbers of *E. coli* present in the water filter samples.

4.6. Gastrointestinal Disease and Water Filter Use. Collectively, fifteen surveyed homes reported diarrhea beginning in the 30 days prior to survey collection; five reports were from La Hicaca and eleven were from other villages ($P < 0.01$).

There was an overall difference in the self-reported incidence of diarrhea between individuals using a filter and those not using a filter ($P < 0.01$). Five of the forty-five respondents using a filter reported diarrhea in their home within the last 30 days (11%), compared to eight of twenty not using a filter (40%). When analyzed by geographic site in either La Hicaca or in the surrounding villages, no difference was observed in self-reported diarrheal illness in homes with and without water filter use (Table 4).

TABLE 4: Filter use and diarrheal illness in La Hicaca and surrounding villages.

	La Hicaca		Surrounding villages	
	Diarrhea	No diarrhea	Diarrhea	No diarrhea
Filter	4	32	3	6
No filter	1	0	8	11
Total	5	32	11	17

The mean number of CFU was also compared between homes in La Hicaca with diarrheal illness and homes with no diarrheal illness. The homes in which no individuals reported diarrheal illness within the past 30 days had a mean CFU of 2954.9, compared to a mean CFU of 6400 in homes reporting recent diarrhea.

5. Discussion

Public health interventions to improve clean drinking water access are a priority for the medical relief trips of HOMBRE as well as the Global Health and Health Disparities Program of the VCU Medical Center. The water filter program began in 2008 and to date over 240 filters have been distributed in the region.

Access to clean water, the use of water filters, and the use of other water treatment methods differed within these geographically proximal communities. Individuals living in La Hicaca demonstrated a higher percentage of respondents with consistent access to a clean water source and a greater use of water filters. The self-reported incidence of diarrheal illness was lower in La Hicaca than in the surrounding villages.

While this water filter project has expanded to include villages surrounding La Hicaca, there may be additional barriers to access to potable water. Previous research suggests that distance is not the sole barrier to healthcare and access to clean water [15].

Topography and a lack of modern roads may limit the ability of villagers to travel by foot to the HOMBRE clinic and water filter distribution sites. For some, the travel time by foot was between 1 and 5 hours, in hot, summer weather. Individuals in La Hicaca have several resource advantages such as a functional dirt road as well as a small public health outpost. Although the region is impoverished, with no plumbing or electricity, compared to the surrounding villages, La Hicaca has a lower burden of poverty. This may consequently result in a heightened ability to obtain filters or employ other water treatment methods (Personal Communication, Olanchito Ministry of Health).

After testing water samples obtained from the filters, eighty-five percent revealed the presence of some bacterial growth. However, of the twenty-eight plates exhibiting bacterial growth, only six were positive for 40-1860 CFU/100 mL of *E. coli*. Enterotoxigenic *E. coli* (ETEC) strains are the principal etiologic pathogens of watery diarrhea and childhood diarrhea in the developing world [16]. ETEC accounts for more than 200 million causes of diarrhea [17].

Low counts of *E. coli* were recorded in the water samples. For water filters distributed in 2010 and 2011, the mean *E. coli* bacterial counts were 16.4 CFU/mL and 140 CFU/mL, respectively. Despite low level recovery of *E. coli* from a minority of filters, these households also did not report diarrheal illness. These data further suggest that clay water filters are microbiologically efficacious for the reduction of *E. coli*, as previously reported [18].

The low frequency of self-reported diarrhea in the study population may be the result of several factors. Studies on the pathogenesis of ETEC suggest that a dose of 10^4–10^{10} bacteria is necessary to cause infection [19]. WHO risk categories for *E. coli* in drinking water are 0/100 mL (compliance), 1–10/100 mL (low risk), 11–100/100 mL (intermediate risk), and 101–1000/100 mL (high risk). Of the six water samples positive for *E. coli*, four were intermediate and two were high risk by WHO risk category. Thus, household based clay water filters may sufficiently reduce microbial burden of enteric pathogens to levels below infectious inoculation.

Enterobacter/Citrobacter/Klebsiella colonies were detected in twenty-two samples, while *Proteus/Salmonella* (nontyphoidal) colonies were detected in twenty samples. *Klebsiella* species in drinking water are generally not enteric pathogens and are unlikely to pose health problems [20]. Similarly, nontyphoidal *Salmonella* species rarely cause waterborne diarrheal outbreaks [20]. It is postulated that their presence may be due in part to inconsistent cleaning of the filters and by environmental contamination. Of the homes undergoing water sampling, only two reported diarrhea in the past thirty days. Neither of these samples cultured positive for *E. coli*. This suggests that the diarrheal infections, if bacterial in origin and water borne, were from a source other than the water filters.

Although the majority of survey respondents lacked direct, piped water to their homes and used a large plastic container for water collection and storage, the questionnaire survey analysis revealed several important trends. First, although La Hicaca and the surrounding villages are geographically proximal and fall under the auspices of the same local Health Ministry, significant differences exist in water use, treatment practices, and self-reported diarrheal incidence. Ninety-seven percent of respondents in La Hicaca consistently used a household-based clay water filter, while only thirty-two percent of respondents from the other villages used a filter. Forty-three percent of respondents from the surrounding villages did not use any method of water treatment. While no respondents from La Hicaca indicated that their main source of drinking water was a river or stream, fourteen percent of respondents from the proximal villages obtained water from a local river. The high percentage of self-reported filter use in La Hicaca suggests that water filter use is a sustainable endeavor.

This study has several strengths. This study to the authors' knowledge is the first to assess the efficacy of household-based clay water filters, on site, in a Central American community. All interviews were performed as structured questionnaires by a trained interviewer limiting bias. Standardized methodology for water sampling and for field bacteriologic assessment of water was employed. Sample size was small and may not be representative of all households in the geographic catchment area. Exclusive use of household-based clay water filters for treatment cannot be confirmed. The heterogeneity in water storage containers and methods may have led to disparities in microbial contamination. Additional limitations include the absence of paired individual level data on diarrheal illness and confirmation of exclusive water filter use by respondents. For respondents using multiple sources of water treatment, it cannot be excluded that another source was used more frequently than the water filter. All of these factors may have impacted the self-reported incidence of diarrheal illness.

This study adds to the body of literature on water filtration systems for potable water in resource poor settings, particularly in Central America. Even within proximal, resource-poor communities, access to potable water varies. In addition, the data suggest that while home-based clay filters may not be completely efficacious in removing bacterial contaminants from drinking water, they may sufficiently reduce coliform bacterial counts to levels below infectious inoculation. Further, for households with home-based clay water filters, self-reported use of the filters was high, suggesting that these water filtration systems may impact diarrheal illness. Thus, simple, inexpensive clay filters may be a sustainable and reliable public health intervention in resource limited settings lacking potable water. Consequently, their use should continue to expand in developing countries as a means to reduce gastrointestinal illness until more permanent solutions are successfully and consistently implemented.

Conflict of Interests

The authors declare that there is no conflict of interests regarding the publication of this paper.

Acknowledgments

The authors thank the VCU Global Health and Health Disparities Program and the Golden Phoenix Foundation for their continued support of the medical brigades and public health efforts.

References

[1] J. M. Brown, S. Proum, and M. D. Sobsey, "*Escherichia coli* in household drinking water and diarrheal disease risk: evidence from Cambodia," *Water Science and Technology*, vol. 58, no. 4, pp. 757–763, 2008.

[2] D. M. Johnson, D. R. Hokanson, Q. Zhang, K. D. Czupinski, and J. Tang, "Feasibility of water purification technology in rural areas of developing countries," *Journal of Environmental Management*, vol. 88, no. 3, pp. 416–427, 2008.

[3] Water for People. Our Work: Honduras, http://www.water-forpeople.org/programs/central-america/honduras.html.

[4] G. Fink, I. Günther, and K. Hill, "The effect of water and sanitation on child health: evidence from the demographic and health surveys 1986–2007," *International Journal of Epidemiology*, vol. 40, no. 5, pp. 1196–1204, 2011.

[5] World Health Organization, *World Health Statistics 2012*, World Health Organization, Geneva, Switzerland, 2012.

[6] V. A. Oyanedel-Craver and J. A. Smith, "Sustainable colloidal-silver-impregnated ceramic filter for point-of-use water treatment," *Environmental Science and Technology*, vol. 42, no. 3, pp. 927–933, 2008.

[7] M. D. Sobsey, *Managing Water in the Home: Accelerated Health Gains from Improved Water Supply*, WHO, Geneva, Switzerland, 2002.

[8] T. F. Clasen, J. Brown, S. Collin, O. Suntura, and S. Cairn-cross, "Reducing diarrhea through the use of household-based ceramic water filters: a randomized, controlled trial in rural Bolivia," *The American Journal of Tropical Medicine and Hygiene*, vol. 70, no. 6, pp. 651–657, 2004.

[9] T. Clasen, W.-P. Schmidt, T. Rabie, I. Roberts, and S. Cairn-cross, "Interventions to improve water quality for preventing diarrhoea: systematic review and meta-analysis," *British Medical Journal*, vol. 334, no. 7597, pp. 782–785, 2007.

[10] La Hicaca, Northern Honduras. Map. N.d. La Hicaca, Honduras Weather Forecast. Web. February 2014.

[11] R. Hemrajani, B. Morehouse, K. Elam et al., "Top health concerns in rural Honduras following the introduction of clay water filters," *International Journal of Infectious Diseases*, vol. 14, no. 1, article e66, 2010.

[12] G. Halder, G. Bearman, K. Sanogo, and M. P. Stevens, "Water sanitation, access, use and self-reported diarrheal disease in rural Honduras," *Journal of Rural and Remote Health*, vol. 13, no. 2413, 2013.

[13] T. F. Clasen, J. Brown, and S. M. Collin, "Preventing diarrhoea with household ceramic water filters: assessment of a pilot project in Bolivia," *International Journal of Environmental Health Research*, vol. 16, no. 3, pp. 231–239, 2006.

[14] *Detection of Waterborne Coliforms and Fecal Coliforms with Coliscan Easygel*, http://bellehavenwatershed.wikispaces.com/file/detail/Coliform+Bacteria+Instructions.pdf.

[15] C. A. Pearson, M. P. Stevens, K. Sanogo, and G. Bearman, "Access and barriers to healthcare vary among three neighboring communities in northern Honduras," *International Journal of Family Medicine*, vol. 2012, Article ID 298472, 6 pages, 2012.

[16] J. B. Kaper, J. P. Nataro, and H. L. T. Mobley, "Pathogenic *Escherichia coli*," *Nature Reviews Microbiology*, vol. 2, no. 2, pp. 123–140, 2004.

[17] M. Tauschek, R. J. Gorrell, R. A. Strugnell, and R. M. Robins-Browne, "Identification of a protein secretory pathway for the secretion of heat-labile enterotoxin by an enterotoxigenic strain of *Escherichia coli*," *Proceedings of the National Academy of Sciences of the United States of America*, vol. 99, no. 10, pp. 7066–7071, 2002.

[18] J. Brown and M. Sobesy, *Use of Ceramic Water Filters in Cambodia*, Water and Sanitation Program. UNICEF, 2007.

[19] H. L. DuPont, S. B. Formal, R. B. Hornick et al., "Pathogenesis of *Escherichia coli* diarrhea," *The New England Journal of Medicine*, vol. 285, no. 1, pp. 1–9, 1971.

[20] World Health Organization, *Microbial Fact Sheets*, http://www.who.int/water_sanitation_health/dwq/gdwq3_11.pdf.

23

Prediction of Optimal Daily Step Count Achievement from Segmented School Physical Activity

Ryan D. Burns,[1] **Timothy A. Brusseau,**[1] **and James C. Hannon**[2]

[1]*Department of Exercise and Sport Science, College of Health, University of Utah, 250 S. 1850 E., HPER North, RM 241,*
  Salt Lake City, UT 84112, USA
[2]*College of Physical Activity and Sport Sciences, West Virginia University, 375 Birch Street, P.O. Box 6116,*
  Morgantown, WV 26505, USA

Correspondence should be addressed to Ryan D. Burns; ryan.d.burns@utah.edu

Academic Editor: Julio Diaz

Optimizing physical activity in childhood is needed for prevention of disease and for healthy social and psychological development. There is limited research examining how segmented school physical activity patterns relate to a child achieving optimal physical activity levels. The purpose of this study was to examine the predictive relationship between step counts during specific school segments and achieving optimal school (6,000 steps/day) and daily (12,000 steps/day) step counts in children. Participants included 1,714 school-aged children (mean age = 9.7 ± 1.0 years) recruited across six elementary schools. Physical activity was monitored for one week using pedometers. Generalized linear mixed effects models were used to determine the adjusted odds ratios (ORs) of achieving both school and daily step count standards for every 1,000 steps taken during each school segment. The school segment that related in strongest way to a student achieving 6,000 steps during school hours was afternoon recess (OR = 40.03; $P < 0.001$) and for achieving 12,000 steps for the entire day was lunch recess (OR = 5.03; $P < 0.001$). School segments including lunch and afternoon recess play an important role for optimizing daily physical activity in children.

1. Introduction

Physical activity has numerous benefits in children including attenuation of chronic disease risk [1], improved motor development [2], improved classroom behavior [3], and improved cognitive functioning leading to better performance in the classroom [4]. Over the past few decades, numerous research studies have examined the correlates of physical activity in children [5]. The pedometer has been and continues to be a popular instrument for physical activity assessment. Recently it has been suggested that 12,000 steps should be a daily step count cut-point used to assess optimal physical activity levels in children [6]. Because children spend a significant proportion of weekdays in school settings, it is reasonable to expect that at least one-half of this daily recommendation should be met during school hours (i.e., 6,000 steps). Given the relative novelty of the aforementioned recommendations, there has been a paucity of research studies examining how various segments of the school day relate to a child achieving these standards.

Even though the majority of school hours are spent in sedentary behaviors, there are various segments throughout the school day where children can engage in physical activity. Research has shown that school segments such as PE, recess, and classroom activity breaks can provide opportunities for the child to engage in active play to increase their daily physical activity levels [7]. Before school and after school are other leisure times to engage in active play; however these segments are not typically considered "school hours" and are highly variable from day to day because of varying after school activities and transportation schedules. Of the school segments specifically included during school hours, recess has shown to have a significant impact on physical activity in children [8, 9]. Various intervention studies have been employed over the last couple of decades and have shown increases in moderate-to-vigorous physical activity (MVPA) during recess, especially when increasing the number of unfixed equipment available on school grounds [10]. Most students have access to at least one recess per school day, but recess times have been cut in some school districts in the USA in favor for academic classes [11].

Classroom activity breaks can also increase physical activity in children [12]. Classroom breaks such as Energizers or implementation of programs such as TAKE 10! have shown to be significantly effective in increasing daily physical activity [13]. However, this specific school segment can also be highly variable from day to day because of classroom teacher's compliance with implementing these breaks in addition to competition with other school priorities [14, 15].

Physical education is a school subject vital for the physical, social, and psychological development of the child. Unfortunately, like recess, PE is being cut to prioritize more time in academic classes [16]. Indeed, most children are lucky to receive 40 minutes per week in PE and only a small proportion of schools in the USA implement daily PE curricula [17]. This significantly limits the amount of time a child can participate in active play to increase their daily physical activity during school hours; thus PE itself may have a small effect on improving the odds that a child achieves the 12,000-step physical activity standard.

Each of the aforementioned school segments has the potential to increase physical activity behaviors of school-aged children. Given the lack of research examining how various school segments influence achievement of optimal school (6,000 steps) and daily (12,000 steps) physical activity levels, examining these relationships is a priority using large population samples of elementary school children. Identifying which school segments relate in strongest way to step count standards will provide information on how to more efficiently optimize physical activity in children during school hours and may provide evidence for future interventions to prioritize increasing physical activity behaviors during specific segments of the school day. Therefore, the purpose of this study was to examine the predictive relationship between school segment step counts and the odds of achieving school and daily step count standards in children. It was hypothesized that school segments such as lunch and afternoon recess will significantly relate to a child achieving the school and daily step count standards.

2. Methods

2.1. Participants. Participants were a convenience sample of 1,714 school-aged children recruited from six elementary schools located in a large metropolitan area in the Southwestern USA. The mean age of the sample was 9.7 ± 1.0 years and there were 926 girls and 788 boys who participated. The racial composition of the sample was 43% Caucasian, 44% Hispanic, 7% African American, 4% American Indian, and 2% Asian or Pacific Islander. Written assent was obtained from the students and written consent was obtained from the parents prior to data collection. The University Institutional Review Board approved the protocols used in this study.

2.2. Instrumentation. The Yamax SW-200 pedometer was used to measure children's physical activity. This model has produced valid and reliable scores in measuring children's physical activity in field settings [18]. Prior to data collection, the pedometers were checked for test-retest reliability using a series of shake tests, developed by Vincent and Sidman [19]. Additionally, all participants completed a walking test [20] to ensure that the pedometers accurately measured steps. Classroom and PE teachers provided opportunities for students to practice wearing the devices before data collection to attenuate risk for behavioral reactivity. On the first day of data collection, a five-minute review of the pedometer protocol was given by a member of the research team addressing how to (a) place pedometers on the body, (b) remove the pedometers before engaging in water activities and sleeping, and (c) reattach the pedometer each morning upon dressing for the school day. Participants were instructed to wear their pedometers at all times before, during, and after school hours while participating in their normal daily activities except during water activities and sleeping.

2.3. Procedures. Parents completed a background questionnaire used to collect demographic information including the child's age, sex, and ethnicity. Height (to the nearest 0.5 cm) and weight (to the nearest 0.1 kg) were measured using a digital scale (Seca 882 Digital BMI Scale, Hanover, MD, USA) and stadiometer (Seca 214, Hanover, MD, USA). At the beginning of the school day, students were prompted to record their pedometer step counts from the previous day and reset their pedometer for the current day. At the beginning and end of each school segment and at the end of each school day students were also prompted to record their step counts. During data collection, research team members actively provided prompts reminding the students how to correctly wear the instrument. Research team members scanned student responses on their recorded step count data and questioned children if step count outliers and extreme scores were detected. After given the information regarding recorded step counts from the previous day, the researchers entered the data into an Excel spreadsheet. If pedometers were lost, broken, or misused, students were prevented from getting another pedometer (<5% of participants). Furthermore, students participated in random daily validation checks by completing a brief survey about their previous day's physical activity. Survey question items required a yes or no response regarding if they wore their pedometer the entire day and if they removed the pedometer for any reason other than showering, swimming, or sleeping. The pedometer data collection process was repeated daily across five days of the school week at each of the six schools.

2.4. Statistical Analysis. Data were screened for outliers using z-scores and boxplots and checked for Gaussian distributions using histograms and k-density plots. Differences between the sexes and grade levels on step counts within each school segment were examined using 2 × 2 Factorial ANOVA tests. Alpha level was adjusted using the Bonferroni method to account for analysis on multiple dependent variables. Effect

TABLE 1: Descriptive statistics for the total sample and within sex and grade groups (means and standard deviations).

	Total sample (N = 1,714)	Girls (n = 926)	Boys (n = 788)	Grade 4 (n = 816)	Grade 5 (n = 898)
BMI[a] (kg/m^2)	19.6 (4.2)	19.1 (4.1)	19.6 (4.3)	19.1 (4.3)	19.6 (4.0)
PE[b] steps	1,897 (808)	1,823 (781)	**1,979* (831)**	1,890 (771)	1,953 (873)
Lunch recess steps	1,537 (523)	1,374 (456)	**1,706* (536)**	1,512 (484)	**1,614* (534)**
Afternoon recess steps	1,281 (541)	1,184 (504)	**1,394* (561)**	1,313 (499)	1,266 (560)
Classroom steps	2,052 (1,566)	1,850 (1,390)	2,261 (1,707)	1,931 (1,540)	2,037 (1,560)
School steps	5,625 (1,855)	5,242 (1,712)	**6,018* (1,915)**	5,139 (1,687)	**6,106* (1,865)**
Total day steps	13,048 (4,248)	10,218 (3,195)	**12,088* (3,895)**	12,403 (4,306)	**13,578* (4,071)**

Note. [a]BMI stands for Body Mass Index; [b]PE stands for physical education; bold denotes statistical significance between sexes or between grade levels, *$P < 0.001$.

sizes were also calculated for each pair-wise comparison using Cohen's d. Effect sizes were considered small if $d < 0.20$, medium if $d \approx 0.50$, and large if $d \geq 0.8$ [21].

The primary analysis consisted of employing generalized linear mixed effects models with a logit link function to examine the odds of achieving school and daily step count standards per unit change in a school segment step count. The daily standard was 12,000 steps per day as recommended by Colley et al. [6], and the school standard was 6,000 steps per day. School segment step count data was converted from absolute steps to thousands of steps in order to interpret the predictor variables in meaningful units. The student unit of measurement was clustered within individual classrooms; therefore classrooms were a higher level and treated as a random effect. Although there were multiple schools in the data set, it was not treated as a higher level with an additional random effect because of the small number clusters. This decision was supported by a nonsignificant likelihood ratio chi-square statistic that tested if the model including a school-level and teacher-level random effect was statistically different compared to a model with a teacher-level random effect only. Additional variables that were entered into each model included sex, grade, and ethnicity to control for any modifying effects. The reported results included an adjusted odds ratio for meeting the school day or total day step count standard per every one thousand step increase within a specific school segment. All analyses had an initial alpha level set at $P \leq 0.05$ and were carried out using STATA v14.0 statistical software package (College Station, TX, USA).

3. Results

The descriptive statistics for the total sample and within each sex and grade level are presented in Table 1. Boys took statistically more steps than girls during PE (mean difference = 156 steps, $P < 0.001$, Cohen's $d = 0.18$), lunch recess (mean difference = 332 steps, $P < 0.001$, Cohen's $d = 0.62$), and afternoon recess (mean difference = 210 steps, $P < 0.001$, Cohen's $d = 0.37$) and took more steps during the school day (mean difference = 776 steps, $P < 0.001$, Cohen's $d = 0.40$) and during the entire day (mean difference = 1,870 steps, $P < 0.001$, Cohen's $d = 0.48$). Children in the fifth grade took more steps than children in the fourth grade during lunch recess (mean difference = 102 steps, $P < 0.001$, Cohen's $d = 0.19$)

TABLE 2: Parameter estimates from the final fixed effects model solution using the school step target criterion (6,000 steps).

	Adjusted odds ratio	95% CI[b]	P value
PE[a] steps	**3.39***	(1.82, 6.29)	<0.001
Lunch recess steps	**26.90***	(6.03, 119.89)	<0.001
Afternoon recess steps	**40.03***	(9.90, 161.75)	<0.001
Classroom steps	**14.21***	(6.43, 31.40)	<0.001
Female	0.72	(0.29, 1.78)	0.475
4th grade	1.15	(0.42, 3.22)	0.779
Hispanic	0.21	(0.04, 1.19)	0.080
African American	1.54	(0.17, 14.41)	0.701
American Indian	0.57	(0.05, 2.61)	0.322
Asian/Pacific Islander	0.38	(0.05, 2.61)	0.322

Note. [a]PE stands for physical education; [b]95% CI stands for the 95% Confidence Interval; bold denotes statistical significance, *$P < 0.001$.

and took more steps during the school day (mean difference = 967 steps, $P < 0.001$, Cohen's $d = 0.50$) and during the entire day (mean difference = 1,175 steps, $P < 0.001$, Cohen's $d = 0.27$). ANOVA tests revealed no statistically significant sex × grade interactions.

The results from the generalized mixed effects models are presented in Tables 2 and 3 for school and daily standards, respectively. The odds of a child achieving school standards were 3.39 times higher if 1,000 more steps were taken during PE, 26.90 times higher during lunch, 40.03 times higher during recess, and 14.21 times higher during classroom activity breaks after controlling for sex, grade, race, and teacher-level clustering ($P < 0.001$). Regarding daily step count standards, the odds of achieving the daily standard were 5.03 times greater for every 1,000 steps taken during lunch, 3.70 times greater during recess, and 1.98 times greater during classroom activity breaks after controlling for sex, grade, race, and teacher-level clustering. Increases in step counts during PE did not yield any significant change in odds in achieving the daily standard during PE days. Figures 1 and 2 display a scatterplot with line of best fit showing the strongest school segment associations between afternoon recess steps and school steps and between lunch recess steps and daily steps, respectively.

TABLE 3: Parameter estimates from the final fixed effects model solution using the daily step target criterion (12,000 steps).

	Adjusted odds ratio	95% CI[b]	P value
PE[a] steps	1.03	(0.72, 1.48)	0.835
Lunch recess steps	**5.03**[†]	(1.85, 13.74)	0.002
Afternoon recess steps	**3.70**[†]	(1.53, 8.78)	0.003
Classroom steps	**1.98**[†]	(1.41, 2.76)	<0.001
Female	0.82	(0.42, 1.61)	0.495
4th grade	0.76	(0.35, 1.67)	0.495
Hispanic	0.40	(0.12, 1.29)	0.126
African American	0.92	(0.19, 4.37)	0.921
American Indian	1.88	(0.90, 3.93)	0.090
Asian/Pacific Islander	3.38	(0.75, 15.19)	0.112

Note. [a]PE stands for physical education; [b]95% CI stands for the 95% Confidence Interval; bold denotes statistical significance, [†]$P < 0.01$.

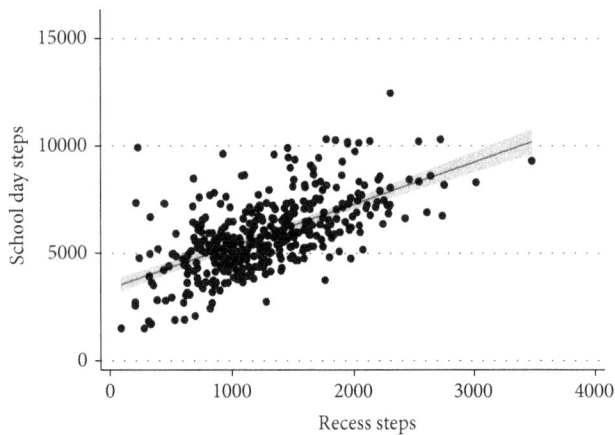

FIGURE 2: Scatterplot and line of best fit showing the linear relationship between lunch recess steps and total daily steps ($r = 0.44$; $P < 0.001$).

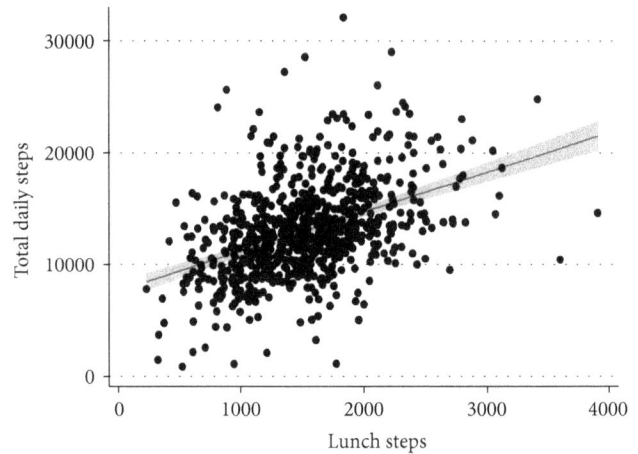

FIGURE 1: Scatterplot and line of best fit showing the linear relationship between afternoon recess steps and school steps ($r = 0.61$; $P < 0.001$).

4. Discussion

The purpose of this study was to examine the predictive relationship between step counts taken during specific school segments and achievement of optimal school and daily physical activity levels. The results indicated that lunch and afternoon recess had the strongest predictive ability for determining the odds of achieving school and daily step count standards. Although all school segments related to achieving 6,000 steps during school and all but PE related to achieving 12,000 steps during the entire day, researchers and practitioners aiming to improve the odds that a child can achieve optimal levels of physical activity may want to prioritize school recess times because of the strong associations found in this study.

The primary finding from the current study was that the recess school segments had the strongest predictive relationship with a child achieving school and daily pedometer step count standards. Recess is considered a school leisure time where girls and boys have opportunities to participate in active play. Structured and semistructured recess times have both been shown to increase physical activity levels in children. Increases in physical activity during recess are most significant when students are given unfixed equipment and are outdoors and upon providing students options to play in their preferred modes of physical activity [22]. It has been shown that urban school-aged girls take on average 976 steps and boys take approximately 1,281 steps during outdoor recess [23]. Brusseau and Kulinna [24] showed that fifth graders achieved the most steps during the entire day on the days they had multiple recess times and the least amount of steps on the days when they had just one recess. Indeed, recess has been shown to account for anywhere between 11% and 21% of their daily step counts and can account for as much as 40% of daily MVPA recommendations [25]. The results from the current study suggest that increasing physical activity by 1,000 steps during this school segment (recess) has the strongest predictive ability that a student will achieve at least 6,000 steps per school day and at least 12,000 steps during the entire day. Possible explanations why recess yielded the greatest odds of achieving physical activity guidelines include the frequency of physical activity exposure, as recess was daily and at multiple times at each school, the amount of play space and available play equipment for the children to use, and the number of other students/peers to interact with, as each recess time period typically involved several classes and grade levels. There may be discordance in the exposure of these factors compared to other school segments including PE or during classroom activity breaks where the frequency of physical activity exposure is more limited (e.g., PE is only once per week), the amount of play space tends to limited to gymnasium or classroom space, certain play equipment may be unavailable to use, and the number of other students to interact with is limited to peers within a child's respective classroom.

Other school leisure times that associated with the odds of achieving school and daily step count standards included classroom activity breaks. Classroom activity breaks have been shown to have a positive effect not only on physical activity but also on classroom behaviors and improving academic performance [26, 27]. Unfortunately, studies have shown that individual teacher compliance with implementing activity breaks varies widely not only among different schools but also within the same school [14, 15]. However, the results from this study clearly show that, even after controlling for demographic information and the effect of other school segments, classroom activity breaks still have a significant relationship with predicting if a student achieved step count standards. The results indicated that additional 1,000 steps from classroom activity breaks associate with 14 times higher odds that a child achieved 6,000 steps during the school day and almost doubled the odds that a child achieved 12,000 steps during the entire day. Despite these very strong associations, previous research interventions employing classroom activity breaks increase step counts, on average, between approximately 600 and 800 steps [12, 13]. This study clearly showed that children took a significantly greater number of steps during classroom breaks (approximately 2,000 steps) compared to past research. This may be because most of the teachers in the current study implemented more than one 10-minute break throughout the school day, as opposed to only one activity break per school day implemented in previous intervention work. Teachers in this study were recommended to employ at least two classroom activity breaks per day (one in the morning and one in the afternoon). Therefore, given the results from this and past studies, using classroom activity breaks to increase a child's step count by 1,000 steps, although certainly feasible, may not be the norm within a day-to-day context if only implementing one activity break per school day.

Although steps taken during PE did associate with students achieving school step count standards, it did not associate with achievement of daily standards after accounting for demographic information and the effect of the other school segments. In this study, PE was given once per week for 40 minutes. The number of steps taken during PE was approximately 2,000 steps for both sexes, which is more than what has been previously reported using population samples of similar age where steps ranging from approximately 1,200 to 1,400 steps were taken [28]. In the current study, the number of steps taken during PE was similar to those taken during classroom breaks and more than those taken during both recess times; however its relationship with achievement of daily levels was not statistically significant. One possible explanation for this was that there might have been a compensatory effect where children became inactive during other school segments as well as after school during the days that they had PE. It has been suggested that on restricted physical activity days (i.e., days without PE or recess times) there may be increased physical activity during other school segments and leisure times to achieve a balanced energy homeostasis [29]. It is therefore plausible that the opposite is true, where increased activity in PE may lead to decreased energy expenditure (i.e., decreased step counts) during recess or after school hours to maintain this energy homeostasis. However, the authors do not know of any other studies examining this phenomenon and therefore may be a priority for future research.

There are limitations to this study that must be considered before generalizations can be made. Because of the cross-sectional nature of the current study, no casual links can be established, only correlational and predictive relationships. Also, only fourth and fifth grade students were examined; therefore the results cannot be generalized to younger or older age groups. This study used PE curriculum that was administered just one day per week at each of the six schools; therefore the results do not generalize to schools offering daily PE curricula. Finally, physical activity was monitored using pedometers; therefore physical activity of specific intensities was not examined in addition to physical activity modes nonambulatory in nature such as swimming, cycling, and resistance training.

In conclusion, school segments including lunch and afternoon recess most strongly relate to the odds that a child achieves 6,000 steps during school hours and achieves 12,000 steps during the entire day. Other school segments that relate to achieving the school step count standard include PE and classroom activity breaks and those relating to achieving the daily step count standard include classroom activity breaks. The results indicate that increasing school physical activity during most of the examined school segments has the potential to significantly increase the odds that a child can achieve optimal school and daily levels; however the recess times tended to have the strongest effect. Interventions aiming to increase school and daily physical activity levels in children may want to prioritize increasing these behaviors during recess because of the strong relationships seen in the current study. Indeed, optimizing physical activity levels in children is important for optimal physical and psychological development, and this study provides unique insights into how varying levels of physical activity during specific school segments relate to achieving current step count standards to improve their overall health and well-being.

Conflict of Interests

The authors declare that there is no conflict of interests regarding the publication of this paper.

Acknowledgments

The authors would like to thank the teachers and students who participated in this study.

References

[1] L. M. Boddy, M. H. Murphy, C. Cunningham et al., "Physical activity, cardiorespiratory fitness, and clustered cardiometabolic risk in 10- to 12-year-old school children: the REACH Y6 study," *American Journal of Human Biology*, vol. 26, no. 4, pp. 446–451, 2014.

[2] D. F. Stodden, Z. Gao, J. D. Goodway, and S. J. Langendorfer, "Dynamic relationships between motor skill competence and health-related fitness in youth," *Pediatric Exercise Science*, vol. 26, no. 3, pp. 231–241, 2014.

[3] M. T. Mahar, "Impact of short bouts of physical activity on attention-to-task in elementary school children," *Preventive Medicine*, vol. 52, supplement 1, pp. S60–S64, 2011.

[4] D. M. Castelli, C. H. Hillman, S. M. Buck, and H. E. Erwin, "Physical fitness and academic achievement in third- and fifth-grade students," *Journal of Sport & Exercise Psychology*, vol. 29, no. 2, pp. 239–252, 2007.

[5] J. F. Sallis, J. J. Prochaska, and W. C. Taylor, "A review of correlates of physical activity of children and adolescents," *Medicine and Science in Sports and Exercise*, vol. 32, no. 5, pp. 963–975, 2000.

[6] R. C. Colley, I. Janssen, and M. S. Tremblay, "Daily step target to measure adherence to physical activity guidelines in children," *Medicine & Science in Sports & Exercise*, vol. 44, no. 5, pp. 977–982, 2012.

[7] T. L. McKenzie, N. C. Crespo, B. Baquero, and J. P. Elder, "Leisure-time physical activity in elementary schools: analysis of contextual conditions," *Journal of School Health*, vol. 80, no. 10, pp. 470–477, 2010.

[8] A. Beighle, C. F. Morgan, G. Le Masurier, and R. P. Pangrazi, "Children's physical activity during recess and outside of school," *Journal of School Health*, vol. 76, no. 10, pp. 516–520, 2006.

[9] J. Mota, P. Silva, M. P. Santos, J. C. Ribeiro, J. Oliveira, and J. A. Duarte, "Physical activity and school recess time: differences between the sexes and the relationship between children's playground physical activity and habitual physical activity," *Journal of Sports Sciences*, vol. 23, no. 3, pp. 269–275, 2005.

[10] N. D. Ridgers, J. Salmon, A.-M. Parrish, R. M. Stanley, and A. D. Okely, "Physical activity during school recess: a systematic review," *American Journal of Preventive Medicine*, vol. 43, no. 3, pp. 320–328, 2012.

[11] Center on Educational Policy, *Instructional Time in Elementary Schools: A Closer Look at Changes for Specific Subjects*, Center on Educational Policy, Washington, DC, USA, 2008.

[12] M. T. Mahar, S. K. Murphy, D. A. Rowe, J. Golden, A. T. Shields, and T. D. Raedeke, "Effects of a classroom-based program on physical activity and on-task behavior," *Medicine and Science in Sports and Exercise*, vol. 38, no. 12, pp. 2086–2094, 2006.

[13] T. L. Goh, J. Hannon, C. A. Webster, L. W. Podlog, T. Brusseau, and M. Newton, "Effects of a classroom-based physical activity program on children's physical activity levels," *Journal of Teaching in Physical Education*, vol. 33, no. 4, pp. 558–572, 2014.

[14] J. E. Donnelly, J. L. Greene, C. A. Gibson et al., "Physical Activity Across the Curriculum (PAAC): a randomized controlled trial to promote physical activity and diminish overweight and obesity in elementary school children," *Preventive Medicine*, vol. 49, no. 4, pp. 336–341, 2009.

[15] M. W. Martin, S. Martin, and P. Rosengard, "PE2GO: program evaluation of a physical activity program in elementary schools," *Journal of Physical Activity and Health*, vol. 7, no. 5, pp. 677–684, 2010.

[16] Centers for Disease Control and Prevention, *The Association Between School-Based Physical Activity, Including Physical Education, and Academic Performance*, US Department of Health and Human Services, Atlanta, Ga, USA, 2010.

[17] S. M. Lee, C. R. Burgeson, J. E. Fulton, and C. G. Spain, "Physical education and physical activity: results from the school health policies and programs study 2006," *Journal of School Health*, vol. 77, no. 8, pp. 435–463, 2007.

[18] J. P. Barfield, D. A. Rowe, and T. J. Michael, "Interinstrument consistency of the Yamax Digi-Walker pedometer in elementary school-aged children," *Measurement in Physical Education and Exercise Science*, vol. 8, no. 2, pp. 109–116, 2004.

[19] S. D. Vincent and C. L. Sidman, "Determining measurement error in digital pedometers," *Measurement in Physical Education and Exercise Science*, vol. 7, no. 1, pp. 19–24, 2003.

[20] C. Tudor-Locke, "Taking steps toward increase physical activity, using pedometers to measure and motivate," *Research Digest*, vol. 3, no. 7, pp. 1–8, 2002.

[21] J. Cohen, *Statistical Power Analysis for the Behavioral Sciences*, Lawrence Erlbaum Associates, Hillsdale, NJ, USA, 1998.

[22] J. N. Larson, T. A. Brusseau, B. Chase, A. Heinemann, and J. C. Hannon, "Youth physical activity and enjoyment during semi-structured versus unstructured school recess," *Open Journal of Preventive Medicine*, vol. 4, no. 8, pp. 631–639, 2014.

[23] I. Tran, B. R. Clark, and S. B. Racette, "Physical activity during recess outdoors and indoors among urban public school students, St. Louis, Missouri, 2010-2011," *Preventing Chronic Disease*, vol. 10, Article ID 130135, 2013.

[24] T. A. Brusseau and P. H. Kulinna, "An examination of four traditional physical activity models on children's step counts and MVPA," *Research Quarterly for Exercise and Sport*, vol. 86, pp. 88–93, 2015.

[25] N. D. Ridgers, G. Stratton, and S. J. Fairclough, "Physical activity levels of children during school playtime," *Sports Medicine*, vol. 36, no. 4, pp. 359–371, 2006.

[26] J. R. Best, "Effects of physical activity on children's executive function: contributions of experimental research on aerobic exercise," *Developmental Review*, vol. 30, no. 4, pp. 331–351, 2010.

[27] D. McNaughten and C. Gabbard, "Physical exertion and immediate mental performance of sixth-grade children," *Perceptual and Motor Skills*, vol. 77, part 2, no. 3, pp. 1155–1159, 1993.

[28] B. L. Alderman, T. Benham-Deal, A. Beighle, H. E. Erwin, and R. L. Olson, "Physical education's contribution to daily physical activity among middle school youth," *Pediatric Exercise Science*, vol. 24, no. 4, pp. 634–648, 2012.

[29] D. Dale, C. B. Corbin, and K. S. Dale, "Restricting opportunities to be active during school time: Do children compensate by increasing physical activity levels after school?" *Research Quarterly for Exercise and Sport*, vol. 71, no. 3, pp. 240–248, 2000.

24

Factors Associated with Home Delivery in West Pokot County of Kenya

Jared Otieno Ogolla

Department of Public Health, School of Health Sciences, Mount Kenya University, P.O. Box 2591-30100, Eldoret, Kenya

Correspondence should be addressed to Jared Otieno Ogolla; jotienoogolla@gmail.com

Academic Editor: Gudlavalleti Venkata Murthy

Background. This paper sought to estimate the percentage of women who deliver at home in West Pokot County and establish the factors associated with home delivery in the area. *Design and Methods.* The cross-sectional survey targeted 18,174 households between the months of April and July 2013. Six hundred mothers participated in the study. Association between predictors and the place where the delivery took place was analysed by chi-square test (χ^2) at 95% confidence interval. Factors with P value < 0.05 were considered statistically significant. These factors were entered into multivariate logistic regression model after controlling for confounding to ascertain how each one influenced home delivery. Odds ratio was used to determine the extent of association. *Results.* Based on the mother's most recent births, 200 (33.3%) women delivered in a health facility while 400 (66.7%) delivered at home. Factors associated with home delivering were housewives (OR: 4.5, 95% CI: 2.1–9.5; $P = 0.001$) and low socioeconomic status of 10 km (OR: 0.5, 9.5% CI: 0.3–0.7; $P = 0.001$). *Conclusions.* The findings of this study provide novel information for stakeholders responsible for maternal and child health in West Pokot County.

1. Introduction

Pregnancy and childbirth related complications contribute to a significant number of pregnancy and childbirth related deaths and disabilities in the world especially in developing countries [1]. The major causes of these deaths are prolonged/obstructed labour, complications from unsafe abortion, haemorrhage, malaria during pregnancy, anaemia, and sepsis [1–3]. Notably, most of these deaths and disabilities are preventable if women make good use of the available maternal health services [1]. Despite the Government of Kenya (GoK) and other stakeholders' efforts to curb pregnancy related deaths and disabilities, maternal mortality rates (MMRs) have remained soaring high in country [2].

Safe motherhood initiatives such as the provision of free maternity services are still being underutilised by many women in Kenya especially those in poor, rural, and remote settings of the country [1, 3, 4]. This has led to extremely high rates of MMRs in some parts of Kenya [1, 3]. One such area is West Pokot County. It is estimated that 565 deaths per 100,000 births occur in West Pokot County alone annually [5]. This is a sharp contrast to the reported national rate of 488 deaths per 100,000 live births [3]. However, County MMR is likely to

be an underestimation, considering that there is inadequate community-based maternal mortality data in the area [5].

The high MMR in West Pokot is mainly attributed to obstructed labour, high rate of infibulations (type III), and cephalopelvic disproportion (CPD) due to early marriages [5]. It is estimated that 74% of women in West Pokot County give birth at home with traditional birth attendants (TBAs) attending most of these deliveries [3–5]. Only 10% of these women receive postpartum care within 2 days [1–3, 5]. Since most maternal deaths occur in the first week after birth, this means missed opportunity in terms of recognition and responding to danger signs after delivery.

Safe motherhood interventions are thus crucial in reducing maternal deaths and pregnancy associated morbidity in the County. This paper sought to estimate the proportion of women who deliver at home in West Pokot County and establish the factors associated with home delivery in the area.

2. Material and Methods

2.1. Study Area. West Pokot County is a poor, rural, and marginalized County with poorly developed infrastructure.

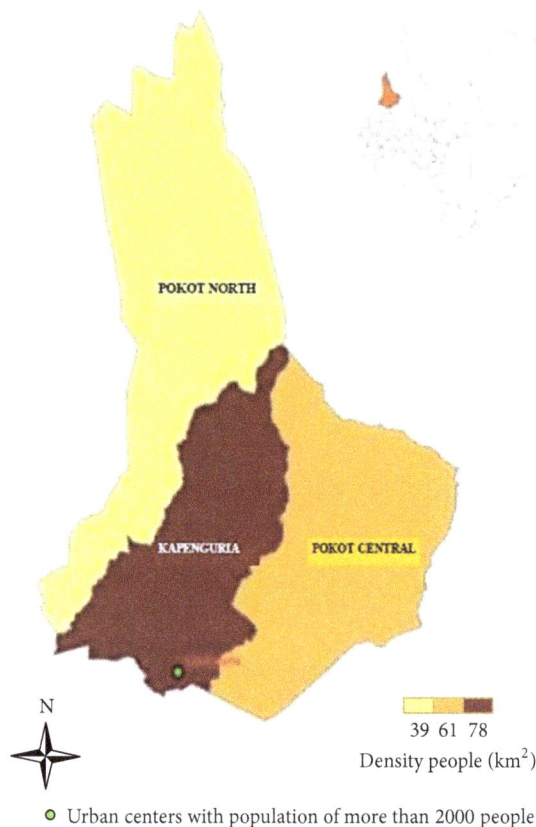

FIGURE 1: A map of West Pokot County.

The female genital mutilation (FGM) rate in the area is about 97%, a figure that is markedly higher than the average national prevalence of 32.2%. The health problems in the County are gross as manifested by the recurrent malaria episodes, ever increasing HIV/AIDS prevalence, and high maternal and neonatal mortality. The combination of harsh climatic condition, cultural practices, difficult terrain, and poor infrastructure has left the County trailing in health and development with devastating consequences on both economic, social, and health statuses of its residents. Figure 1 shows the map of West Pokot County.

2.2. Study Design and Participants. The household survey targeted all the 18,174 households in the study area between the months of April and July 2013. Participants targeted in these households were women of reproductive age who had given birth within six months prior to the study or their immediate family members in case of deceased mothers. Inclusion of underage girls was due to early marriages and pregnancies, which are too rampant in the County, and the fact that early pregnancies also contribute to significant number of pregnancy and childbirth related deaths and disability worldwide [2, 5]. Of the 18,174 targeted households, 56 (8.5%) refused to participate, leaving 18,118 households. Out of the 18,118 households, 1,679 households were located in conflict and banditry areas. These households were inaccessible to the researcher. This left 16,439 households for the survey. One

thousand seven hundred and thirty-five households located in bandit prone areas were inaccessible to the interviewers due to security reasons. Only 600 mothers in the 16,439 households visited met the inclusion criteria.

2.3. Data Collection. Forty-three community health workers with a basic undergraduate degree in community health did data collection. They were trained for two days on data collection procedures and other aspects related to the study. A structured interviewer administered questionnaire was used to collect data. Deliveries that took place in a health facility were verified by GoK approved documents such as birth notification cards, birth certificates, and immunization cards. It was assumed that the birth had taken place at home in cases where the mother or families members of the deceased mother failed to produce any of these documents.

2.4. Data Management and Analysis. The study employed Statistical Package for Social Scientists (SPSS) Software version 20.0 for Windows in data analysis. Association between predictors and the place where the delivery took place was analysed by chi-square test (χ^2) at 95% confidence interval (CI). Factors with P value < 0.05 were considered statistically significant. These factors were entered into multivariate logistic regression model after controlling for confounding to ascertain how each influenced home delivery. Odds ratio (OR) was used to determine the extent of association. Factors analysed included maternal age and education, marital status, occupation, socioeconomic status, distance from the nearest health facility, possession of an insurance cover, and parity. Criteria used in evaluating the socioeconomic status of the mothers are reported elsewhere [6].

2.5. Ethical Consideration. The study obtained ethical approval from Mount Kenya University. It also sought written consent from all the study participants. Ethical issues (including plagiarism, informed consent, misconduct, data fabrication and/or falsification, double publication and/or submission, redundancy, etc.) have been completely observed by the author.

3. Results

3.1. Characteristics of the Respondents. Based on the mother's most recent births, 200 (33.3%) women gave birth in a health facility while 400 (66.7%) delivered at home. Sixty-five percent ($n = 390$) of the respondents were <20 years, 21.7% were 20–35 years ($n = 130$), and 13.3% were above 35 years of age ($n = 80$). In terms of the mothers level of education, 1.3% ($n = 8$) were illiterate, 97.8% were educated ($n = 587$) up to primary level, 0.5% were up to secondary level ($n = 3$), and 0.3% were up to tertiary level ($n = 2$). Most of the women who gave birth at home were either illiterate or had basic education (86.7%). Majority of the women interviewed were single mothers (63.8%; $n = 383$), 114 were married (19%), and 103 were divorced (17.2%). 66.7% of women in the County were found to be giving birth at home. Table 1 shows

TABLE 1: Sociodemographic correlates for choice of place of childbirth.

Variables	Place of delivery				OR	95% CI	P
	Facility		Home				
	N (200)	%	N (400)	%			
Age (in years)							
<20	152	39.0	238	61.0	2.2 ref	1.5–3.2	<0.001
20–35	36	27.7	94	72.3	0.6	0.4–1.0	0.02
>35	12	15.0	68	85.0	0.3	0.1–0.6	<0.001
Level of education							
Illiterate	4	50.0	4	50.0	2.0	0.5–8.2	0.5
Primary	196	33.4	391	66.6	0.5	0.1–2.0	0.5
Secondary	0	0.0	3	100.0	—		
Tertiary	0	0.0	2	100.0	—		
Marital status							
Single	154	40.2	229	59.8	2.5 ref	1.7–3.7	<0.001
Married	33	28.9	81	71.1	0.6	0.4–1.0	0.03
Divorced	13	12.6	90	87.4	0.2	0.1–0.4	<0.001
Occupation							
Housewife	52	70.3	22	29.7	6.0	3.5–10.3	<0.001
Employed	148	28.1	378	71.9	—		
Socioeconomic status (Sh.)							
<5000	72	54.1	61	45.9	3.1 ref	2.1–4.7	<0.001
5000–10000	60	30.6	136	69.4	0.4	0.2–0.6	<0.001
>10000	68	25.1	203	74.9	0.3	0.2–0.5	<0.001
Distance from the nearest health facility (km)							
>10	169	37.1	287	62.9	0.5 ref	0.3–0.7	0.001
<5	21	29.2	51	70.8	0.7	0.4–1.2	0.2
5–10	10	13.9	62	86.1	0.3	0.1–0.6	<0.001
Possession of a medical insurance cover							
No	161	40.7	235	59.3	2.9	1.9–4.3	<0.001
Yes	39	19.1	165	80.9			
Parity							
1	31	68.9	14	31.1	5.1 ref	2.6–9.8	<0.001
2	105	29.9	246	70.1	0.2	0.1–0.4	0.001
>3	64	31.4	140	68.6	0.2	0.1–0.4	0.001

sociodemographic characteristics of the women by place of delivery.

3.2. Bivariate Analyses.
Mothers aged <20 years were twice more likely to give birth at home compared to those aged 20–35 and >35 years (OR, 2.2, 95% CI, 1.5–3.2; $P < 0.001$). Similarly, single mothers were three times likely to deliver at home compared to their married or divorced counterparts (OR, 2.5, 95% CI, 1.7–3.7; $P < 0.001$) while housewives were six times more likely to deliver at home compared to those who were employed (OR, 6.0, 95% CI, 3.5–10.3; $P < 0.001$). Women of low socioeconomic status (<Sh. 5000) were three times more likely to deliver at home compared to those of medium (Sh. 5000–10000) or high (Sh. >10000) socioeconomic status (OR, 3.1, 95% CI, 2.1–4.7, $P < 0.001$). Mothers who had no medical insurance cover were 3 times more likely to deliver at home compared to those who had none (OR, 2.9, 95% CI, 1.9–4.3; $P < 0.001$) while first time

mothers were five times more likely to give birth at home compared to those who had two or more children (OR, 5.1, 95% CI, 2.6–9.8; $P < 0.001$). Level of education was comparable among women who delivered at home and at the facility ($P = 0.5$ and $P = 0.5$, resp.) (Table 1).

3.3. Multivariate Analysis.
Of the factors considered in bivariate analysis, housewives, women of socioeconomic status <Sh. 5000, and those located >10 km to the nearest health facility were factors associated with giving birth at home. Compared to employed mothers, mothers who were housewives were 5 times more likely to deliver at home (OR, 4.5, 95% CI, 2.1–9.5; $P = 0.001$). Mothers whose socioeconomic status was <Sh. 5000 were 4 times more likely to deliver at home compared to mothers who had a higher socioeconomic status (OR, 4.4, 9.5% CI, 2.4–8.1; $P = 0.001$). Those located >10 km to the nearest health facility were once more likely to give birth at home as opposed to 5–10 km (OR,

TABLE 2: Multivariate analysis of predictors of place of delivery.

Variables	Place of delivery				OR	95% CI	P
	Facility		Home				
	N	%	N	%			
Age (in years)							
<20	152	39.0	238	61.0	0.7	0.4–1.3	0.23
Marital status							
Single	154	40.2	229	59.8	1.3	0.6–2.5	0.5
Occupation							
Housewife	52	70.3	22	29.7	4.5	2.1–9.5	0.001
Socioeconomic status (Sh.)							
<5000	72	54.1	61	45.9	4.4	2.4–8.1	0.001
Distance from the nearest health facility (Km)							
>10	169	37.1	287	62.9	0.5 ref	0.3–0.7	0.001
Possession of a medical insurance cover							
No	161	40.7	235	59.3	1.7	0.96–3.0	0.07
Parity							
1	31	68.9	14	31.1	1.5	0.5–4.6	0.51

0.5, 9.5% CI, 0.3–0.7; $P = 0.001$). Mothers who aged <20 (OR, 0.7, 95% CI, 0.4–1.3; $P = 0.23$), single mothers (OR, 1.3, 95% CI, 0.6–2.5; $P = 0.5$), lack of a medical insurance cover (OR, 1.7, 95% CI, 0.96–3.0; $P = 0.07$), and first time mothers (OR, 1.5, 95% CI, 0.5–4.6; $P = 0.51$) were comparable between mothers who gave birth at facility and home (Table 2).

4. Discussion

This study has documented the percentage of women who deliver at home in West Pokot County of Kenya. It found out that 66.7% of women in the County give birth at home. This figure is 6.3% lower than the previously estimated levels of 74% [1, 3, 5]. The increase in the number of women giving birth in the health facility could be because of various safe motherhood interventions instituted by the Government of Kenya and other stakeholders aimed at reducing maternal and child mortality rates in the County. Such interventions include but not limited to provision of free maternity services.

However, maternal deaths rate in West Pokot County is still arguably higher when compared to other similar rural areas in the country [7]. This finding reflects a huge variation in the utilization of maternal health services across the country. It also shows that many women still prefer to give birth at home than in the health facilities. This is not only a trend in Kenya but also in other developing countries [1–3, 5, 8, 9]. Hence, there is a need to implement new and noble interventions that can help improve maternal health in the area. In particular, the interventions should encourage women to deliver in the health facilities. This will help support the existing interventions such as free maternal health care including maternity services [1, 3, 4].

The study also provides an insight into some factors associated with the utilisation of maternity health services in West Pokot County. As the study depicted, most women in the study area are either illiterate or have basic education. A

number of studies conducted in developing world that have linked marital status with home delivery [10, 11]. Being a housewife coupled with poor or no education, harsh climatic conditions, inadequate public utilities including healthcare services, and transport system impacts negatively on women in West Pokot County ability to access maternal services.

Most often, women who are purely housewives have limited or no access to resources and at the same time lack ability to make decision in their marital homes; they are therefore entirely compelled to rely on their mothers' in-law perception of their pregnancy including delivery care needs [12]. Socioeconomic status is another factor that was found to influence women to home delivery. This can be attributed to the unavailability of cash for transport even in a case of free maternal services, which bias decisions towards home deliveries [13]. Lack of income is a known barrier to delivery at health facility [14–19]. This finding is in agreement with a similar finding of a study conducted in rural and marginalised community in Tanzania [20]. However, it contradicts another in Nepal, which showed that economic factors insignificantly influence place of birth [21]. These calls for simple interventions that can help empower women economically in West Pokot. For instance, women in the County should be encouraged to form Women Groups and other Self-Help Groups. Through such forums, they can help them pull resources together and exchange maternal health related information [5].

The study has also shown that distance to the nearest health facility is a factor that determines where delivery will take place, a finding that is in agreement with a similar finding in Nepal [22] and in rural Malawi [23]. Most often, pregnant women consider not seeking maternity services in health facilities located far from their home areas [24]. It is nearly impossible or difficult to do so especially when labor begins at night. Women who make such effort often fail while those with severe complications end up with pregnancy related mortalities or even death. The situation becomes even grimmer when means of transport such as in West Pokot County is poor or unavailable. Intervention such as "waiting homes" near health facilities to accommodate the expectant mothers located far from the nearest health facilities days before delivery day can be helpful in this regard [5].

Although it is carried out in West Pokot County, this study finding may be generalised to other remote and rural parts of the country. However, it suffers from a major limitation in that it solely relied on quantitative techniques. This calls for more studies employing both quantitative and qualitative approaches to corroborate these findings.

5. Conclusions

The findings of this study provide information for stakeholders responsible for maternal and child health in West Pokot County. It identified factors associated with women giving birth at home in West Pokot County. These include housewives, women of low socioeconomic status (<Sh. 5000), and situation of a health facility >10 km. These findings will assist in the formulation of safe motherhood initiatives to forestall the high maternal mortality in West Pokot County.

Significance for Public Health

Pregnancy and childbirth related complications contribute to a significant number of pregnancy and childbirth related deaths and disabilities in the world especially in developing countries. This paper sought to estimate the proportion of women who delivers at home in West Pokot County and establish the factors associated with home delivery in the area.

Conflict of Interests

The author declares that there is no conflict of interests.

Acknowledgments

The author would like to thank Mr. Joash O. Ogada and Mrs. Margaret A. Ogolla for funding the study. Appreciation also goes to the West Pokot County Health Management Team for their invaluable support during the study. Finally, the authors thank local administration, all research assistants, and mothers who participated in the study.

References

[1] NCAPD, "Maternal deaths on the rise in Kenya: a call to save women's lives," *Policy Brief*, vol. 9, pp. 1–9, 2010.

[2] UNFPA, *Continental Review of Progress towards the Implementation of the Maputo Plan of Action (MPOA) on Sexual and Reproductive Health and Rights (SRHR)*, UNFPA/African Union Commission Liaison Office, Addis Ababa, Ethiopia, 2010.

[3] Kenya National Bureau of Statistics and ICF Macro, *Kenya Demographic and Health Survey 2008-09*, Kenya National Bureau of Statistics and ICF Macro, Calverton, Md, USA, 2010.

[4] Government of Kenya, *Kenya Vision 2030: A Globally Competitive and Prosperous Kenya*, Ministry of Planning and National Development and the National Economic and Social Council (NESC), Nairobi, Kenya, 2007.

[5] B. Kavita, W. Rebekah, D. Rozalin et al., *Partnership for Maternal and Neonatal Health—West Pokot District Child Survival and Health Program*, Doctors of the World USA, 2007.

[6] D. Filmer and L. H. Pritchett, "Estimating wealth effects without expenditure data—or tears: an application to educational enrollments in states of India," *Demography*, vol. 38, no. 1, pp. 115–132, 2001.

[7] D. Hodgkin, "Household characteristics affecting where mothers deliver in rural Kenya," *Health Economics*, vol. 5, no. 4, pp. 333–340, 1996.

[8] A. N. Hazemba and S. Siziya, "Choice of place for childbirth: prevalence and correlates of utilization of health facilities in Chongwe district, Zambia," *Medical Journal of Zambia*, vol. 35, pp. 53–57, 2008.

[9] K. Cotter, M. Hawken, and M. Temmerman, "Low use of skilled attendant's delivery services in rural Kenya," *Journal of Health, Population and Nutrition*, vol. 24, no. 4, pp. 467–471, 2006.

[10] P. Y. Katung, "Socio-economic factors responsible for poor utilisation of the primary health care services in a rural community in Nigeria," *Nigerian Journal of Medicine*, vol. 10, no. 1, pp. 28–29, 2001.

[11] S. Yanagisawa, S. Oum, and S. Wakai, "Determinants of skilled birth attendance in rural Cambodia," *Tropical Medicine and International Health*, vol. 11, no. 2, pp. 238–251, 2006.

[12] B. Simkhada, M. A. Porter, and E. R. van Teijlingen, "The role of mothers-in-law in antenatal care decision-making in Nepal: a qualitative study," *BMC Pregnancy and Childbirth*, vol. 10, article 34, 2010.

[13] E. A. Envuladu, H. A. Agbo, S. Lassa, J. H. Kigbu, and A. I. Zoakah, "Factors determining the choice of a place of delivery among pregnant women in Russia village of Jos North, Nigeria: achieving the MDGs 4 and 5," *International Journal of Medicine and Biomedical Research*, vol. 2, no. 1, pp. 23–27, 2013.

[14] B. Amooti-Kaguna and F. Nuwaha, "Factors influencing choice of delivery sites in Rakai district of Uganda," *Social Science and Medicine*, vol. 50, no. 2, pp. 203–213, 2000.

[15] L. D'Ambruoso, M. Abbey, and J. Hussein, "Please understand when I cry out in pain: women's accounts of maternity services during labour and delivery in Ghana," *BMC Public Health*, vol. 5, article 140, 2005.

[16] National Bureau of Statistics & Macro International, *Tanzania Demographic Health Survey Key Findings*, National Bureau of Statistics, Dares Salaam, Tanzania, ORC Macro, Calverton, Md, USA, 2005.

[17] J. Borghi, T. Ensor, A. Somanathan, C. Lissner, and A. Mills, "Mobilising financial resources for maternal health," *The Lancet*, vol. 368, no. 9545, pp. 1457–1465, 2006.

[18] M. Koblinsky, Z. Matthews, J. Hussein et al., "Going to scale with professional skilled care," *The Lancet*, vol. 368, no. 9544, pp. 1377–1386, 2006.

[19] W. R. Brieger, K. J. Luchok, E. Eng, and J. A. Earp, "Use of maternity services by pregnant women in a small Nigerian community," *Health Care for Women International*, vol. 15, no. 2, pp. 101–110, 1994.

[20] M. Mrisho, J. A. Schellenberg, A. K. Mushi et al., "Factors affecting home delivery in rural Tanzania," *Tropical Medicine & International Health*, vol. 12, no. 7, pp. 862–872, 2007.

[21] A. Bolam, D. S. Manandhar, P. Shrestha, M. Ellis, K. Malla, and A. M. Costello, "Factors affecting home delivery in the

Kathmandu Valley, Nepal," *Health Policy and Planning*, vol. 13, no. 2, pp. 152–158, 1998.

[22] S. K. Shrestha, B. Banu, K. Khanom et al., "Changing trends on the place of delivery: why do Nepali women give birth at home?" *Reproductive Health*, vol. 9, no. 1, article 25, 2012.

[23] T. Kulmala, *Maternal health and pregnancy outcomes in rural Malawi [Ph.D. dissertation]*, Medical School, University of Tempere, Acta Electronica Universitatis Temperenasis 76, 2000.

[24] S. Thaddeus and D. Maine, "Too far to walk: maternal mortality in context," *Social Science and Medicine*, vol. 38, no. 8, pp. 1091–1110, 1994.

25

Improving Adult ART Clinic Patient Waiting Time by Implementing an Appointment System at Gondar University Teaching Hospital, Northwest Ethiopia

Asmamaw Atnafu,[1,2] Damen Haile Mariam,[3] Rex Wong,[4] Taddese Awoke,[1] and Yitayih Wondimeneh[1]

[1]*School of Biomedical and Laboratory Science, College of Medicine and Health Sciences, University of Gondar, Gondar, Ethiopia*
[2]*Graduate School of Public Health, Seoul National University, Seoul, Republic of Korea*
[3]*School of Public Health, College of Health Sciences, Addis Ababa University, Addis Ababa, Ethiopia*
[4]*School of Public Health, Yale University, New Haven, CT, USA*

Correspondence should be addressed to Asmamaw Atnafu; asme2002@gmail.com

Academic Editor: Julio Diaz

Background. Long waiting time has been among the major factors that affect patient satisfaction and health service delivery. The aim of this study was to determine the median waiting time at the Anti-Retroviral Therapy (ART) Clinic before and after introduction of an intervention of the systematic appointment system. *Methods.* Patient waiting time was measured before and after the introduction of an intervention; target population of the study was all adult HIV patients/clients who have visited the outpatient ART Clinic in the study period. 173 patients were included before and after the intervention. Systematic patient appointment system and health education to patients on appointment system were provided as an intervention. The study period was from October 2011 to the end of January 2012. Data were analyzed using SPSS software version 17.0. Independent sample *t*-test at 95% confidence interval and 5% significance level was used to determine the significance of median waiting time difference between pre- and postintervention periods. *Results and Conclusion.* The total median waiting time was reduced from 274.8 minutes (IQR 180.6 minutes and 453.6 minutes) before intervention to 165 minutes (IQR 120 minutes and 377.4 minutes) after intervention (40% decrease, $p = 0.02$). Overall, the study showed that the introduction of the new appointment system significantly reduces patient waiting time.

1. Introduction

Long waiting time has been among the major factors that affect patient satisfaction and health service delivery, efficiency, quality, transparency, and accountability [1–4]. In many health care facilities in Ethiopia as well as in other countries, waiting time could exceed two hours [5–7]. In 2001, a study conducted by the Health Care Financing Secretariat of the Federal Ministry of Health showed the average outpatient clinic waiting time in health facilities in Ethiopia as being 6.4 hours [8]. Another study at Jimma Hospital in 1998 has indicated an average of 4.5 hours' waiting time [5].

Long waiting time is among the several factors that can negatively impact the outcome of ART treatment [6, 8]. It was regarded as a barrier for accessing ART services and the cause of high dropout rate [7]. In Ethiopia, as well as in many sub-Saharan African countries, Human Immunodeficiency Virus/Acquired Immune Deficiency Syndrome (HIV/AIDS) remains the greatest challenge to the health care system [9]. In response, the ART coverage of Ethiopia has increased from 46% to 55% from 2008 to 2010 [9, 10]. And the number of people receiving ART has continued to increase since 2005.

Shortage of medical staff and medical and laboratory supplies and lack of systematic appointment system are among the factors that contribute to long waiting time [6]. In a poor setting with heavy workload, a doctor may examine 40–60 patients per day compared to the very low number of patients a day by American physicians; therefore, it leads to lack of time specific appointment and causes long waiting time [11]. Moreover, the majority of cases are rooted in the inefficiency of the ART Clinic management system, which can be manifested in lack of scheduling, inefficient registration and triage procedures, misfiling of cards, delay in consultations, and simultaneous break times [6, 12]. Various interventions targeting these root causes have shown successes in reducing waiting time, including addition or reallocation of human resources, changing work processes, and scheduling follow-up visits for less busy times [6, 13]. However, there are no intervention studies conducted in Ethiopia to observe the various factors that affect waiting time at facilities providing ART services.

Therefore, this project was undertaken in an effort to apply quality improvement technique to address the long waiting service time at the ART Clinic of the Gondar University Hospital. Hence, the aim of this project was to improve patient waiting time by strengthening scheduling system and providing continuing health education. The hospital senior management team, the head of the ART Clinic, the nursing director, and some front line health professionals, including nurses, health officers, and nursing assistants working at the ART Clinic, were engaged in planning, implementing, and evaluating stages of the new patient schedule management system for the ART Clinic.

2. Methods

2.1. Setting and Preintervention. Gondar University Hospital, teaching referral hospital in northwest Ethiopia, has 400 beds and 14 outpatient clinics. It serves approximately 110,000 outpatients every year. The ART Clinic provides ART care and HIV counseling and testing. During the study period, the clinic had 4 physicians, 1 health officer, 6 nurses, 4 medical laboratory technologists, 3 pharmacists, 2 case managers, 2 data clerks, and 3 medical record workers. Over 9,565 adults and pediatric cases have been enrolled in HIV care, with 6,022 newly initiated and 3,899 already in the course of ART (3,543 adults and 356 children). Patients usually visited the clinic every three months.

During the preintervention period, all ART patients used to be informed to return on a specific day for follow-up. Neither an upper limit on the number of patients to be scheduled nor proper documentation of appointment existed. Due to lack of a coordinated appointment system, the number of patients scheduled on any given appointment day frequently exceeds the capacity of the ART Clinic which, as a result, causes long waiting time. Additionally, in the absence of calendar or appointment book, patients frequently were told to return during holiday and weekends by mistake, resulting in an unnecessary long waiting time and confusion.

2.2. Study Design and Data Collection. This study utilized pre- and postintervention design to measure the impact of the appointment system on patient waiting time for services at the ART Clinic.

Time motion collection formats were designed by the team, to collect basic demographic information: arriving and departing time for each service point and the reason for the visit. Five data collectors and one supervisor were recruited to conduct the time collection. To ensure quality, one-day training on the data collection procedure, the objectives of the assessment, ethical issues, techniques, supervision, and the use of the time motion form were given by the principal investigator. The time motion collection forms were checked for completeness and accuracy by data collectors and supervisors. Waiting time for all segmented services, total waiting from arrival at ART Clinic to finish all services, and the percentages of preintervention and postintervention patients wrongly scheduled on weekends and holidays were also collected.

Data entry errors were minimized by performing double checking entry into the computer by two separate data clerks. Ethical clearance was obtained from Addis Ababa University, College of Health Sciences, and School of Public Health as the study was conducted as part of master's thesis for the first author. Respondents were briefed about the confidentiality of their responses and the importance of providing true and accurate information. Verbal consent was obtained from all study participants prior to data collection.

2.3. Sample Size Determination. Both pre- and postintervention samples were collected using a systematic sampling method. By using mean difference formula, 173 patients before and after intervention were included. Every 6th patient at the adult ART outpatient clinic was selected over a period of 2 weeks. The preintervention sample was collected in October 1–15, 2011; the intervention period was from November 2011 to January 20, 2012, and patients with appointment date starting from January 21, 2012, comprised the postintervention sample. Only HIV positive patients who were 18 years old or older were included in this study, with the exclusion of seriously ill patients who had compromised mental capacity and pediatric patients.

2.4. Intervention. In October 2011, a project team was formed with members from senior management team and ART Clinic managers and supervisors. Focus interviews were conducted with five health professionals to identify the root causes. The team developed the implementation strategy and decided to establish a centralized appointment system for ART follow-up patients and agreed that a daily quota should be set to limit and regulate the ART Clinic patient volume.

The new patient appointment system included setting a daily patient limit for each clinical day, centralizing the appointment process, using an appointment book, and educating patient on adherence to appointment. There were 3,543 adult patients actively on ART. The maximum number of patients per day was calculated by dividing the total number of patients by the number of working days in a 3-month cycle (3543/66 = 54) and adding the estimated number of new patients per day (16) giving a total of 70 patients per day.

A centralized appointment system was created in which patients, after completing their clinical visit, go to the central appointment room to make an appointment. Health care providers were no longer allowed to give appointments individually. Appointments were given by a scheduler and were recorded in an appointment calendar. Weekends and holidays were crossed off from the calendar and no appointment would be given on those days. Patients were given appointment cards and reminded to adhere to their scheduled appointments. The importance of adhering to the appointment schedule was also incorporated into the health education sessions given by nursing staff and case managers.

2.5. Data Analysis and Statistical Consideration. The preintervention and postintervention median waiting service times were analyzed using independent sample t-tests and the preintervention and postintervention percentages of patients wrongly scheduled on weekends and holidays were compared using chi-square test. Both tests used confidence level at <0.05 to determine the statistical significance. All data analyses were performed using SPSS version 17.0 (SPSS, Inc., Chicago) and log transformation was used because the data were skewed.

2.6. Operational Definitions. Operational definitions are as follows:

Total waiting time: the time spent to get all the services and the time spent with the service provider.

OPD (Out Patient Department) services waiting time: the time spent for those services which are only examinations at OPD (not including other services like laboratory and pharmacy and the time spent in OPD).

Pharmacy waiting time: the time spent for pharmacy services.

Laboratory waiting time: the time spent for the laboratory services.

3. Results

Both preintervention and postintervention samples had 173 patients each. The preintervention and postintervention samples did not differ significantly by sex, age, visit type, and type of services received (Table 1).

There was a significant decrease in waiting time. The median waiting time was reduced from 274.8 minutes (IQR 180.6 minutes and 453.6 minutes) before intervention to 2.75 hours (IQR 120 minutes and 377.4 minutes) after intervention (40% decrease, $p = 0.02$).

Two services showed significant decrease in waiting time; the card retrieval time decreased from 60 minutes before intervention to 40 minutes after intervention (33% decrease, $p = 0.001$). The medication refill time was reduced from 60 minutes before intervention to 20 minutes after intervention (67% decrease, $p = 0.04$).

Two other services also showed decrease in waiting time, although these were not statistically significant. Waiting time for pharmacy services decreased from 55 minutes before intervention to 38 minutes after intervention (30% decrease, $p = 0.942$), while that for laboratory services decreased

TABLE 1: Patient sample characteristics (preintervention and postintervention).

Sample size (N = 173)	Preintervention N (%)	Postintervention N (%)
Age (mean ± SD)	36.2 ± 10.3	37.6 ± 9.4
Sex		
Male	62 (35.8%)	70 (40%)
Female	111 (64.2%)	103 (60%)
Visit types		
New	19 (11%)	26 (15%)
Repeat	154 (89%)	147 (85%)
Coming for specific services		
OPD	22 (12.7%)	15 (8.7%)
Pharmacy	88 (50.9%)	92 (53.2%)
Laboratory	19 (11%)	31 (19.7%)
Pharmacy and laboratory	27 (15.6)	27 (15.6%)
OPD, laboratory, and pharmacy	11 (6.4%)	6 (3.5%)

Key. OPD: Out Patient Department; N = total sample size of the study.

from 315 minutes before intervention to 285 minutes after intervention (10% decrease, $p = 0.534$).

The median waiting time for health education increased from 15 minutes before intervention to 20 minutes after intervention (32% increase, $p < 0.001$, Table 2).

There was a significant decrease in the percentage of patients wrongly scheduled on weekends and holidays. Wrong scheduling decreased from 4.4% before intervention to 0.1% after intervention ($p < 0.000$, Table 2).

4. Discussion

The result of the study showed that our intervention has reduced the overall patient waiting time at the ART Clinic by 40% from 274.8 minutes to 165 minutes ($p = 0.02$). It has also significantly reduced the wrong scheduling error by 4.3%. Two services at the ART Clinic (card retrieval and medical refill) particularly contributed to the overall reduced waiting time: The median time for card retrieval decreased from 60 to 40 minutes ($p = 0.001$) and that for medication refill decreased from 60 minutes to 20 minutes ($p = 0.04$). In line with this, different studies have shown reduction of waiting time after introduction of simple intervention, community health center in East Bronx, NY (91.9 minutes to 78.3 minutes), and at the Specialist Hospital, Bauchi, Nigeria (6.48 h–4.35 h). On the other hand, the median total waiting time found in this study was lower than the study done in Ethiopia in 2001 (6 hrs). This difference might be due to the fact that the focus of the present study was only on one special clinic of the hospital. The increase in time for patient health education might be due to additional contents of the health education and the health educator may be aware of the study.

Despite the significant reduction in waiting time for services, this study has its own limitations: the appointment system was limited to only giving appointment dates to

TABLE 2: Preintervention and postintervention waiting time and schedule error comparison.

Waiting service time (minutes)	Preintervention		Postintervention		Change	p value
	Median	IQR (25th and 75th)	Median	IQR (25th and 75th)		
Card retrieval	60	45 and 84.6	40	25 and 60	−33%	0.001*
Pharmacy	55.2	30 and 60	38	30 and 50	−30%	0.942
Refilling	60	30 and 60	20	15 and 30	−67%	0.04*
Laboratory	315	212 and 570	285	240 and 480	−10%	0.534
Health education	15	15 and 15	20	15 and 25	+32%	0.000*
Overall waiting service time	274.8	180.6 and 453.6	165	120 and 377	−40%	0.02*
Schedule error	N	%	N	%	Change	p value
Correct appointment	1634	95.6%	1714	99.9%	—	
Wrong appointment	76	4.4%	2	0.1%	−4.3%	<0.000*

*Significant at p = 0.05.
*IQR: interquartile range at the 25th and 75th percentile.

patients without specific time. It was only the first phase of the new appointment system. Although reduction in waiting time was observed, its full impact has not been achieved as it only addressed a small portion of a complex issue. Long waiting time could be due to a combination of factors and this study was only focused on the appointment system. In addition to the above limitation as time is a variable which is not normal, we used log transformation to make it normal. However, nonparametric alternatives should have been used. Finally, the authors believed that the new appointment system reduced the patient waiting time. However, we recommended that it would be better to conduct further studies by using control groups.

5. Conclusion

Our study has shown that the introduction of the new appointment system significantly reduces patient waiting time at the ART Clinic. The intervention was inexpensive and effective. Long term follow-up is needed to assess the sustainability of the intervention. Quality improvement projects of this approach should be encouraged to be applied in other areas of hospital management in Ethiopia to enhance the quality of health care services.

Conflict of Interests

All authors declare that they have no competing financial or any other interest in relation to the work.

Authors' Contribution

Asmamaw Atnafu conceived the study, undertook statistical analysis, and drafted the paper. Damen Haile Mariam, Rex Wong, Taddese Awoke, and Yitayih Wondimeneh initiated the study and made major contributions to the study design, data collection, and statistical analysis. All authors contributed to the writing of the paper and approved its submitted version.

Acknowledgments

The authors appreciate the management of Gondar University Hospital and the health workers and patients in the ART Clinic that were involved in the survey. They would also like to extend their thanks to Dr. Jeph Herin, Professor Elizabeth Bradley, Zahirah McNatt, and Ato Dawit Tatek, for their inspiration and technical support in many ways.

References

[1] O. Lowe, *An Assessment of Patient Waiting Times at Clinics in Tygerberg, Western District in Cape Town, Metropolitan*, Public Health Program, Faculty of Community Health Sciences, University of the Western Cape, Western Cape, South Africa, 2000.

[2] X.-M. Huang, "Patient attitude towards waiting in an outpatient clinic and its applications," *Health Services Management Research*, vol. 7, no. 1, pp. 2–8, 1994.

[3] P. Lynam, "COPE: helping to improve the quality of family planning services in Africa," *QA Brief*, vol. 2, no. 1, pp. 7–8, 1993.

[4] S. Kuguoglu, F. E. Aslan, and G. Icli, "Are patients in Western Turkey contented with healthcare services? A quality assessment study," *Journal of Nursing Care Quality*, vol. 21, no. 4, pp. 366–371, 2006.

[5] A. Addissie, C. Jira, and F. Bekele, "Patient waiting and service time in the outpatient department of Jimma hospital," *Ethiopian Journal of Health Sciences*, vol. 8, no. 1, pp. 15–21, 1998.

[6] H. Mahomed and M. O. Bachmann, "Block appointments in an overloaded South African health centre: quantitative and qualitative evaluation," *International Journal of Health Care Quality Assurance*, vol. 11, no. 4, pp. 123–126, 1998.

[7] M. O. Bachmann and P. Barron, "Why wait so long for child care? An analysis of waits, queues and work in a South African urban health centre," *Tropical Doctor*, vol. 27, no. 1, pp. 34–38, 1997.

[8] Federal Ministry of Health, *Estimating Willingness to Pay for Health Care in Ethiopia: Research Results and Analysis*, edited by: HCF Secretariat, Federal Ministry of Health, Addis Ababa, Ethiopia, 2001.

[9] HIV/AIDS Prevention and Control Office, *Scaling up in Ethiopia Success and Challenge*, HIV/AIDS Prevention and Control Office, Addis Ababa, Ethiopia, 2009.

[10] Federal HIV/AIDS Prevention and Control Office (HAPCO), *Reports on Progress towards Implementation of the UN Declaration of Commitment on HIV/AIDS*, edited by: Federal HIV/AIDS Prevention and Control Office (HAPCO), 2010.

[11] I. O. Ajayi, "Patients' waiting time at an outpatient clinic in Nigeria—can it be put to better use?" *Patient Education and Counseling*, vol. 47, no. 2, pp. 121–126, 2002.

[12] R. Colebunders, T. Bukenya, N. Pakker et al., "Assessment of the patient flow at the infectious diseases institute out-patient clinic, Kampala, Uganda," *AIDS Care*, vol. 19, no. 2, pp. 149–151, 2007.

[13] D. Andrew, A. Racine, and G. Davidson, "Peadiatric clinic waiting time," *Archives of Pediatrics and Adolescent Medicine*, vol. 156, pp. 1203–1220, 2002.

26

Infection and Foot Care in Diabetics Seeking Treatment in a Tertiary Care Hospital, Bhubaneswar, Odisha State, India

Sonali Kar,[1] Shalini Ray,[2] and Dayanidhi Meher[3]

[1]Department of Community Medicine, Kalinga Institute of Medical Sciences, KIIT University, Patia, Bhubaneswar 751024, India
[2]Kalinga Institute of Medical Sciences, KIIT University, Patia, Bhubaneswar 751024, India
[3]Department of Medicine, Kalinga Institute of Medical Sciences, KIIT University, Patia, Bhubaneswar 751024, India

Correspondence should be addressed to Sonali Kar; sonsam72@yahoo.co.uk

Academic Editor: Gudlavalleti Venkata Murthy

Diabetes mellitus is a major public health problem that can cause a number of serious complications. Foot ulceration is one of its most common complications. Poor foot care knowledge and practices are important risk factors for foot problems among diabetics. The present study was undertaken in the diabetes outpatient department of a tertiary care hospital to assess the practices regarding foot care in diabetes, find out the determinants of foot ulcer in diabetics, and offer suggestions to improve care. After informed consent, a total of 124 diabetics were interviewed to collect all relevant information. The diabetic foot care practice responses were converted into scores and for the sake of analysis were inferred as poor (0–5), fair (6-7), and good (>7) practices. Of the study population, 68.5% (85/124) consisted of men. The disease was diagnosed within the last 5 years for 66% (81/124) of the study participants. Of the study subjects, 83% (103/124) were on oral hypoglycemic agents (OHAs), 15.3% (19) on insulin, and 2 on diet control only. Among them about 18.5% had a history of foot ulcer. 37.9% reported using special slippers, 12% diabetics used slippers indoors, and 66.9% used slippers while using toilet. Of the study subjects, 67.8% said that feet should be inspected daily. 27.4% said they regularly applied oil/moisturizer on their feet. There is a need on part of the primary or secondary physician and an active participation of the patient to receive education about foot care as well as awareness regarding risk factors, recognition, clinical evaluation, and thus prevention of the complications of diabetes.

1. Introduction

Diabetes mellitus (DM) is a major public health problem depicting a rising prevalence worldwide. Currently, there are an estimated 366 million people affected with diabetes mellitus globally. India is estimated to have 61.3 million diabetics, which is projected to cross 100 million by the year 2030 [1]. Diabetes mellitus is a multifaceted disease and foot ulceration is one of its most common complications. Foot ulcers can cause severe disability and hospitalization to patients and considerable economic burden to families and health systems [1, 2]. Infection occurring in about half of the diabetic foot ulcers is a further complication. Of all the complications of diabetes, those that occur in the foot are considered the most preventable [3]. Poor knowledge of foot care and poor foot care practices were identified as important risk factors for foot problems in diabetes. Evidence suggests that consistent patient education with prophylactic foot care for those judged to be at high risk may reduce foot ulceration and amputations.

State of Odisha in India has a remarkable prevalence of diabetes with urban prevalence of 15.7% [4]. The capital of the state, that is, Bhubaneswar, has four tertiary care hospitals, with one being government and the remaining three private. Kalinga Institute of Medical Sciences (KIMS) is a state-of-the-art private center which harbors a medical college along with facilities for super specialist care. It has an actively functional diabetic clinic with a trained diabetologist. There is a dearth of studies in Odisha, which assessed the diabetic foot care practice of patients, especially in tertiary care setting. With this background the current study was planned in the Diabetes OPD of tertiary care hospital KIMS.

2. Methodology

The study was a hospital based study conducted as a part of a bigger study on skin infections wherein diabetic foot care assessment was undertaken among the attendees of the diabetes OPD of KIMS (conducted in October–December 2014, i.e., one quarter of a year). As specified the assessment aimed at knowing the current foot care practices among the diabetics attending the clinic and through a detailed questionnaire also finds out the determinants of foot ulcer in this population. Ethical clearance was sought from the Institutional Ethics and Research Committee to undertake the study.

The inclusion criteria were set as known cases of type 2 diabetes aged 30 years and above, diagnosed with the disease since at least one-year duration and visiting the diabetic outpatient clinic. Those with cognitive impairment and disability that could affect the functions of the nervous system affect independent self-care behavior, and those who had amputations of the lower limbs [4] and not willing to participate were excluded from the study. All such eligible patients were taken as the study subjects after due informed consent till the desired sample size was achieved. Assuming that 50% of the diabetics had reasonable knowledge about various factors associated with the disease and that we require a precision of 10%, the sample size is calculated as

$$N = \frac{4pq}{d^2} = \frac{(4 * 0.5 * 0.5)}{(0.1 * 0.1)} = 100. \tag{1}$$

Considering 10% as nonresponse rate, total study subjects interviewed were 124.

A predesigned pretested semistructured questionnaire certified by the diabetologist at KIMS and translated in local languages like Oriya and Hindi was used, which consisted of sections pertaining to socioeconomic details, awareness regarding diabetes, treatment modalities and compliance, practice of self-care of feet, and feet examination details. Survey instrument regarding diabetic foot care practices was modified and adapted from questionnaire used in previous studies [4–8].

The operational definition of foot ulcer for this study was taken as "a breakdown in the skin below the ankle that may extend to involve the subcutaneous tissue or even to the level of muscle or bone which is non-healing or poorly healing" [9, 10].

The diabetic foot care practice responses were converted into scores and for the sake of analysis were inferred as poor (0–5), fair (6-7), and good (>7) practices. Association between poor diabetic foot care practices, knowledge and health seeking behavior, and history of foot ulcer was explored. Patients were asked if they were ever counseled by doctor regarding footcare and use of educational charts for the same by the health provider was also explored. Data was collated and subsequently analyzed using Epi info 7.

3. Results

Table 1 depicts the mean age of the study participants was 60.6 ± 9.13 years, with nearly 58% of them having a higher secondary level education and above. Of the study population, 68.5% consisted of male participants, hinting at a male

TABLE 1: Sociodemographic profile of the respondent diabetics ($n = 124$).

Parameters	Number	Percentage/mean ± sd
Age in years	124	60.6 ± 9.13
Gender		
Male	85	68.5
Female	39	31.4
Education		
Illiterate	07	5.6
Primary	43	34.6
Secondary	2	1.6
Higher secondary	54	43.5
Graduate and above	18	14.5
Occupation		
Unemployed	2	1.6
Unskilled	13	10.4
Semiskilled and skilled	35	28.2
Clerical, shop owner, and farmer	12	9.6
Semiprofessional	12	9.6
Housewife	22	17.7 (56.4% of female subjects)
Retired	28	22.5

TABLE 2: Details of disease and treatment among study subjects.

Demographic details	Categories	Number ($n = 124$)	Percentage
Duration of illness (diabetes)	<5 years	82	66.1
	>5 years	42	33.8
Age at diagnosis	<50 years	84	67.7
	>50 years	40	32.2
Treatment	Diet control	2	1.6
	Drugs	103	83
	Insulin	19	15.3
Treatment regularity	Regular	90	72.5
	Irregular	34	27.4
Foot ulcer (past/present)	Yes	23	18.5
	No	101	81.4
Physical activity/exercise	Yes	52	41.9
	No	72	58.1

predominance of the disease, though the underreporting among females or hesitance to seek health care on their behalf cannot be ruled out. Of the study participants, 5.6% had not received any formal education. Housewives accounted for 56.4% (22/39) of the female study participants, unskilled workers 10.4%, and farmers, shop owners, and clerical job holders 9.6% of study participants.

Table 2 shows that the disease was diagnosed within the last five years for 66% of study population. Of the study

TABLE 3: Possible determinants of foot ulcer in diabetics.

Determinants of foot care in diabetics	Hx of foot ulcer/current ulcer	No foot ulcer	Odds ratio (95% CI)
Duration of diabetes			
<5 years	12	70	0.48 (0.19–1.21)
>5 years	11	31	
Treatment compliance			
Yes	8	82	0.12* (0.04–0.33)
No	15	19	
Foot care practice			
Poor (0–5)	19	58	
Fair and above (6–10)	04	43	3.52* (1.11–11.1)
Counseling on foot care			
Received	9	76	0.21* (0.08–0.54)
Not received	14	25	

*Significant odds ratio.

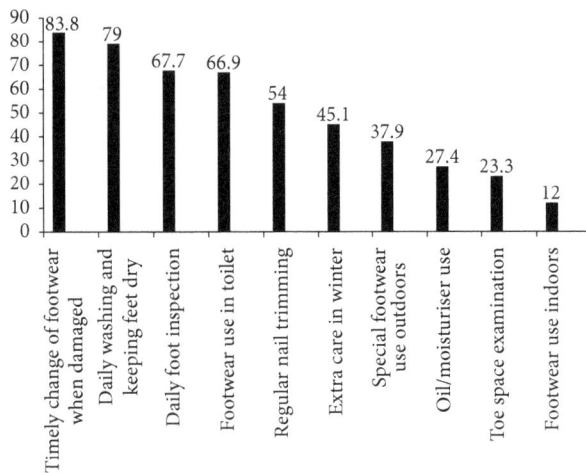

FIGURE 1: Foot care practices among study subjects.

subjects, 83% (103/124) were on oral hypoglycemic agents (OHAs), 15.3% (19) were on insulin, only 41.9% of the study subjects were involved in regular exercise or physical activity, and 72.5% of the diabetics were having good treatment compliance. Among the study subjects 18.5% (23/124) had a history/current foot ulcer.

Figure 1 shows that, out of the total study population, only 37.9% reported using special slippers (extra cushioned, thick soled) outdoors, and only 12% diabetics used footwear indoors though 66.9% used slippers while using toilet. Of the study subjects, 67.7% said that feet should be inspected daily. 27.4% said they regularly applied oil/moisturizer on their feet. Among them, 83.8% reported change of footwear when damaged or ill-fitted and 45.1% reported taking extra care in winter. 54% and 23.3% of subjects reported regular nail trimming and toe space examination regularly, respectively. However 79% of the subjects reported daily washing and drying of feet.

After cumulative scoring, 61.6%, 32%, and only 5.6% of the patients had a poor, fair, and good diabetic foot care practice.

Table 3 shows that poor foot care practice (OR 3.52, 95% CI 1.11–11.1), treatment noncompliance (OR 0.12, 95% CI 0.04–0.33), and absence of counseling regarding foot care (OR 0.21, 95% CI 0.08–0.54) in diabetes were significantly associated with occurrence of foot ulcer in diabetics.

4. Discussion and Conclusion

The important findings of the study are that the majority of the participants were males (68.5%). This could be attributed to the fact that perhaps males have a comparatively better health seeking behavior as compared to females. Nearly 58% participants were with higher secondary level education and above and this could be explained as the study was undertaken in a tertiary care centre in a city. Nearly 18.5% of the study subjects reported having foot ulcer. 67.7% reported daily foot inspection and 37.9% reported using special slippers outdoors. However, only 12% of the participants used slippers indoors which could be because of cultural practices. The deficiency in foot care practices in the present study is comparable to similar studies in India and other developing countries where daily inspection of the feet is reported by less than 70% and special care in winters is taken by less than 50% of patients [4–6]. In our study, absence of counseling and poor foot care practices were significant determinants of presence of foot ulcer

Regular blood glucose monitoring and compliance to diet and life-style advice were found to be comparatively better in the present study. This is in line with an earlier finding that foot care and health education were least suggested by doctors [11]. This suggests a tip of the iceberg as the study is being undertaken in a city based tertiary care center and now India has become the largest diabetic load country in the world where nearly 70% of the population are from the rural background.

Findings can be used to guide a health education program on foot care for diabetics. Emphasis should be laid on such deficient areas by health education and misconceptions should be cleared. This study has few limitations. This is a hospital based study, the results of which do not reflect the awareness and practices in the community. There is a need on part of the doctor and an active participation of the patient to receive education about foot care as well as awareness regarding risk factor recognition, clinical evaluation, and prevention of complications of diabetes.

Conflict of Interests

The authors declare that there is no conflict of interests regarding the publication of this paper.

References

[1] World Health Organization, *Diabetes Fact Sheet N0312*, World Health Organization, Geneva, Switzerland, 2009.

[2] F. Crawford, M. Inkster, J. Kleijnen, and T. Fahey, "Predicting foot ulcers in patients with diabetes: a systematic review and meta-analysis," *QJM*, vol. 100, no. 2, pp. 65–86, 2007.

[3] V. Viswanathan, R. Shobhana, C. Snehalatha, R. Seena, and A. Ramachandran, "Need for education on footcare in diabetic patients in India," *Journal of Association of Physicians of India*, vol. 47, no. 11, pp. 1083–1085, 1999.

[4] G. Hanu, P. S. Rakesh, K. Manjunath et al., "Foot care knowledge and practices and the prevalence of peripheral neuropathy among people with diabetes attending a secondary care rural hospital in southern India," *Journal of Family Medicine and Primary Care*, vol. 2, no. 1, pp. 27–32, 2013.

[5] S. Hasnain and N. H. Sheikh, "Knowledge and practices regarding foot care in diabetic patients visiting diabetic clinic in Jinnah Hospital, Lahore," *Journal of the Pakistan Medical Association*, vol. 59, no. 10, pp. 687–690, 2009.

[6] S. Saurabh, S. Sarkar, K. Selvaraj, S. Kar, S. Kumar, and G. Roy, "Effectiveness of foot care education among people with type 2 diabetes in rural Puducherry, India," *Indian Journal of Endocrinology and Metabolism*, vol. 18, no. 1, pp. 106–110, 2014.

[7] N. Unwin, D. Whiting, L. Guariguata, G. Ghyoot, and D. Gan, Eds., *Diabetes Atlas*, International Diabetes Federation, Brussels, Belgium, 5th edition, 2011.

[8] American Diabetes Association, "Economic costs of diabetes in the U.S. in 2012," *Diabetes Care*, vol. 36, pp. 1033–1046, 2013.

[9] B. R. Mehra, A. P. Thawait, S. S. Karandikar, D. O. Gupta, and R. R. Narang, "Evaluation of foot problems among diabetics in rural population," *Indian Journal of Surgery*, vol. 70, no. 4, pp. 175–180, 2008.

[10] http://www.hopkinsguides.com/hopkins/view/Johns_Hopkins_Diabetes_Guide/547054/all/Foot_Ulcers.

[11] V. N. Shah, P. K. Kamdar, and N. Shah, "Assessing the knowledge, attitudes and practice of type 2 diabetes among patients of saurashtra region, Gujarat," *International Journal of Diabetes in Developing Countries*, vol. 29, no. 3, pp. 118–122, 2009.

27

Sexual Coercion and Associated Factors among Female Students of Madawalabu University, Southeast Ethiopia

Abulie Takele[1] and Tesfaye Setegn[2]

[1]*Department of Nursing, College of Medicine & Health Sciences, Madawalabu University, 302 Bale Goba, Ethiopia*
[2]*Department of Reproductive Health, College of Medicine and Health Sciences, School of Public Health,*
 Bahir Dar University, 3008 Bahir Dar, Ethiopia

Correspondence should be addressed to Abulie Takele; abuletakele@yahoo.com

Academic Editor: Ronald J. Prineas

Introduction. Violence against women, in its various forms, is an important social and public health problem in different communities around the world. Although violence against women is against the inalienable human right and resulted in physical, sexual, and psychological harm or suffering to women, little has been documented regarding its factors and distribution among youth population such as university students. Therefore, the objective of this study was to assess factors associated with sexual coercion among female students at Madawalabu University. *Methods.* This was a cross-sectional institution based study conducted on 411 female students which were selected by systematic random sampling from the list of female students. Data were collected in April 2012 using structured-interview administered questionnaire. Descriptive, binary, and multivariable logistic regression analysis were carried out using SPSS version 16. *Result.* In this study, the mean (±SD) age at first sex was 18.19 (+1.83) years. Lifetime and coercion in last twelve months were 163 (41.1%) and 101 (25.4%), respectively. Twenty-one (5.9%) of the respondents were raped. Being influenced/forced into unwanted sexual act 74 (18.6%) and having their genitalia/breast unwillingly touched 44 (11.1%) were reported as the commonest mechanisms of coercion. Age at first sex (17–19 years) (AOR = 0.241, 95% CI: 0.074, 0.765) and occasional alcohol use (AOR = 4.161, 95% CI: 1.386, 12.658) were significantly associated with coercion in the last twelve months. *Conclusion.* The overall lifetime sexual coercion was found to be 41.1%. In this study 6.8% of female students were raped and majority have had trial of rape. But 93.75% did not report to any legal body. With the existing prevalence and identified factors, the university should work towards minimizing the risk of sexual coercion through intensifying life skill peer education and assertiveness trainings.

1. Introduction

Gender based violence (GBV) is a pervasive problem for most women all over the world [1–3]. Violence against women, in its various forms, is endemic in all communities and countries around the world. It affects all race, age, religious, and national boundaries [1]. According to the United Nations Declaration, violence against women includes any act of gender based violence that results in physical, sexual, and psychological harm or suffering to women, including threats or such acts as coercion or durable deprivation of liberty, whether occurring in public or private life [4].

Over the past 25 years, there is recognition of gender based violence under reporting. In addition, there are high prevalence and increased acknowledgment that it can affect women at any stage of their lives and can occur in various forms that may involve physical, psychological sexual, and/or economic abuse. Violence against women is a crucial violation of human right to liberty and freedom from fear, and now it is recognized as a priority public health and human rights issue [5]. Abuse by intimate male partners and coerced sex were the most common forms of violence against women, whether it takes place in childhood, adolescence, or adulthood [6]. This problem is more severe among young adolescents and could affect their health in different aspects including physical, mental, and social wellbeing of the victim.

Intimate partner violence and sexual violence are serious and widespread problems worldwide. In addition to violations of human rights, violence profoundly damages the physical, sexual, reproductive, emotional, mental, and social wellbeing of individuals and families [7]. Sexual violence thus appears to be a major challenge of school life for many adolescent females in Ethiopia and elsewhere [8].

Sexual violence is the act of forcing (or attempting to force) a female through physical body harm or any means to engage in a sexual behavior against her will. Sexual coercion exists along a continuum, from forcible rape to nonphysical forms of pressure that compels girls and women to engage in sex against their will. In some forms of coercion a woman lacks choice and faces several physical or social consequences if she resists sexual advances. Around the world, at least one woman in every three has been beaten, coerced into sex, or otherwise abused in her lifetime [6]. Much sexual coercion takes place against children or adolescents in both industrial and developing countries whereby between one-third and two-thirds of women that are sexual assault victims are young [9]. The experience of sexual coercion leads to a greater likelihood of risky sexual behavior such as early sexual debut, many sexual partners, and inconsistent condom use. Alcohol increases the likelihood of sexual assault occurring among acquaintances during social interactions. These pathways include beliefs about alcohol, deficits in higher order cognitive processing, and motor impairment induced by alcohol and peer group norms that encourage heavy drinking leading to forced sex. Studies on sexual coercion in higher learning institutions/universities in Ethiopia are limited and the problem was not well studied.

The level of sexual coercion and its factors among female students were not studied in Madawalabu University. Therefore, this study tried to assess sexual coercion among female students and associated factors as a crucial step to improve sexual health of female students in Madawalabu University. The finding from this study can be used as a baseline for further studies and as an input for policy makers and program designers. Thus the general objective of this study was to determine the prevalence and consequences and assess factors associated with it among female Madawalabu University students in southeast Ethiopia.

2. Materials and Methods

2.1. Study Setting and Sample. Institution based cross-sectional quantitative study was conducted in April 2012 in order to assess sexual coercion and its associated factors. The study was conducted in Madawalabu University that is located in Bale Zone, Oromia National Regional State, 430 km from the capital of the country, Addis Ababa, in the southeast direction. Madawalabu University is one of the public higher learning institutions established in Ethiopia in 2007. The university currently has two campuses (Goba and Robe). In the two campuses there were 3,211 regular students of which 2,484 males and 727 females were in the second year and above. The source population for the study was all female students registered in the 2nd year and above in the academic year of 2011/12. The study excluded all newly registered students that came from preparatory programs.

The study used a single population proportion to determine the sample size. The study considered a 41.8% proportion of sexual coercion that was used from a study conducted in Addis Ababa University female students [10] at 95% certainty and margin of error 0.05. Contingency of 10% was added to increase power and compensate for possible nonresponse. And the final sample size is 411 female students. The study follows the university's nine schools, one institute, and one college. Sample size for each school was distributed according to proportion of population female students. Sampling frame was prepared by taking a list of all second year and above students from the university registrar and alumni directorate office, and systematic random sampling was employed in each school to obtain a proportionally allocated number of participants from each school/college.

2.2. Measurement. For meeting the objectives of the study the following variables were included. Dependent variable is sexual coercion including rape, assault, and harassment. The independent variables for the study wereage, previous residence, religion, ethnicity, year of study, parent marital status, student's marital status, family background including family income and money sent (provided by family member), previous sexual activity, history of coercion, and student habits (khat chewing, alcohol use, and/or smoking).

A structured questionnaire was prepared first in English and translated to Amharic and finally back-translated to English in order to ensure its consistency for self-administration. The questionnaire was pretested in one of the departments of the university, which was not included in the study. Appropriate modification was made based on the findings of the pretest.

Data was collected by five diploma holder nurses who were trained for one day on the data collection process and the instrument for data collection. The principal investigators and two supervisors were assigned to lead the data collection, to check for completeness and consistency of a questionnaire, and to assist data collectors. Before data collection started, directors and student deans of the respective campuses and schools were approached using a letter written by the academic vice president. List of female students and selection of eligible students and questionnaire administration halls/rooms were arranged and prepared in these schools and colleges. The selected students were made to seat separately and the purpose of the study was well explained. Following a self-administered response to the questions, completed questionnaire was collected in a collection box.

2.3. Data Analysis. Data were checked for completeness, sorted, entered, cleaned, and processed by Statistical Packages for Social Science (SPSS) version 16. Analysis of association for selected exposure variables was done with the outcome variables. Logistic regression was performed using SPSS version 16. The results were presented using figures, frequencies, proportions, odds ratio, and confidence interval.

In order to see the association between lifetime sexual coercion and explanatory variable, binary logistic regression was carried out. Those variables found to be statistically significant within the binary logistic regression model based on the COR and their P value ($P < 0.05$) were entered into the multivariable logistic regression model to come up with final predictors of lifetime sexual coercion with their respective adjusted odds ratios.

In the interest of common understanding the operational definitions of the following words and phrases are given.

Attempted rape: it is defined as a trial to have sexual intercourse without consent of the girl but without penetration of the vagina or anus or mouth.

Consequences of sexual coercion: they include social, physical, economical, educational, and psychological status of the victim women or girl after coercion.

Economic implication: sometimes parents are forced to take their daughter out of school because they are afraid of rape or girls drop out of school after being raped or abducted which results in improper education and unemployment or poverty.

Performed rape: it is defined as any nonconsensual penetration of the vagina or anus or mouth. It is done physically or by threatening of body harm, or when the victim is incapable of giving consent.

Physical consequences: raped victims reported problems of lacerations, pregnancy/abortion, and sexually transmitted diseases (STDs) and other injuries.

Rape: it is the act of forcing a female student through violent threats and deception to engage in sexual behaviors with penetration of the vagina.

Sexual coercion: it is the act of forcing (or attempting to force) a female student through physical body harm or any means to engage in a sexual behavior against her will.

Sexual harassment: it is unwanted sexual behavior such as physical contact or verbal comments, jokes, questions, and suggestions.

3. Results

Three hundred ninety-seven (96.6%) respondents completed the questionnaire administered. About two-thirds of the respondents, 242 (61%), were in the age group of 20–24 years and the mean age of the study subjects was 21.08 ± 1.40 SD; the majority, 358 (90.2%), of the respondents were not married. Two hundred twenty-four (56.4%) were Oromo ethnic group. More than half of the respondents, 255 (64.2%), were Orthodox; two hundred ninety-six (74.6%) were from urban areas and the majority of the respondents, 383 (96.5%), lived in the campus (Table 1).

The mean of the last semester cumulative GPA of the respondents was 2.78 ± 0.50 SD. One hundred thirteen (28.5%) of respondents' fathers' education levels were college/university. And eighty-two (20.7%) of mothers of study subjects were able to read and write. Two hundred sixty (65.8%) of respondents' mothers and fathers lived together

Table 1: Sociodemographic characteristics of the respondents in Madawalabu University, southeast Ethiopia, April 2012.

Variable	Number	Percent
Age of the respondent		
<20	146	36.8
20–24	242	61.8
>24	9	2.3
Currently married		
Yes	39	9.8
No	358	90.2
Ethnicity		
Oromo	224	56.4
Amhara	105	26.4
Gurage	28	7.1
Tigre	20	5.0
Sidamo	16	4.0
Others*	4	1.0
Religion		
Orthodox	255	64.2
Protestant	86	21.7
Muslim	44	11.1
Catholic	9	2.3
Others**	3	0.8
Residence before joining university		
Urban	296	74.6
Rural	101	25.4
Residence		
In the campus	383	96.5
Out of campus	14	3.5
Year of study		
Second	229	57.7
Third	162	40.8
Fourth	6	1.5

*Kembata and Somali; **Kale Hiwot and Missionary.

and 12 (3.0%) did not have both mother and father. Three-fourths, 297 (75.2%), of the respondents were living with their family (mother and father) before joining university (Table 2).

The mean age at first sex was 18.19 years ± 1.83 SD. One hundred ninety (47.9%) of the respondents had constant sexual partner. And 96 (24.2%) responded that they had had sex. Sixty-one (64.9%) of those sexually active had started sex in their late adolescent (17–19 years). About two-thirds, 62 (64.6%), of the respondents who were sexually active had started sex before joining university. Seventeen (50%) of the respondents who started sex after joining university started sex in the second year of their study. About one-third (36.8%) of the sexually active respondents started sex within marriage and 27 (28.4%) started sex by their interest (Table 3).

Thirty-six (9.1%) of the respondents were using any of the substances always. Among the substances used were alcohol 23 (5.8%), khat 11 (2.8%), hashish 6 (1.5%), cigarettes (2.3%), and others 13 (3.3%). Eighty-eight (22.2%) of the respondents were using different substances sometimes. The substances

TABLE 2: Family educational status, mother and father living situation, and students' living arrangement before joining university in Madawalabu University, southeast Ethiopia, April 2012.

Variable	Frequency	Percentage
Fathers' educational status		
Illiterate	38	9.6
Read and write	79	19.9
1–6	60	15.1
7-8	52	13.1
9–12	55	13.9
College/university	113	28.5
Mothers' educational status		
Illiterate	75	18.9
Read and write	82	20.7
1–6 grades	68	17.1
7-8 grades	36	9.1
9–12 grades	78	19.6
College/university	58	14.6
Family living situation		
Live together	260	65.8
Divorced	46	11.6
Father alive	21	5.3
Mother alive	56	14.2
Both died	12	3.0
Living with whom before university		
Family	297	75.2
Mother only	33	8.4
Father only	9	2.3
Relatives	24	6.1
Husband	17	4.3
Others*	15	3.8
Last semester grade		
<2.00	20	6.1
2.01–2.50	95	29.1
2.51–3.00	121	37.1
3.01–3.50	59	18.1
3.51–4.00	31	9.5

*Nonrelatives and alone.

TABLE 3: Sexual history and characterises of sexual initiation respondents in Madawalabu University, southeast Ethiopia, April 2012.

Variable	Frequency	Percent
Have constant sexual partner		
Yes	190	47.9
No	207	52.1
Ever had sex		
Yes	96	24.2
No	306	75.8
Age at first sex in years		
10–16	14	14.9
17–19	61	64.9
≥20	19	20.2
When sex started		
Before joining university	62	64.6
After joining university	34	35.4
At which year of study sex started		
First	16	47.0
Second	17	50.0
Third	1	3.0
How sex started		
Within marriage	35	36.8
Self-interest	27	28.4
Peer pressure	13	13.7
Friend promise	23	24.2
For money	6	6.3
To pass examinations	8	8.4
Forced	5	5.3
Intoxicated with alcohol	1	1.1

As a result of coercion the study subjects experienced frequent headache, poor appetite, sleeplessness, fear, self-blaming, blaming others, loss of self-value, the thought of coercion as end of life, the thought of death as being better than being coerced, and other consequences.

From the total study subjects 27 (6.8%) had faced rape and nearly half (48.1%) of the rape was committed in the perpetrators' home. The time of rape was in the afternoon 12 (44.4%), evening 11 (40.7%), and early morning 4 (14.8%). Surprisingly, only 2 (6.25) of the victims of rape reported the event to legal bodies (Table 4). Boyfriends account for the highest percentage of perpetrators followed by brother's friend and neighbors (Figure 1). Following rape attack eight (28.6%) became pregnant; four (14.3%) faced abortion; six (21.4%) faced genital trauma; six (21.4%) experienced unusual vaginal discharge; four (14.3%) developed genital swelling; and four (14.3%) suffered from other problems.

For 14 (51.9%) of rape victims the way of forcing was beating them (physical force). Moreover, nine (32.1%) were raped after they were given alcohol. Fifty-six (49.1%) of the mechanisms used to escape rape were by cheating with false promise. Seventeen (47.2%) of the victims of rape did not report the event to anyone. Fear of families was the main

used were alcohol 73 (18.4%), khat 23 (5.8%), hashish 7 (1.8%), cigarettes 11 (2.8%), and others 10 (2.8%).

Lifetime coercion for the study subjects was 163 (41.1%). The mechanisms of forcing were by influencing them in unwanted sexual acts 121 (30.5%), having their genitalia/breast unwillingly touched 86 (21.7%), having faced trial of rape 20 (5.0%), being forced into sex 13 (3.3%), and using force for sex by frightening 8 (2.6%). In the past twelve months 101 (25.4%) of the respondents were coerced. The mechanisms of coercion were being influenced to unwanted sexual act 74 (18.6%), having their genitalia/breast unwillingly touched 44 (11.1%), having faced trial of rape 10 (2.5%), and being forced into sexual act 8 (2.0%).

TABLE 4: Ever raped, where rape was committed, time of rape event, number of rape events, and reporting rape to legal body, Madawalabu University, May 2012.

Variable	Frequency	Percent
Ever raped		
Yes	27	6.8
No	370	93.8
Where rape was committed		
Victim's home	2	7.4
Perpetrators' home	13	48.1
Hotel	5	18.5
Outside of home	7	25.9
The time of rape		
Afternoon	12	44.4
Evening	11	40.7
Early morning	4	14.8
Number of trial/complete rape events		
Once	33	71.7
Twice	7	15.2
Three times	5	10.9
Four times	1	2.2
Rape events reported to legal body		
Yes	2	6.25
No	30	93.75

TABLE 5: Ways of raping, mechanism used to escape, to whom rape was reported, and reason for not reporting rape, Madawalabu University, May 2012.

Variable	Frequency	Percent
Way of force used for rape		
Biting	14	51.9
Showing knife	2	7.1
Giving alcohol	9	32.1
Giving drugs with alcohol	2	7.4
Making pass examinations	2	7.4
Giving money	2	7.4
Mechanisms used to escape rape by those who escaped rape		
Crying to call for help	9	7.9
Just escaped	27	23.7
By cheating with promise	56	49.1
Fighting	15	6.1
Others	7	13.2
To whom rape was reported		
Anyone	17	47.2
Friend	10	27.8
Sisters	3	8.3
Health professionals	8	22.2
Others	1	2.9
Reason for not disclosing rape		
Did not know what to do	7	28.0
Afraid of families	12	48.0
Afraid of community	5	20.0
Afraid of perpetrator	6	24.0
Think legal bodies do not function	2	8.0
Others	1	4.0

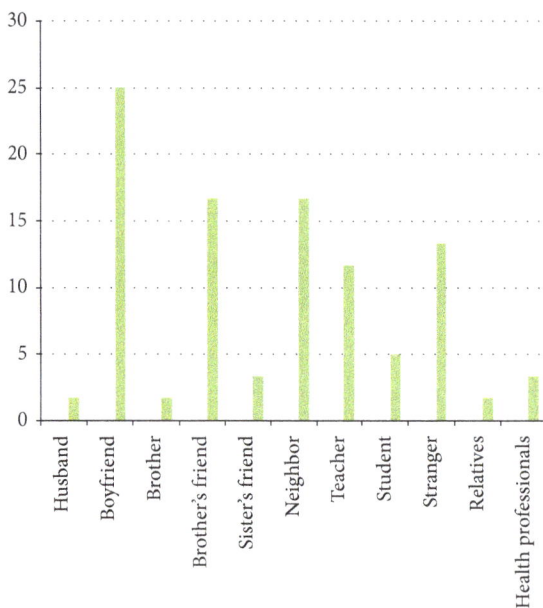

FIGURE 1: Percentage distribution of perpetrators of rape, Madawalabu University, May 2012.

on the COR and their P value ($P < 0.05$) were entered into the multivariable logistic regression model to come up with final predictors of lifetime sexual coercion with their respective adjusted odds ratios.

Variables which were associated with lifetime sexual coercion were having constant sexual partner (COR = 0.556, 95% CI: 0.371, 0.833), having had sex (COR = 0.618 (95% CI: 0.399, 0.982)), being in the age group between 17–19 years at first sex (COR = 0.249, 95% CI: 0.061, 0.560), using substances sometimes (COR = 3.102, 95% CI: 1.899, 5.068), having money sent enough (COR = 1.627, 95% CI: 1.069, 2.477), and using alcohol sometimes (COR = 3.102, 95% CI: 1.899, 5.068). Considering the AOR it was found out that only age of between 17 and 19 years at first sex (AOR = 0.241, 95% CI: 0.074, 0.765) and use of alcohol sometimes (AOR = 4.161 (1.386, 12.658)) were predictors of lifetime sexual coercion (Table 6). All the other variables were checked for their association and did not show statistically significant association (Table 6).

reason for not disclosing rape 12 (48.0%), followed by not knowing what to do 7 (28.0%) (Table 5).

In order to see the association between lifetime sexual coercion and explanatory variable, binary logistic regression was carried out. Those variables found to be statistically significant within the binary logistic regression model based

TABLE 6: Association of lifetime coercion and behavioral characteristics of respondents in Madawalabu University, southeast Ethiopia, May 2012.

Variable	Lifetime coercion		Crude OR with 95% CI	Adjusted OR with 95% CI
	No (%)	Yes (%)		
Have constant sexual partner				
No	98 (51.6)	92 (48.4)	1.00	1.00
Yes	136 (65.7)	71 (34.3)	**0.556 (0.371, 0.833)**	1.409 (0.463, 4.298)
Ever had sex				
No	48 (50.0)	48 (50.0)	1.00	1.00
Yes	186 (61.8)	115 (38.2)	**0.618 (0.399, 0.982)**	0.534 (0.289, 1.102)
Age at first sex				
10–16	43 (57.3)	32 (42.7)	**1.00**	**1.00**
17–19	5 (26.3)	14 (73.7)	**0.249 (0.061, 0.560)**	**0.241 (0.074, 0.765)**
Using substance always				
No	214 (59.3)	147 (40.7)	1.00	1.00
Yes	20 (55.6)	16 (44.4)	1.165 (0.584, 2.322)	0.455 (0.093, 2.229)
Using substance sometimes				
No	201 (65.0)	108 (35.0)	1.00	1.00
Yes	33 (37.5)	55 (62.5)	**3.102 (1.899, 5.068)**	3.230 (0.277, 2.229)
Money sent enough				
No	165 (63.0)	97 (37.0)	1.00	1.00
Yes	69 (51.1)	66 (48.9)	**1.627 (1.069, 2.477)**	0.995 (0.380, 2.603)
Using alcohol sometimes				
No	25 (33.8)	49 (66.2)	**1.00**	**1.00**
Yes	209 (64.7)	114 (35.3)	**3.102 (1.899, 5.068)**	**4.161 (1.386, 12.658)**

4. Discussion

This study identified sexual coercion and its associated factors. The lifetime prevalence of coercion in this study was found to be 41.1%. This finding was less than the finding in Uganda, 31.1% (94), but very much less than prevalence of sexual harassment in high schools of Addis Ababa [2]. This difference could be due to the difference in the setting of the study area [11].

The study tried to show the forms of coercion as physical, sexual, and psychological. As a result of coercion the study subjects experienced frequent headache, poor appetite, sleeplessness, easy fear, self-blaming, blaming others, loss of self-value, the thought of coercion as end of life, equating of coercion to death, and other consequences. These were also the consequences identified in Addis Ababa University [10]. The perpetrators of sexual coercion were relatives, husbands, teachers, strangers, boyfriends, and health professionals which is similar to the finding of Nigerian university [12]. The coercion was perpetrated by both intimate and nonintimate persons using physical force, psychological influence, and intoxication by alcohol [3].

Intimate partner violence is worldwide [7] and the consequences of sexual violence are a serious problem worldwide whether it is caused by intimate partner or stranger [13]. In this study 6.8% of the respondents reported they were raped which is higher than the finding in Nigerian university (3.2%) [12] and lower than the finding of Addis Ababa University (12.7%) [10]. Only 3.2% had reported the rape event to legal

bodies and 28.3% of the victims were raped more than two times. The prevalence of rape among Jijiga and Addis Ababa Universities students was 15.1% and 12.7%, respectively [10, 14]. In Addis Ababa University 6.4% of the victims had reported the event to legal body. In Nigeria University only 3.2% of rape victims had reported the event to police [15]. After rape attack the victims faced unwanted pregnancy, abortion, genital trauma, unusual vaginal discharge, genital swelling, and other problems. These are also similar to the findings of other studies [10, 12, 15].

In this study, 24.2% of the respondents were sexually active but in Addis Ababa University and Jijiga University 25.8% and 35.9, respectively, were sexually active [10, 14]. This may indicate that in our study area students' sexual practice was less or they may not tell that they are sexually active. In this study, the age of initiating sex (sexual debut) was 18.19 years. In a study conducted in northeast Nigeria and Cameroon the mean age at first sex was 16.1 and 15.3 years, respectively [15, 16], whereas in Addis Ababa and Jijiga Universities the mean age at first sex was 18.75 and 17.59 years, respectively [10, 14]. In a study on high school students in Addis Ababa, the mean age at first sex was 18.5 years [2]. Studies conducted on sexual behavior of youth in Ethiopia revealed that the mean age at first sex in Dessie town was 17.18 years [17], in Nekemte town in western Ethiopia was 15.2 years [18], and in high schools in Harar (east Ethiopia) was 16 years [19]. These differences could be due to difference in factors for starting sex early such as perception of the respondents about early sexual practice and knowledge of the effects of early sexual initiation. Early initiation of sexual practice could lead to early pregnancy, thereby predisposing the girl to unwanted pregnancy, its complication such as sexually transmitted infection including HIV/AIDS, and physical injuries such as laceration of the genital tract.

In this study 64.9% of the respondents have started sex in the late adolescent 17–19 years. More than one-third (35.4%) of the respondents started sex after joining university which is much higher than the proportion of students who started sex after joining university in Haramaya University (22.8%) [20]. In this study 50.0% of those who started sex after joining university started sex in the first year of study. In a study conducted in Jijiga University 92.2% of sexually active students who had sex had started sex before joining university [14]. In this study 65.2% of those sexually active had started sex willingly whereas 37.9% had started sex by the pressure from their peers and friends. This finding was inconsistent with the findings of Jijiga University [14]. This is indicative of the need for providing intensive education for students joining university by designing different approaches like life skill and peer education training [21]. And this could be due to lack of assertiveness and the fact that they are unable to negotiate safe sex and decide responsibly.

The other impressive finding of this study was 38.9% transactional sex, which is sex to any benefit from the partner at the time of initiating sex. The benefits mentioned in this study were friend promise (24.2%), gain of money (6.3%), and passing of examinations (8.4%). Transactional sex was a problem as it may open the gate to risky sexual relation.

From those who were sexually active only 36.8% started sex with marriage, while for 63.2% of them sexual activity was premarital. The high prevalence of premarital sex would likely increase the risk of sexually transmitted infections including HIV/AIDS and unwanted pregnancy. In Addis Ababa University the reasons mentioned for initiating sex before marriage were self-interest, peer influence, friend promise, getting money, being forced, and others [10]. These were also the reasons mentioned for the initiation of sexual intercourse by adolescents in Nekemte town [18]. Peer influences have significant effect on early initiation of sex which is risk behavior [6, 8].

The study shows that 9.1% of the respondents use substance always whereas 22.2% use only sometimes. Alcohol and khat were the most widely used by the respondents. Using such substances was a risk for problems of unsafe sexual practices that predispose them to sexually transmitted infections including unwanted pregnancy, HIV/IDS, and other consequences of unsafe sex. These problems were also the problems faced by university students in China and Sweden [22, 23]. In Addis Ababa 22.0% use alcohol and 8.0% chew khat [10]. In Jijiga University 29.5% use alcohol sometimes and 16.6% chew khat [10, 14]. Substance use including alcohol is a risk factor for risky sexual behavior [24, 25]. If the students and/or their partner/s were using alcohol it may result in altered behavior that leads to violence.

Following coercion the victims faced sexual and reproductive health problems such as unwanted pregnancy, abortion, genital trauma, genital swelling, and unusual vaginal discharge. This is similar to the finding of Addis Ababa and Jijiga Universities [10, 14]. These adolescents need help and support in order to protect them from such health risks of risky sexual relation [26]. Such violence is a violation of sexual rights of a person and a human right violation at large. These consequences have an impact on the physical, mental, and psychosocial wellbeing of the victim.

5. Conclusion and Recommendation

In conclusion, the study has found that coercion is prevalent in the study area and has illustrated the contribution of several factors to sexual coercion. The educational approach to life skills and peer education for students could avert the problem. Therefore the university should strengthen the sexual and reproductive health services. Using substances including alcohol needs to be avoided in order to reduce the risk of sexual coercion and mitigate its impact.

Madawalabu University is expected to work towards minimizing the risk of sexual coercion and its consequences by implanting strategies like life skill, peer education, and assertive training and strengthening youth friendly services through different outlets.

Ethical Approval

Before the actual data collection process, ethical clearance was obtained from the Ethical Review Committee of Madawalabu University. Informed consent was obtained from the study participants after brief explanation of the purpose of the study was made. Name of the respondent was excluded from the questionnaire to ensure confidentiality and anonymity of the participants' information.

Conflict of Interests

The authors declare that there is no conflict of interests regarding the publication of this paper.

Authors' Contribution

Abulie Takele and Tesfaye Setegn have taken a leading role in writing the proposal, submission, and follow-up for ethical review, data collection, data entry and analysis, and writing of the preliminary results. All authors read and approved the final paper.

Acknowledgments

The authors would like to acknowledge Madawalabu and Bahir Dar Universities and respective Medical and Health Science Colleges where they are based for their technical support. They also would like to thank Dr. Alemu Disasa for language editing and data collectors and participants.

References

[1] WHO, *Putting Women First Ethical and Safety Recommendation for Research on Domestic Violence Against Women*, WHO, Geneva, Switzerland, 2001.

[2] G. Lelissa and L. Yusuf, "A cross sectional study on prevalence of gender based violence in three high schools, Addis Ababa, Ethiopia," *Ethiopian Journal of Reproductive Health*, vol. 2, no. 1, 2008.

[3] National of Institute Justice, *The Campus Sexual Assault Study Final Report*, National of Institute Justice, Washington, DC, USA, 2005–2007.

[4] United Nation General Assembly, *Declaration on the Elimination of Violence Against Women*, 1993.

[5] WHO, *Violence Against Women: Aphordis Health Issue*, WHO, Geneva, Switzerland, 1997.

[6] "Ending Violence against Women: 2003 Series," Population Reports 11, 2003.

[7] WHO, *Preventing Intimate Partner and Sexual Violence Against Women. Taking Action and Generating Evidence*, WHO, Geneva, Switzerland, 2010.

[8] A. Bleached, *Determinants of Sexual Violence Among Ethiopian Secondary School Students*, BV. Ridderkerk, Ridderkerk, The Netherlands, 2012.

[9] L. Heise, J. Pitanguy, and A. German, "Violence against women: the hidden health burden," *Social Science & Medicine*, vol. 39, pp. 233–245, 1994.

[10] S. Tadesse, *Assessment of sexual coercion among Addis Ababa university students [Masters thesis]*, Addis Ababa University, Medical Faculty Department of Public Health, Addis Ababa, Ethiopia.

[11] Chemonics International, "Women's Legal Rights Initiative: Regional Centre for Africa (RCSA) Assessment and Analysis Report August 19-September 11, 2003, Jan. 14, 2004," http://www.usaid.gov/our_work/cross-cutting_programs/wid/pubs/wlr_rcsa.pdf.

[12] Z. Iliyasu, I. S. Abubakar, M. H. Aliyu, H. S. Galadanci, and H. M. Salihu, "Prevalence and correlates of gender-based violence among female university students in Northern Nigeria," *African Journal of Reproductive Health*, vol. 15, no. 3, pp. 111–119, 2011.

[13] Population Council, "Sexual and gender based violence in Africa: issues for programming 2008," http://www.popcouncil.org/.

[14] A. T. Jema, *Sexual experiences and their correlate3s among Jijiga University students [M.S. thesis]*, Addis Ababa University, Addis Ababa, Ethiopia, 2011.

[15] A. Abby, *Alcohol-Related Sexual Assault: A Common Problem among College Students*, Department of Community Medicine, Wayne State University, Detroit, Mich, USA, 2002.

[16] P. Foumane, A. Chiabi, C. Kamdem, F. Monebenimp, J. S. Dohbit, and R. E. Mbu, "Sexual activity of adolescent school girls in an urban secondary school in cameroon," *Journal of Reproduction and Infertility*, vol. 14, no. 2, pp. 85–89, 2013.

[17] F. Mazengia and A. Worku, "Age at sexual initiation and factors associated with it among youths in North East Ethiopia," *Ethiopian Journal of Health Development*, vol. 23, no. 2, 2009.

[18] A. Seme and D. Wirtu, "Premarital sexual practice among school adolescents in Nekemte Town, East Wollega," *Ethiopian Journal of Health Development*, vol. 22, no. 2, pp. 167–173, 2008.

[19] A. J. Mason-Jones, C. Crisp, M. Momberg, J. Koech, P. de Koker, and C. Mathews, "A systematic review of the role of school-based healthcare in adolescent sexual, reproductive, and mental health," *Systematic Reviews*, vol. 1, no. 1, article 49, 2012.

[20] T. Dingeta, L. Oljira, and N. Assefa, "Patterns of sexual risk behavior among undergraduate university students in Ethiopia: a cross-sectional study," *Pan Africa Medical Journal*, vol. 12, article 33, 2012.

[21] R. Adhikari and J. Tamang, "Premarital sexual behavior among male college students of Kathmandu, Nepal," *BMC Public Health*, vol. 9, article 241, 2009.

[22] Q. Ma, M. Ono-Kihara, L. Cong et al., "Early initiation of sexual activity: a risk factor for sexually transmitted diseases, HIV infection, and unwanted pregnancy among university students in China," *BMC Public Health*, vol. 9, article 111, 2009.

[23] C. Gunby, A. Carline, M. A. Bellis, and C. Beynon, "Gender differences in alcohol-related non-consensual sex; cross-sectional analysis of a student population," *BMC Public Health*, vol. 12, article 216, 2012.

[24] A. Agardh, K. Odberg-Pettersson, and P.-O. Östergren, "Experience of sexual coercion and risky sexual behavior among Ugandan university students," *BMC Public Health*, vol. 11, article 527, 2011.

[25] S. E. Toscano, "A grounded theory of female adolescents' dating experiences and factors influencing safety: the dynamics of the Circle," *BMC Nursing*, vol. 6, article 7, 2007.

[26] H. D. Boonstra, "Young people need help in preventing pregnancy and HIV; how will the world respond?" *Guttmacher Policy Review*, vol. 10, no. 3, 2007.

28

A Tool to Improve Accuracy of Parental Measurements of Preschool Child Height

Meredith Yorkin,[1] Kim Spaccarotella,[1,2] Jennifer Martin-Biggers,[1] Carolina Lozada,[1] Nobuko Hongu,[3] Virginia Quick,[4] and Carol Byrd-Bredbenner[1]

[1]*Department of Nutritional Sciences, Rutgers, The State University of New Jersey, New Brunswick, NJ 08901, USA*
[2]*Department of Biological Sciences, Kean University, Union, NJ 07083, USA*
[3]*Department of Nutritional Sciences, University of Arizona, Tucson, AZ 85721, USA*
[4]*Department of Health Sciences, James Madison University, Harrisonburg, VA 22807, USA*

Correspondence should be addressed to Jennifer Martin-Biggers; jmartin@njaes.rutgers.edu

Academic Editor: Livio Pagano

Background. Parent-reported measurement of child height is common in public health research but may be inaccurate, especially for preschoolers. A standardized protocol and tools to improve measurement accuracy are needed. The purpose of this study was to develop and test materials to improve parents' accuracy when measuring their preschooler's height. *Methods.* In Phase A, 24 parents were observed measuring child height using written instructions and an easy-to-read tape measure; after each of 3 testing rounds, instructions were refined based on observed errors and parent versus researcher measurements. In Phase B, a video replaced written instructions and was refined over 4 rounds with 37 parents. *Results.* The height kit with written instructions, tape measure, plumb line, and explanatory video helped parents accurately measure child height. Compared to written instructions alone, parents rated the video as having significantly greater clarity and likelihood of improving measurements. Although no significant differences in accuracy were found between paper and video instructions, observations indicated written instructions were more difficult for parents with less education to use with fidelity. *Conclusions.* The kit may improve parent measurement of preschooler height, thereby improving accuracy of body mass index calculations, tracking of obesity prevalence, and obesity prevention and treatment.

1. Introduction

Body mass index (BMI) is calculated using body weight and height measurements. Parent-reported measurement of child's height and weight is often used in public health research because this data collection method is efficient and cost-effective [1, 2]. However, parent reports of child height may not be accurate, especially for young children [3, 4]. In a study of parent-reported weights and heights of themselves and their obese children, a fifth of children's heights were overestimated by more than 2.5 cm (~1 in) [5]. Similarly, a more recent study of 837 children reported that 16.5% of parents underestimated and 25% overestimated child height by at least 2.5 cm (~1 in) [6]. Another study found that mothers' overestimation of both child weight and height

resulted in an overestimation of the percentage of overweight children by more than 3% in a sample of 1,549 4-year-olds [7].

Inaccuracies in parent reports of child height may be due to difficulty measuring young children due to their small size, children's difficulty in standing still during measurement procedures, parent use of incorrect measuring techniques, parent reliance on recall of height data from a doctor's visit, and parent reporting bias [4]. In addition, parents may incorrectly report their own height, which causes errors in calculations of their children's target height. A study of 241 families found that only about half of the parents reported their height within ±2 cm of their measured height, and only 70% of the midparental target heights calculated with the parent-reported data were accurate within ±2 cm of the target heights (i.e., the predicted height of the child based on height of both parents) calculated from measured data [8]. Clinicians often used target height calculations when assessing children's growth trajectories, making height an important component of pediatric anthropometric assessment [8].

Although these inaccuracies make it difficult to have confidence in parent-reported child height data when tracking individual children, parental reports of child height and weight may be acceptably accurate for estimating obesity prevalence in populations. A comparison of measured obesity prevalence in 1,497 school children with overweight prevalence estimated from parent-reported height and weight data found that both were similar, despite the tendency of parents to overestimate overweight by about 17% in boys and 10% in girls [9].

The obesity epidemic has spawned increased parent interest in child growth as well as obesity prevention intervention studies using BMI as an outcome measure [10–12]. Due to logistical issues associated with geographic distances between intervention participants and researchers, increased use of Internet-based interventions and data collection methods, funding limitations, and participant convenience, a standardized child height measurement protocol and tools designed for parents that could improve measurement accuracy are needed [13]. Improved height measurement tools would also increase the confidence in obesity prevention intervention results. Thus, the purpose of this study was to develop and pilot-test materials to help parents improve the accuracy with which they measured their preschool child's height.

2. Materials and Methods

This study was approved by the Institutional Review Boards at Rutgers University and the University of Arizona. All participants gave informed consent.

2.1. Sample. Parents of 2- to 5-year-old children were recruited via flyers posted at community sites and emails sent through workplace listservs at Rutgers University and the University of Arizona. Recruitment notices invited parents to review materials, participate in an interview, and implement instructions for measuring their own and their preschool child's height. Each participating parent received $25 compensation, and children received a sheet of stickers to compensate them for their time. No parent-child dyad participated in more than one round of testing.

2.2. Development of Height Measurement Kit. An iterative process was used to develop materials to improve the accuracy with which parents measured and reported child height. The height protocol for parents was created in two phases. Participants in both phases completed a brief survey to gather demographic data (e.g., age, highest education level achieved).

2.3. Phase A. Brief, written instructions for measuring height were developed by nutrition researchers with extensive experience conducting anthropometric measurements. Drafts were iteratively reviewed, tested, and refined by a panel of experts in anthropometric measurements ($n = 3$) to ensure accuracy and nonexperts ($n = 8$) to ensure comprehension by inexperienced audiences. The instructions described how to hang the tape measure and how to measure height accurately (Figure 1). Research staff then prepared height kits that contained a measuring tape, plumb line (called a weighted string in the instructions, made by tying a 1.27 cm (1/2 in) flat washer to a length of mason's line), removable tape for hanging the tape measure and plumb line, and written instructions.

A vast array of commercially available tape measures were reviewed to determine which would have the greatest likelihood of yielding the most accurate measurements. Most were narrow (less than 2.5 cm or 1 in wide) and had measurements (tick marks) in increments of 1/16th in (0.16 cm). These were judged by the research staff as cost-effective but difficult to read accurately when hanging on a wall and had a precision level beyond that needed to calculate body mass index (BMI) percentile. Thus, a 7.6 cm wide (3 in) tape measure similar to those used by visually impaired individuals with increments marked at 1/4th in (0.63 cm) was created using a poster printer; these dimensions and precision level were selected to make it easier for parents to read and differentiate between fractions. In addition, this tape measure labeled foot increments and restarted numbering of inches at each foot marker (i.e., the measurements were 1, 2, 3, 4, 5, 6, 7, 8, 9, 10, and 11 inches, 1 foot, 1, 2, 3, 4, 5, 6, 7, 8, 9, 10, and 11 inches, 2 feet, and so on) so that parents could report height in feet and inches (e.g., 3 feet, 2 inches), which is customary in the United States.

The height kits were subjected to three rounds of testing in Phase A. In all rounds, researchers explained to parents that they planned to mail the height kits to parents in an upcoming Internet-based study and wanted to be certain the instructions for measuring height were clear. The researchers further explained that the purpose of parents' participation was to help researchers improve the kits; thus parents should act as though they were in their own homes and the researchers were not there to answer questions. Each parent then was asked to read and follow the instructions and report the height measurements they obtained for their preschool child who accompanied them to the testing site. Then, with the parent watching, the researcher removed the measuring tape and plumb line, rehung the tape measure and plumb line in the same location used by the parent (if appropriate) or another location (if necessary to avoid obstacles that would result in erroneous measurements such as baseboards and carpet), and measured the child in duplicate. Finally, parents were asked for suggestions for improving the instructions and to use a 5-point scale, with 5 being the best score, to rate the instructions' clarity, readability, and likelihood that they would improve the way they measure their children's height.

Two trained researchers observed each parent as they operationalized the instructions to identify errors made in height measurement procedures. These errors were analyzed and used to refine the height kit prior to the next round of testing.

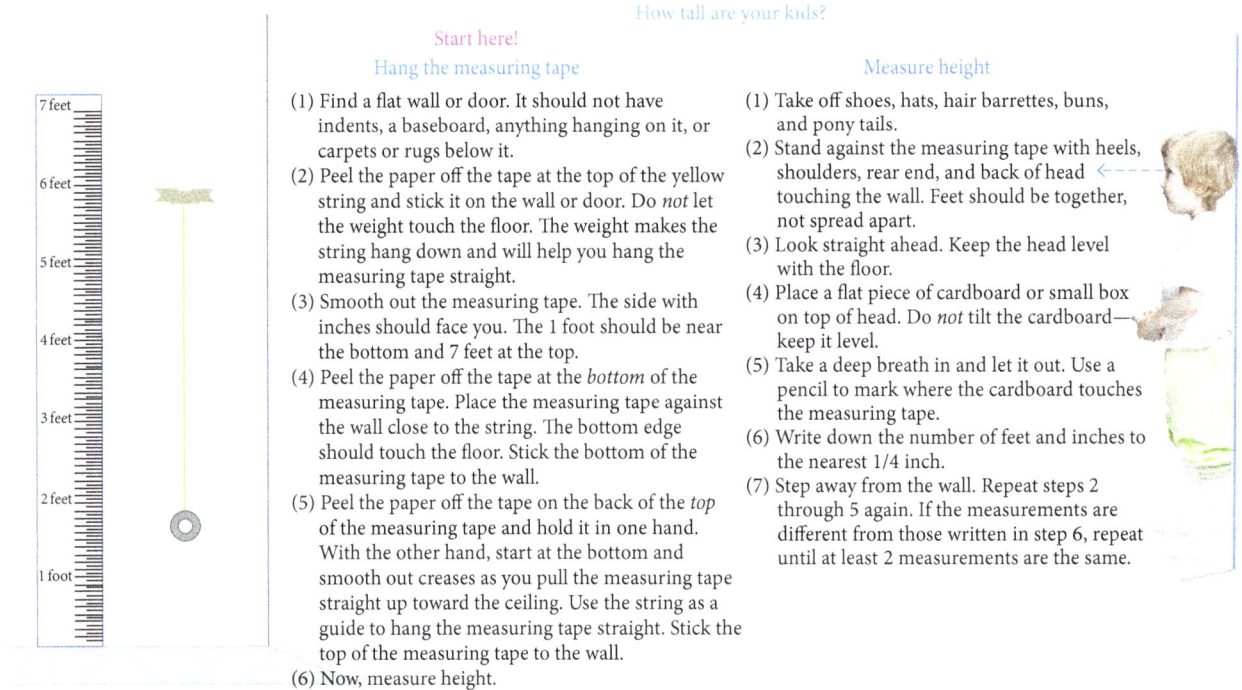

How tall are your kids?

Start here!
Hang the measuring tape

Measure height

(1) Find a flat wall or door. It should not have indents, a baseboard, anything hanging on it, or carpets or rugs below it.

(2) Peel the paper off the tape at the top of the yellow string and stick it on the wall or door. Do *not* let the weight touch the floor. The weight makes the string hang down and will help you hang the measuring tape straight.

(3) Smooth out the measuring tape. The side with inches should face you. The 1 foot should be near the bottom and 7 feet at the top.

(4) Peel the paper off the tape at the *bottom* of the measuring tape. Place the measuring tape against the wall close to the string. The bottom edge should touch the floor. Stick the bottom of the measuring tape to the wall.

(5) Peel the paper off the tape on the back of the *top* of the measuring tape and hold it in one hand. With the other hand, start at the bottom and smooth out creases as you pull the measuring tape straight up toward the ceiling. Use the string as a guide to hang the measuring tape straight. Stick the top of the measuring tape to the wall.

(6) Now, measure height.

(1) Take off shoes, hats, hair barrettes, buns, and pony tails.

(2) Stand against the measuring tape with heels, shoulders, rear end, and back of head touching the wall. Feet should be together, not spread apart.

(3) Look straight ahead. Keep the head level with the floor.

(4) Place a flat piece of cardboard or small box on top of head. Do *not* tilt the cardboard—keep it level.

(5) Take a deep breath in and let it out. Use a pencil to mark where the cardboard touches the measuring tape.

(6) Write down the number of feet and inches to the nearest 1/4 inch.

(7) Step away from the wall. Repeat steps 2 through 5 again. If the measurements are different from those written in step 6, repeat until at least 2 measurements are the same.

FIGURE 1: Height measurement protocol.

2.4. Phase B. The need for Phase B became apparent with the findings from Phase A (see Results and Discussion). In Phase B, the research team created a brief (8-minute) narrated video (http://healthyhomestyles.com/height/). The video was developed using Phase A's written instructions and was reviewed by a panel of experts in anthropometric measurements ($n = 3$) and nonexperts ($n = 5$). The video had components that described and depicted how to select a suitable location for hanging the tape measure, purpose and importance of the weighted string, how to ensure the tape measure was hung straight on the wall, how to prepare the child for being measured (e.g., remove shoes, hats, and hair decorations), positioning the child for measurement (having child's head, shoulders, buttocks, and heals touch the wall while child looks straight ahead), importance of child inhaling and exhaling before measurement, recording height to the nearest 1/4 in (0.63 cm), and importance of taking measurements twice.

The video and height kits were iteratively tested and refined in a series of four rounds of testing in Phase B. The video, played at research sites on a standalone laptop computer, was accompanied by a height kit developed and refined in Phase A. The procedures mirrored those used in Phase A. In addition, the survey completed at the start of the data collection protocol asked parents to report their child's height and indicate how sure they were of the reported height using a 5-point scale. Parents also were interviewed by trained researchers at the end of the session to identify questions that arose as they watched each component of the video and suggestions for improving the understandability of the video. Finally, parents used a 5-point scale, with 5 being the best score, to rate the clarity of the instructions in the video, how

well the video held their attention, and likelihood that the video would improve their measurement of child height.

2.5. Statistical Analysis. For each participant, the difference between mean height as measured by the parent and the researcher "gold standard" was calculated and compared. t-tests were used to compare height measurements made by research staff with those made by parents. Differences were considered significant at $P < 0.05$. Values are reported as means and standard deviations (SD) unless otherwise noted.

3. Results and Discussion

3.1. Results: Phase A. Table 1 describes participating parents' mean ages, education level, and number of children living in their households. Six parent-child dyads recruited from a university-based preschool participated in Round 1 of testing. As shown in Table 2, parents rated the instructions as being clear, easy to read, and likely to improve their measurements of child height. A comparison of height measurements taken by parents with those of researchers revealed close agreement in child heights. Instructions were refined based on parent feedback and consistent errors noted by researchers. The key error noted during this round was that parents did not understand the use of the plumb line and did not always choose a flat wall (many hung the tape measure over a baseboard). Additionally, many parents had difficulty differentiating between the fractions and accurately stating child height.

In Round 2, 13 parent-child dyads recruited from a university-based preschool participated. As in Round 1, parents had a mean age of about 38 years and all had at least some postsecondary education. Similarly, parents rated the clarity

TABLE 1: Characteristics of participants and accuracy of child height measurements.

Phase Round	Parent's age in years	Education		Number of children <18 in household	Absolute mean difference in inches (cm) between parent and researcher measured child heights
	Mean ± SD	Percent with secondary education or less	Percent with postsecondary education	Mean ± SD	Mean ± SD
Phase A					
Round 1 ($n = 6$)	38.80 ± 6.15	0%	100%	2.16 ± 0.41	0.23 ± 0.23 (0.58 ± 0.58)
Round 2 ($n = 13$)	38.38 ± 4.23	0%	100%	2.00 ± 0.82	0.60 ± 0.65 (1.52 ± 1.65)[a]
Round 3 ($n = 5$)	b	100%	0%	b	1.38 ± 2.12 (3.51 ± 5.38)
Phase B					
Round 1 ($n = 9$)	31.78 ± 8.91	44%	66%	2.44 ± 1.33	1.66 ± 1.97 (4.22 ± 5.00)
Round 2 ($n = 13$)	35.67 ± 12.48	54%	46%	1.42 ± 0.51	0.71 ± 0.99 (1.80 ± 2.51)[c]
Round 3 ($n = 5$)	28.60 ± 6.80	40%	60%	3.00 ± 1.58	1.55 ± 1.04 (3.94 ± 2.64)
Round 4 ($n = 10$)	29.11 ± 6.17	50%	50%	1.70 ± 0.82	0.35 ± 0.40 (0.89 ± 1.02)

[a]$n = 11$.
[b]Data unavailable.
[c]$n = 12$.

TABLE 2: Parent rating of height kit.

Phase Round	Clarity of instructions*	Reading ease*[a]	Extent video held viewer's attention*[b]	Likelihood of improving measurement of child's height*
Phase A				
Round 1 ($n = 6$)	4.50 ± 0.55	4.67 ± 0.52	—	4.00 ± 1.55
Round 2 ($n = 13$)[c]	4.50 ± 0.90	4.50 ± 0.90	—	3.92 ± 1.08
Round 3 ($n = 5$)	4.65 ± 0.49	5.00 ± 0.00	—	4.60 ± 0.89
All Phase A rounds combined	4.53 ± 0.72	4.65 ± 0.71		4.09 ± 1.16
Phase B				
Round 1 ($n = 9$)	4.78 ± 0.44	—	3.94 ± 1.07	5.00 ± 0.00
Round 2 ($n = 13$)	4.92 ± 0.28	—	4.54 ± 0.28	5.00 ± 0.00
Round 3 ($n = 5$)	4.80 ± 0.45	—	4.00 ± 1.00	5.00 ± 0.00
Round 4 ($n = 10$)	4.90 ± 0.32	—	4.80 ± 0.42	4.95 ± 0.16
All Phase B rounds combined	4.86 ± 0.35[d]		4.39 ± 0.86	4.98 ± 0.08[e]

*Item rated using a 1-to-5-point scale with 5 being the best score.
[a]Item included in Phase A only.
[b]Item included in Phase B only.
[c]One missing response.
[d]Significantly higher than Phase A ($P = 0.002$).
[e]Significantly higher than Phase A ($P = 0.0004$).

of instructions and reading ease highly but were less positive that the height kit would improve the accuracy of the height measurements they made of their children. A comparison of researcher and parent child height measurements revealed close agreement. Minor refinements were made to the instructions based on parent comments and researcher observations.

In Round 3, 5 parent-child dyads were recruited from a community center. None of these parents had any postsecondary education. Although parents felt the instructions were clear, easy to read, and likely to improve their measurements of child height, researcher observations revealed that written instructions were difficult for parents with less education to use with fidelity. Mean researcher and parent child height measurements differed by 1.38 in (3.51 cm).

3.2. Results: Phase B. In Rounds 1 to 4 of Phase B, 9, 13, 5, and 10 parent-child dyads participated, respectively. Of these, about half had no postsecondary education. Common errors were not verifying tape measure straightness, hanging the tape measure over a baseboard instead of finding a flat wall, adjusting straightness of the tape measure by moving the bottom instead of the top which resulted in the tape not remaining flush with the floor, not removing child shoes, not having child breathe in/out before taking measurements, and misreading fractions. Several parents also suggested that the video should end with a summary of the steps and be accompanied with written instructions (i.e., "*some kind of cue card at the end to remind you of all of the steps*") and that a reminder to start hanging the tape from the bottom should be added ("*more emphasis on remembering to tape the bottom of the measuring tape first*"). The video was refined iteratively after each round to address consistent parent errors and suggestions by emphasizing the importance of procedures, refining text and images appearing in the video, repeating the purpose of procedures (e.g., hanging the plumb line), and adding a summary of procedures. In addition, to improve accuracy in reading fractions, the measuring tape was modified in each round, respectively, by increasing the font size of the numbers, renumbering so that the foot increments were removed and inches ran consecutively, introducing a yellow background to make the increments and numbers more visible, and adding written instructions to the measuring tape itself. To emphasize that the tape measure must touch the floor, a thick black line was added to the bottom of the tape measure and the bottom and top of the tape measure were labeled. Throughout Phase B, parents highly rated the video's clarity, ability to hold viewer attention, and likelihood of improving their measurements of child height. In the final round, mean differences in child height measurements of researchers and parents were approximately 1/3 in (0.85 cm). The final components of the height kit are shown in Figure 2.

Interestingly, on the survey completed at the outset of data collection, 18 (49%) parents reported that they did not know their child's height. Average absolute differences between the values of the parents who reported child height (n = 19) and researchers' measurements were 5.37 ± 4.31 SD in or 13.6 ± 10.9 SD cm (range 0.70 to 15.3 in or 1.8 to 38.9 cm). One

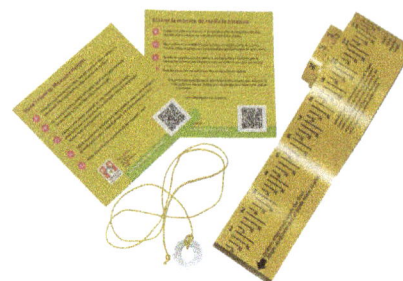

FIGURE 2: Height measurement kit. Video: http://healthyhomestyles .com/height/.

parent in 19 who reported feeling sure about the child height reported underreported the child's height by 1.75 in (4.45 cm).

Comparisons, using t-tests, of instruction clarity ratings for all rounds of Phase A combined with all rounds of Phase B combined revealed that participants rated the video as having significantly greater clarity (P = 0.0204) than written instructions. Similarly, participants rated the video as significantly more likely to improve their measurements of child heights than the written instructions (P = 0.0004). Average absolute differences in child height measurements between researchers and parents for all Phase A and Phase B rounds (i.e., 0.67 ± 1.32 SD and 0.96 ± 1.29 SD in or 1.70 ± 3.34 SD and 2.44 ± 3.28 SD cm, resp.) did not differ significantly (P = 0.1879). Additionally, in Phase B, there were no significant differences between those with high school education levels or less and those with at least some postsecondary education with regard to accuracy of child height measurements compared to those taken by researchers (1.09 ± 1.52 SD versus 0.81 ± 1.00 SD in or 2.77 ± 3.86 SD versus 2.06 ± 2.52 SD cm, P = 0.2533) (sample size was too small to conduct similar comparisons in Phase A).

4. Discussion

This study's findings indicate that a height kit composed of written instructions, an easy-to-read tape measure, plumb line, and explanatory video can help parents accurately measure child height. Compared to written instructions alone, parents rated the video as having significantly greater clarity and likelihood of improving their measurements of child height. Although no significant differences in accuracy were found between the written and video instructions, researcher observations indicated that the written instructions alone were more difficult for parents to use with fidelity, especially those with less formal education.

Self-report data are considered to be an accurate representation only when the data collection instrument has undergone formative testing such as reliability and validity analysis [14]. Adults are generally accurate when providing their own height and weight to calculate BMI [15, 16] (with the exception of overweight and obese women tending to underreport weights) [17]; however, preschool-aged children are rapidly growing and parents frequently misreport both height and weight [6, 7]. Even if a child recently had a pediatric or well-child visit, substantial amounts of growth can happen in a relatively short time frame, and reporting of this data may not be sufficiently accurate for tracking individual differences in growth [3]. The height kit designed and refined in this study can help researchers cost-effectively gather more accurate parent-reported data on child height. Kits cost less than $2.00US each and can be mailed to study participants.

The small sample sizes in this study indicate that statistical comparison should be interpreted with caution. In addition, parents took measurements while under observation and may not be as careful in taking measurements when at home. However, the study has numerous strengths. An iterative process was used to continually modify and refine the measuring tape and written and video instructions and a mixed methods approach was taken for data collection. Quantitative measures of height measurements taken by parents were compared to the researcher "gold standard" and qualitative data collection from parents was used to identify specific areas of confusion and areas for improving and refining the written instructions and video. Future research should investigate the effectiveness of the height kit in improving parental height measurements of older children and determine its utility in more diverse population groups. Pairing the height measurements taken with the kit and child weight could further clarify usefulness of the height kit and video in reporting BMI.

5. Conclusions

Study findings suggest that an instructional video is perceived by parents as clear, easy to use, and likely to improve their measurements of child height. The height measuring kit developed and validated in this study has the potential to improve parent reports of child height, thereby improving the accuracy of BMI calculations, tracking of childhood obesity prevalence, and confidence in obesity prevention and treatment program outcomes based on parent-reported data.

Conflict of Interests

The authors declare that they have no competing interests.

Authors' Contribution

The following coauthors contributed to the work: Meredith Yorkin to study design, data collection, paper preparation, and paper review; Kim Spaccarotella to paper preparation, data analysis, and paper review; Jennifer Martin-Biggers to study design, data collection, data analysis, and paper review; Carolina Lozada to study design, data collection, and paper review; Nobuko Hongu to data collection and paper preparation and review; Virginia Quick to data analysis, paper preparation, and paper review; Carol Byrd-Bredbenner to study design and paper preparation and paper review. All authors read and approved the final paper.

Funding

This work was funded through USDA NIFA #2011-68001-30170.

Acknowledgment

Meredith Yorkin, Kim Spaccarotella, Jennifer Martin-Biggers, Virginia Quick, and Carol Byrd-Bredbenner received funding from the United States Department of Agriculture, National Institute of Food and Agriculture, Grant no. 2011-68001-30170.

References

[1] I. Huybrechts, J. H. Himes, C. Ottevaere et al., "Validity of parent-reported weight and height of preschool children measured at home or estimated without home measurement: a validation study," BMC Pediatrics, vol. 11, article 63, 2011.

[2] N.-L. Yao and M. M. Hillemeier, "Weight status in Chinese children: maternal perceptions and child self-assessments," World Journal of Pediatrics, vol. 8, no. 2, pp. 129–135, 2012.

[3] A. C. Skinner, D. Miles, E. M. Perrin, T. Coyne-Beasley, and C. Ford, "Source of parental reports of child height and weight during phone interviews and influence on obesity prevalence estimates among children aged 3–17 years," Public Health Reports, vol. 128, no. 1, pp. 46–53, 2013.

[4] L. J. Akinbami and C. L. Ogden, "Childhood overweight prevalence in the United States: the impact of parent-reported height and weight," Obesity, vol. 17, no. 8, pp. 1574–1580, 2009.

[5] R. R. Wing, L. H. Epstein, and D. Neff, "Accuracy of parents' reports of height and weight," Journal of Behavioral Assessment, vol. 2, no. 2, pp. 105–110, 1980.

[6] D. P. O'Connor and J. J. Gugenheim, "Comparison of measured and parents' reported height and weight in children and adolescents," Obesity, vol. 19, no. 5, pp. 1040–1046, 2011.

[7] L. Dubois and M. Girad, "Accuracy of maternal reports of preschoolers' weights and heights as estimates of BMI values," International Journal of Epidemiology, vol. 36, no. 1, pp. 132–138, 2007.

[8] I. Braziuniene, T. A. Wilson, and A. H. Lane, "Accuracy of self-reported height measurements in parents and its effect on midparental target height calculation," BMC Endocrine Disorders, vol. 7, article 2, 2007.

[9] A. Banach, T. J. Wade, J. Cairney, J. A. Hay, B. E. Faught, and D. D. O'Leary, "Comparison of anthropometry and parent-reported height and weight among nine year olds," Canadian Journal of Public Health, vol. 98, no. 4, pp. 251–253, 2007.

[10] C. Byrd-Bredbenner, J. Worobey, J. Martin-Biggers et al., "HomeStyles: shaping home environments and lifestyle practices to prevent childhood obesity: a randomized controlled trial," Journal of Nutrition Education and Behavior, vol. 44, no. 4, supplement, p. S81, 2012.

[11] J. Emerson, B. Husaini, P. Hull, R. Levine, and V. Oates, "Nashville children eating well (CHEW) for health," Journal of Nutrition Education and Behavior, vol. 44, no. 4, supplement, p. S81, 2012.

[12] O. Seaver and R. Mullis, "Family food and fitness fun pack: a pilot study," Journal of Nutrition Education and Behavior, vol. 44, no. 4, supplement, pp. S27–S28, 2012.

[13] M. Yorkin, K. Spaccarotella, J. Martin-Biggers, V. Quick, and C. Byrd-Bredbenner, "Accuracy and consistency of weights provided by home bathroom scales," *BMC Public Health*, vol. 13, article 1194, 2013.

[14] C. Redding, J. Maddock, and J. Rossi, "The sequential approach to measurement of health behavior constructs: issues in selecting and developingmeasures," *Californian Journal of Health Promotion*, vol. 4, no. 1, pp. 83–101, 2006.

[15] W. Willett, *Nutritional Epidemiology*, Oxford University Press, New York, NY, USA, 2nd edition, 1998.

[16] M. F. Kuczmarski, R. J. Kuczmarski, and M. Najjar, "Effects of age on validity of self-reported height, weight, and body mass index: findings from the third National Health and Nutrition Examination Survey, 1988–1994," *Journal of the American Dietetic Association*, vol. 101, no. 1, pp. 28–34, 2001.

[17] M. J. Kretsch, A. K. H. Fong, and M. W. Green, "Behavioral and body size correlates of energy intake underreporting by obese and normal-weight women," *Journal of the American Dietetic Association*, vol. 99, no. 3, pp. 300–306, 1999.

Permissions

The contributors of this book come from diverse backgrounds, making this book a truly international effort. This book will bring forth new frontiers with its revolutionizing research information and detailed analysis of the nascent developments around the world.

We would like to thank all the contributing authors for lending their expertise to make the book truly unique. They have played a crucial role in the development of this book. Without their invaluable contributions this book wouldn't have been possible. They have made vital efforts to compile up to date information on the varied aspects of this subject to make this book a valuable addition to the collection of many professionals and students.

This book was conceptualized with the vision of imparting up-to-date information and advanced data in this field. To ensure the same, a matchless editorial board was set up. Every individual on the board went through rigorous rounds of assessment to prove their worth. After which they invested a large part of their time researching and compiling the most relevant data for our readers.

The editorial board has been involved in producing this book since its inception. They have spent rigorous hours researching and exploring the diverse topics which have resulted in the successful publishing of this book. They have passed on their knowledge of decades through this book. To expedite this challenging task, the publisher supported the team at every step. A small team of assistant editors was also appointed to further simplify the editing procedure and attain best results for the readers.

Apart from the editorial board, the designing team has also invested a significant amount of their time in understanding the subject and creating the most relevant covers. They scrutinized every image to scout for the most suitable representation of the subject and create an appropriate cover for the book.

The publishing team has been an ardent support to the editorial, designing and production team. Their endless efforts to recruit the best for this project, has resulted in the accomplishment of this book. They are a veteran in the field of academics and their pool of knowledge is as vast as their experience in printing. Their expertise and guidance has proved useful at every step. Their uncompromising quality standards have made this book an exceptional effort. Their encouragement from time to time has been an inspiration for everyone.

The publisher and the editorial board hope that this book will prove to be a valuable piece of knowledge for researchers, students, practitioners and scholars across the globe.

List of Contributors

S. Pooransingh
Department of Paraclinical Sciences, Faculty of Medical Sciences, The University of the West Indies, St. Augustine, Trinidad and Tobago

K. Ramgulam
South West Regional Health Authority, San Fernando, Trinidad and Tobago

I. Dialsingh
Department of Mathematics and Statistics, The University of the West Indies, St. Augustine, Trinidad and Tobago

Najlaa Aljefree and Faruk Ahmed
Public Health, School of Medicine and Griffith Health Institute, Griffith University, Gold Coast Campus, QLD 4222, Australia

Jeffrey Le, Sarah Alyouha, Michael Bezuhly, and Jason Williams
Division of Plastic and Reconstructive Surgery, Dalhousie Department of Surgery, Dalhousie University, Halifax, NS, Canada

Lihui Liu
Department of Mathematics and Statistics, Dalhousie University, Halifax, NS, Canada

Suhailah Samsudin and Siti Nor Sakinah Saudi
Department of Community Health, Faculty of Medicine and Health Sciences, Universiti Putra Malaysia (UPM), 43400 Serdang, Selangor, Malaysia

Siti Norbaya Masri, Tengku Zetty Maztura Tengku Jamaluddin and Malina Osman
Department of Medical Microbiology and Parasitology, Faculty of Medicine and Health Sciences, Universiti Putra Malaysia (UPM), 43400 Serdang, Selangor, Malaysia

Umi Kalsom Md Ariffin
Department of Urban Services and Health, Ampang Jaya Municipal Council (MPAJ), Jalan Pandan Utama, Taman Pandah Indah, 55100 Ampang, Selangor, Malaysia

Fairuz Amran
Institute of Medical Research, Jalan Pahang, 50588 Kuala Lumpur, Malaysia

Andrew J. Macnab
Department of Pediatrics, University of British Columbia, RoomC323, 4500 Oak Street, Vancouver, BC, Canada V6H 3N
Stellenbosch Institute for Advanced Study, Wallenberg Research Centre, 10 Marais Street, 7600 Stellenbosch, South Africa

Lu Shi
Department of Public Health Sciences, Clemson University, Clemson, SC 29634-0745, USA

Yuping Mao
Department of Media & Communication, Erasmus University Rotterdam, 3000DR, Netherlands

Alemu Tamiso Debiso and Behailu Merdekios Gello
Department of Public Health, College of Medicine and Health Science, Arba Minch University, Arba Minch, Ethiopia

Marelign Tilahun Malaju
Department of Public Health, College of Health Sciences, Debre Tabor University, Debre Tabor, Ethiopia

Anisa M. Durrani and Waseem Fatima
Department of Home Science, Aligarh Muslim University, India

Atef Y. Bakhoum and Max O. Bachmann
Norwich Medical School, University of East Anglia, Norwich, UK

Ehab El Kharrat
Freedom Drugs and HIV Program, Cairo, Egypt

Remon Talaat
Ipsos Healthcare, 35A Saray El Maadi Tower, Cairo, Egypt

Onyemocho Audu and Ishaku Bako Ara
Department of Epidemiology & Community Health, Benue State University, PMB 10 2119, Makurdi, Benue, Nigeria

Abdujalil Abdullahi Umar
Department of Public Health, Ministry of Health, Katsina, Katsina State, Nigeria

Victoria Nanben Omole
Department of Community Medicine, Kaduna State University, Kaduna, Nigeria

Solomon Avidime
Department of Obstetrics/Gynaecology, Ahmadu Bello University Teaching Hospital, Zaria, Kaduna State, Nigeria

Said Usman, Kintoko Rochadi and Fikarwin Zuska
Faculty of Public Health, University of North Sumatra, Medan 20155, Indonesia

Soekidjo Notoadmodjo
Indonesia Respati University, Jakarta 13890, Indonesia

Sheikh Mohammed Shariful Islam
Center for Control of Chronic Disease (CCCD), International Center for Diarrhoeal Disease Research, Bangladesh (ICDDR,B), 68 Shaheed Tajuddin Ahmed Sarani, Mohakhali, Dhaka 1212, Bangladesh
Center for International Health (CIH), Ludwig-Maximilians-Universität (LMU), Leopoldstraße 7, 80802 Munich, Germany

Vikas Bajpai
Centre for Social Medicine and Community Health, Jawaharlal Nehru University, New Delhi, India

Shweta Sharma, Nirmaljit Kaur, Shalini Malhotra, Preeti Madan and Charoo Hans
Department of Microbiology, Dr. Ram Manohar Lohia Hospital & PGIMER, Baba Kharak Singh Marg, New Delhi 110001, India

Evans Danso, Isaac Yeboah Addo and Irene Gyamfuah Ampomah
Department of Population and Health, Faculty of Social Sciences, University of Cape Coast, Cape Coast, Ghana

Eskezyiaw Agedew
Department of PublicHealth, Arba Minch University, Southern Ethiopia, Ethiopia

Tefera Chane
Department of Public Health, Wolaita Sodo University, 251 138 Southern Ethiopia, Ethiopia

Nadira Mallick and Subha Ray
Department of Anthropology, University of Calcutta, 35 Ballygunge Circular Road, Kolkata 700 019, India

Susmita Mukhopadhyay
Biological Anthropology Unit, Indian Statistical Institute, 203 B.T. Road, Kolkata 108, India

Asrat Agalu Abejew and Abebe Zeleke Belay
Department of Pharmacy, College of Medicine and Health Sciences,Wollo University, P.O. Box 1145, Dessie, Ethiopia

Mirkuzie Woldie Kerie
Department of Health Services Management, College of Public Health and Medical Sciences, Jimma University, P.O. Box 1637, Jimma, Ethiopia

Wei-Chen Lee
Center to Eliminate Health Disparities, University of Texas Medical Branch, Galveston, TX, USA

Luohua Jiang
Department of Epidemiology and Biostatistics, School of Rural Public Health, Texas A&M Health Science Center, College Station, TX, USA

Charles D. Phillips and Robert L. Ohsfeldt
Department of Health Policy and Management, School of Rural Public Health, Texas A&M Health Science Center, College Station, TX, USA

Nene Ernest Khalema
Human Sciences Research Council, Private Bag X41, Pretoria 0001, South Africa
School of Public Health, University of Alberta, Edmonton, AB, Canada T6G 2R3
School of Built Environment and Development Studies, University of KwaZulu-Natal, Durban 4041, South Africa

Janki Shankar
Faculty of Social Work, University of Calgary, No. 444, 11044-82 Avenue, Edmonton, AB, Canada T6G OT2

Sudha Xirasagar and Yi-Jhen Li
Department of Health Services Policy and Management, University of South Carolina, Arnold School of Public Health, 915 Greene Street, Columbia, SC 29208, USA

Thomas G. Hurley
South Carolina Statewide Cancer Prevention & Control Program, University of South Carolina, 915 Greene Street, Columbia, SC 29208, USA

James R. Hébert
South Carolina Statewide Cancer Prevention & Control Program, University of South Carolina, 915 Greene Street, Columbia, SC 29208, USA
Department of Epidemiology and Biostatistics, University of South Carolina, Arnold School of Public Health, 915 Greene Street, Columbia, SC 29208, USA

James B. Burch
South Carolina Statewide Cancer Prevention & Control Program, University of South Carolina, 915 Greene Street, Columbia, SC 29208, USA
Department of Epidemiology and Biostatistics, University of South Carolina, Arnold School of Public Health, 915 Greene Street, Columbia, SC 29208, USA
WJB Dorn Department of Veterans Affairs Medical Center, 6439 Garners Ferry Road, Columbia, SC 29209-1639, USA

Virginie G. Daguisé
Division of Cancer Prevention and Control, South Carolina Department of Health and Environmental Control, 2100 Bull Street, Columbia, SC 29201, USA

Michael P. Stevens, Jean M. Rabb, Kakotan Sanogo and Gonzalo M. L. Bearman
Virginia Commonwealth University Medical Center, Richmond, VA 23284, USA

Jaclyn Arquiette
Virginia Commonwealth University Medical Center, Richmond, VA 23284, USA
Virginia Commonwealth University, School of Medicine, Richmond, VA 23284, USA

PatrickMason
Quest Diagnostics Nichols Institute, Chantilly, VA 20153, USA

Ryan D. Burns and Timothy A. Brusseau
Department of Exercise and Sport Science, College of Health, University of Utah, 250 S. 1850 E., HPER North, RM 241, Salt Lake City, UT 84112, USA

James C. Hannon
College of Physical Activity and Sport Sciences, West Virginia University, 375 Birch Street, P.O. Box 6116, Morgantown, WV 26505, USA

Jared Otieno Ogolla
Department of Public Health, School of Health Sciences, Mount Kenya University, P.O. Box 2591-30100, Eldoret, Kenya

Taddese Awoke and Yitayih Wondimeneh Asmamaw Atnafu
School of Biomedical and Laboratory Science, College of Medicine and Health Sciences, University of Gondar, Gondar, Ethiopia
Graduate School of Public Health, Seoul National University, Seoul, Republic of Korea

Damen Haile Mariam
School of Public Health, College of Health Sciences, Addis Ababa University, Addis Ababa, Ethiopia

Rex Wong
School of Public Health, Yale University, New Haven, CT, USA

Sonali Kar
Department of Community Medicine, Kalinga Institute of Medical Sciences, KIIT University, Patia, Bhubaneswar 751024, India

Shalini Ray
Kalinga Institute of Medical Sciences, KIIT University, Patia, Bhubaneswar 751024, India

Dayanidhi Meher
Department of Medicine, Kalinga Institute of Medical Sciences, KIIT University, Patia, Bhubaneswar 751024, India

Abulie Takele
Department of Nursing, College of Medicine & Health Sciences, Madawalabu University, 302 Bale Goba, Ethiopia

Tesfaye Setegn
Department of Reproductive Health, College of Medicine and Health Sciences, School of Public Health, Bahir Dar University, 3008 Bahir Dar, Ethiopia

Meredith Yorkin, Jennifer Martin-Biggers, Carolina Lozada and Carol Byrd-Bredbenner
Department of Nutritional Sciences, Rutgers, The State University of New Jersey, New Brunswick, NJ 08901, USA

Kim Spaccarotella
Department of Nutritional Sciences, Rutgers, The State University of New Jersey, New Brunswick, NJ 08901, USA
Department of Biological Sciences, Kean University, Union, NJ 07083, USA

Nobuko Hongu
Department of Nutritional Sciences, University of Arizona, Tucson, AZ 85721, USA

Virginia Quick
Department of Health Sciences, James Madison University, Harrisonburg, VA 22807, USA

www.ingramcontent.com/pod-product-compliance
Lightning Source LLC
Chambersburg PA
CBHW080622200326
41458CB00013B/4476